Energy Balance and Cancer

Volume 13

Series editor:

Nathan A. Berger
Case Western Reserve University
School of Medicine
Cleveland, OH, USA

More information about this series at http://www.springer.com/series/8282

Nathan A. Berger • Ann H. Klopp • Karen H. Lu
Editors

Focus on Gynecologic Malignancies

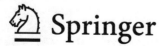 Springer

Editors
Nathan A. Berger
Center for Science, Health and Society
Case Western Reserve University
Cleveland, OH, USA

Ann H. Klopp
Department of Radiation Oncology
MD Anderson Cancer Center
Houston, TX, USA

Karen H. Lu
Department of Gynecologic Oncology
  and Reproductive Medicine
MD Anderson Cancer Center
Houston, TX, USA

ISSN 2199-2622   ISSN 2199-2630   (electronic)
Energy Balance and Cancer
ISBN 978-3-319-87569-9   ISBN 978-3-319-63483-8   (eBook)
DOI 10.1007/978-3-319-63483-8

Printed on acid-free paper

This Springer imprint is published by Springer Nature
The registered company is Springer International Publishing AG
The registered company address is: Gewerbestrasse 11, 6330 Cham, Switzerland

Preface

Among the growing number of malignancies associated with obesity, endometrial cancer risk and prognosis has long been identified with overweight and obesity, and ovarian cancer has more recently been identified as having a positive association. Endometrial cancer has, in fact, been recognized as having the greatest obesity-associated increase in risk and the most alarming obesity-associated increase (sixfold) for death among all cancers in women. Endometrial cancer is the fourth most common cancer in women with an estimated 61,380 new cases and 10,920 deaths in 2017. Ovarian cancer is less common, estimated at 22,440 cases in 2017, but higher in mortality with 14,080 deaths expected in 2017. Almost all aspects of uterine and ovarian cancers, across the spectrum from etiology, epidemiology, diagnosis, selection, and response to intervention, survivorship, and impact of lifestyle on survivorship, as well as effects of ethnic background and age are affected by obesity as well as by other components of energy balance, especially physical activity and exercise.

The overall goal of this volume is to examine the intersection of these factors, their impact on disease progression, and the important influence of research on modifying energy balance to better understand and improve disease prevention, management, and prognosis. The volume is divided into three sections. The first section on epidemiology reviews relation of obesity to endometrial cancer and to ovarian cancer and provides insight into public understanding of the importance of obesity as a risk factor for gynecologic malignancies. The second section describes major aspects of biology and the linkages connecting obesity to gynecologic cancers including hormonal status, adipokines, adipose stromal cells, and in particular, use of model systems to study the impact of energy balance on gynecologic malignancies. Section three focuses on prevention strategies including hormonal and lifestyle interventions to disrupt the linkage between obesity and gynecologic malignancies. The volume concludes with chapters focused on management strategies for obese patients with gynecologic malignancies and their precursors.

The contributors to this volume are drawn from the world's leading physicians and scientists seeking to better understand the relation between energy balance and gynecologic malignancies and improve their outcomes. In Chap. 1, Melissa Merritt, Imperial College London, UK, and Marc Gunter, International Agency for Research on Cancer, Lyon, France, review epidemiologic evidence for the association of obesity with endometrial cancer and its modulation by factors affecting circulating estrogens. In Chap. 2, Carmen Jochem, Inga Schlecht, and Michael Leitzmann, University of Regensburg, Regensburg, Germany, review the epidemiologic evidence relating obesity to ovarian cancer. Chapter 3, written by Shannon Armbruster and Pamela Soliman, University of Texas MD Anderson Cancer Center, Houston, TX, deals with the public awareness, or lack thereof, of the relation between obesity and gynecologic malignancies. In Chap. 4, Louise Brinton and Britton Trabert, National Cancer Institute, Bethesda, MD, explore the important contributions of estrogen and progesterone as modulators of the impact of obesity on gynecologic malignancies. Jaclyn Watkins, Harvard University, Brigham and Women's Hospital, Boston, MA, in Chap. 5, describes the relation of obesity to precursors of endometrial cancer and potential interventions. Starting the section on mechanisms linking obesity to gynecologic cancer, Elizabeth Connor, Ofer Reizes, and Caner Saygin, Lerner College of Medicine at Case Western Reserve University and Cleveland Clinic, Cleveland, Ohio, in Chap. 6, describe the potential role of adipokines as mediators of this relation. Chapter 7 by Ann H. Klopp, University of Texas MD Anderson Cancer Center, describes the contribution of adipose-derived stromal cells to gynecologic cancers. In Chap. 8, Rosemarie Schmandt and Katherine Naff, University of Texas MD Anderson Cancer Center, discuss the use of rodent model systems to study the effects of obesity, diet, and exercise for prevention of gynecologic malignancies. The third section of this volume, focused on prevention strategies, begins with Chap. 9 written by Faina Linkov, Sharon Goughnour, Shalkar Adambekov, Robert Edwards, Nicole Donnellan, and Dana Bovbjerg, University of Pittsburgh, Pittsburgh, PA, who survey lifestyle interventions to reduce the risk of obesity-associated endometrial cancer. Chapter 10 by Sarah Kitson and Emma Crosbie, University of Manchester and St. Mary's Hospital, Manchester, UK, focuses on a mechanistic approach to overcome insulin resistance and prevent endometrial cancer using hormone and metabolic strategies.

The fourth section of this volume is composed of chapters focused on treatment strategies to most effectively address the issues associated with energy balance and to improve outcomes in patients with gynecologic malignancies. In Chap. 11, Joseph Dottino, Karen Lu, and Melinda Yates, University of Texas MD Anderson Cancer Center, Houston, TX, discuss strategies and unique considerations for management of endometrial cancer precursors in obese women. Nora Nock, Case Western Reserve University, Cleveland, OH, in Chap. 12, reviews impact of trials involving exercise, diet, and behavioral counseling in women with gynecologic cancers. In Chap. 13, Tianyi Huang and Shelley Tworoger, Harvard University, Boston, MA, analyze the complex and controversial relation of physical activity with ovarian cancer risk and survival. In Chap. 14, Amanika Kumar and William A. Cliby, Mayo Clinic, Rochester, MN, discuss important aspects of understanding the nuances of intraoperative and perioperative management of gynecologic malignancies in the obese patient. Terri Woodard, University of Texas MD Anderson Cancer Center and Baylor College of Medicine, Houston, TX, and Jessica Robin, Baylor College of Medicine, Houston, TX, in Chap. 15, discuss unique challenges and strategies for preserving fertility while treating women with gynecologic malignancies. In Chap. 16, Leslie Clark and Victoria Bae-Jump, University of North Carolina, Chapel Hill, NC, review the biologic mechanisms and possible therapeutic use of metformin as adjuvant therapy for ovarian and endometrial cancers.

Overall, this volume provides a comprehensive treatise on the latest studies concerning the intersection of gynecologic malignancies with energy balance, which together constitute a major challenge and opportunity for research scientists and clinicians, especially those dealing with the expanding population of women confronted by challenges in energy balance. This volume should be a valuable resource to physicians, oncologists, gynecologists, nurses, nutritionists, dieticians, and exercise therapists dealing with women with challenges and/or questions regarding the linkage between energy balance and cancer. Moreover, because of the magnitude and severity of these problems, this volume should serve as an important resource for cancer researchers, especially for scientists studying lifestyle modification and prevention strategies as well as more fundamental aspects of genetics, pharmacology, and endocrinology.

Cleveland, OH, USA   Nathan A. Berger
Houston, TX, USA   Ann H. Klopp
Houston, TX, USA   Karen H. Lu

Contents

Contributors

Shalkar Adambekov Magee-Womens Research Institute, University of Pittsburgh School of Medicine, Pittsburgh, PA, USA

Shannon Armbruster The University of Texas MD Anderson Cancer Center, Houston, TX, USA

Victoria L. Bae-Jump, M.D., Ph.D. University of North Carolina School of Medicine, Chapel Hill, NC, USA

Dana H. Bovbjerg Hillman Cancer Center, University of Pittsburgh Cancer Institute, Pittsburgh, PA, USA

Louise A. Brinton, Ph.D. Division of Cancer Epidemiology and Genetics, National Cancer Institute, Bethesda, MD, USA

Leslie H. Clark, M.D. University of North Carolina School of Medicine, Chapel Hill, NC, USA

William A. Cliby, M.D. Mayo Clinic, Rochester, MN, USA

Elizabeth V. Connor, M.D. Department of Obstetrics/Gynecology and Women's Health Institute, Cleveland Clinic Foundation, Cleveland, OH, USA

Emma J. Crosbie Division of Molecular & Clinical Cancer Sciences, University of Manchester, Manchester, UK

Nicole Donnellan Magee-Womens Hospital of UPMC, Pittsburgh, PA, USA

Joseph A. Dottino Department of Gynecologic Oncology & Reproductive Medicine, University of Texas MD Anderson Cancer Center, Houston, TX, USA

Robert P. Edwards Magee-Womens Hospital of UPMC, Pittsburgh, PA, USA

Sharon L. Goughnour Magee-Womens Research Institute, University of Pittsburgh School of Medicine, Pittsburgh, PA, USA

Marc J. Gunter, Ph.D. Section of Nutritional and Meteabolism, International Agency for Research on Cancer (IARC), Lyon, France

Tianyi Huang Department of Epidemiology, Harvard University, Boston, MA, USA

Carmen Jochem Department of Epidemiology and Preventive Medicine, University of Regensburg, Regensburg, Germany

Sarah Kitson Division of Molecular & Clinical Cancer Sciences, University of Manchester, Manchester, UK

Ann H. Klopp, M.D., Ph.D. Department of Radiation Oncology, MD Anderson Cancer Center, Houston, TX, USA

Amanika Kumar, M.D. Mayo Clinic, Rochester, MN, USA

Michael Leitzmann Department of Epidemiology and Preventive Medicine, University of Regensburg, Regensburg, Germany

Faina Linkov Magee-Womens Research Institute, University of Pittsburgh School of Medicine, Pittsburgh, PA, USA

Karen H. Lu Department of Gynecologic Oncology and Reproductive Medicine, MD Anderson Cancer Center, Houston, TX, USA

Melissa A. Merritt Epidemiology Program, University of Hawaii Cancer Center, Honolulu, HI, USA

Aparna Mitra Department of Experimental Radiation Oncology, M.D. Anderson Cancer Center, Houston, TX, USA

Katherine A. Naff, D.V.M. Unit 63, Department of Veterinary Medicine and Surgery, UT MD Anderson Cancer Center, Houston, TX, USA

Nora L. Nock, Ph.D. Department of Epidemiology and Biostatistics, Case Western Reserve University School of Medicine, Cleveland, OH, USA

Ofer Reizes, Ph.D. Department of Cellular and Molecular Medicine, Lerner Research Institute, Cleveland Clinic, Cleveland, OH, USA

Jessica Rubin, M.D. Division of Reproductive Endocrinology and Infertility, Baylor College of Medicine, Houston, TX, USA

Caner Saygin, M.D. Department of Cellular and Molecular Medicine, Lerner Research Institute, Cleveland Clinic, Cleveland, OH, USA

Inga Schlecht Department of Epidemiology and Preventive Medicine, University of Regensburg, Regensburg, Germany

Rosemarie E. Schmandt, Ph.D. Department of Gynecologic Oncology and Reproductive Medicine, UT MD Anderson Cancer Center, Unit 1362, Houston, TX, USA

Pamela T. Soliman The University of Texas MD Anderson Cancer Center, Houston, TX, USA

Shelley S. Tworoger Department of Epidemiology, Harvard University, Channing Laboratory, Boston, MA, USA

Britton Trabert, Ph.D. Division of Cancer Epidemiology and Genetics, National Cancer Institute, Bethesda, MD, USA

Jaclyn Watkins, M.D., M.S. Department of Pathology, Microbiology, and Immunology, Vanderbilt University Medical Center, Nashville, TN, USA

Terri L. Woodard, M.D. The University of Texas MD Anderson Cancer Center, Houston, TX, USA

Division of Reproductive Endocrinology and Infertility, Baylor College of Medicine, Houston, TX, USA

Melinda S. Yates Department of Gynecologic Oncology & Reproductive Medicine, University of Texas MD Anderson Cancer Center, Houston, TX, USA

Chapter 1
Epidemiologic Evidence for the Obesity-Endometrial Cancer Relationship

Melissa A. Merritt and Marc J. Gunter

Abstract There are convincing epidemiologic evidence that obesity increases endometrial cancer risk and consistent positive associations between body mass index (BMI) and other adiposity parameters and endometrial cancer risk have been observed across different study populations. Indeed, the risk of endometrial cancer is estimated to be 1.54-times higher per 5 kg/m^2 increment increase in BMI—an association with BMI that is the strongest that has been observed for any type of cancer. The higher risk of endometrial cancer among overweight and obese women appears to be restricted to those who have not used postmenopausal hormone therapy, suggesting that the modulation of estrogenic activity may be a possible mechanism that underlies the obesity-endometrial cancer link. Further, circulating estrogen levels are positively associated with endometrial cancer risk and partly explain the obesity endometrial cancer association in mediation models. Another key mechanism that may link obesity with endometrial cancer risk includes hyperinsulinemia as supported by both experimental and observational data. Inflammation and increased exposure to inflammatory cytokines derived from adipose tissue represent additional putative pathways that could contribute to the role of obesity in endometrial cancer development. This review summarizes results from epidemiologic studies on obesity (assessed as BMI, waist circumference and other measures) and endometrial cancer development, highlights mechanisms that may link obesity to endometrial carcinogenesis, and discusses areas of ongoing and future research that could help to develop improved strategies for endometrial cancer prevention.

Keywords Endometrial cancer • Obesity • Body mass index • Waist circumference • Estrogen • Insulin

M.A. Merritt
Epidemiology Program, University of Hawaii Cancer Center,
701 Ilalo Street, Honolulu 96813, HI, USA
e-mail: mamerrit@hawaii.edu

M.J. Gunter, Ph.D. (✉)
Section of Nutrition and Metabolism, International Agency for Research on Cancer (IARC),
150, Cours Albert Thomas, Cedex 08, 69372 Lyon, France
e-mail: GunterM@iarc.fr

© Springer International Publishing AG 2018
N.A. Berger et al. (eds.), *Focus on Gynecologic Malignancies*, Energy Balance and Cancer 13, DOI 10.1007/978-3-319-63483-8_1

Introduction

Cancer of the uterine corpus is often referred to as endometrial cancer because approximately 92% of these cancers originate in the endometrium (epithelial lining of the uterus) [1]. Endometrial cancer is the fifth most common cancer in women and the most recent worldwide estimates identified 319,605 new cases in 2012 [2]. In many parts of the world the incidence of endometrial cancer is rising; for example, in the United Kingdom the age standardised incidence rates have increased by 25% (from 2002–2004 to 2011–2013) [3]. In the United States, endometrial cancer incidence rates have been rising by 1.3 and 1.9% per year in women younger than 50 years of age and in women aged 50 years and older, respectively [1].

Endometrial cancer is more common in industrialized countries and the highest incidence rates are observed in North America, Central and Eastern Europe as compared with lower rates in Central and Western Africa [2]. These geographic differences may be explained in part by the distribution of two major endometrial cancer risk factors, estrogen exposure and obesity. It is hypothesized that endometrial cancers develop under conditions of higher estrogen levels that are simultaneously unopposed by progesterone [4]. A greater body mass index (BMI) has been linked to higher estrogen levels in postmenopausal women where adipose tissue is the main site of estrogen production from androgen precursors [5, 6]. In premenopausal women a different mechanism may operate where obesity-related anovulation has been linked to progesterone deficiency (reviewed by [7]). Notably, the higher risk for developing endometrial cancer with increasing BMI is the strongest BMI risk association observed for any cancer site [8] and it has been estimated that 41% of endometrial cancers are attributable to overweight and obesity [9].

Endometrial cancer is a heterogeneous disease that is comprised of several histologic subtypes including endometrioid (most common), serous, clear cell and mucinous tumors. The majority of endometrial cancers can be classified into two clinicopathologic groups, endometrioid (type I) and non-endometrioid (type II) tumors [10]. Most endometrial cancers (70–80%) are classified as type I tumors and are typically endometrioid histology, are thought to develop by endocrine modulation (exposure to estrogen unopposed by progesterone), harbor molecular alterations in PTEN, KRAS and β-catenin and have relatively indolent tumor behavior [11]. Type II tumors are usually serous or clear cell histologic subtype [12], the most common molecular alteration is p53 mutation [11, 13] and these tumors tend to demonstrate a more aggressive tumor behavior [14, 15]. A recent pooled analysis using individual data from 10 cohort and 14 case-control studies from the Epidemiology of Endometrial Cancer Consortium evaluated whether factors that are associated with increased risk of endometrial cancer overall, including BMI, history of diabetes, nulliparity, non-use of oral contraceptives and an early age at menarche, were similarly associated with risk of developing type I versus type II tumors [16] (Table 1.1). They observed generally similar risk factors associations across type I and type II tumors with the exception that BMI was more strongly associated with increased risk of developing type I as compared with type II

Table 1.1 Selected pooled studies and meta-analyses that have investigated the obesity–endometrial cancer relationship

Reference	Study design	Comparison	Cases and/or publications (n)[a]	Summary risk estimate (95% CI)	Covariates	Comments
Aune et al. [17]	Dose-response meta-analysis of 30 prospective cohort studies (28 publications) from North America, Asia and Europe	BMI [per 5 kg/m²] -Overall	22,320	1.54 (1.47–1.61)	Specific to individual studies (detailed in [17] supplementary table S2)	Observed high heterogeneity across studies for most of the adiposity-related analyses, which was attributed to differences in the strength of the association rather than the directionality of the effect
		-Never users of menopausal hormones	6 publications	1.65 (1.33–2.05)		
		-Ever users of menopausal hormone	5 publications	1.10 (1.06–1.14)		
		-Premenopause	6 publications	1.41 (1.37–1.45)		Significant heterogeneity was observed for the BMI association by menopausal hormone use (P-heterogeneity = 0.005)
		-Postmenopause	15 publications	1.54 (1.42–1.67)		
		-Age 18–25 years	9 publications	1.45 (1.28–1.64)		
		Weight gain, Per 5 kg from early adulthood to baseline	7 publications	1.16 (1.12–1.20)		
		Waist circumference, Per 10 cm	4 publications	1.27 (1.17–1.39)		
		Waist-hip ratio, Per 0.1 unit	5 publications	1.21 (1.13–1.29)		

(continued)

Table 1.1 (continued)

Reference	Study design	Comparison	Cases and/or publications (n)[a]	Summary risk estimate (95% CI)	Covariates	Comments
Setiawan et al. [16]	Pooled analysis of individual data from 10 cohort and 14 case-control studies from the epidemiology of endometrial cancer consortium (studies from the United States, Canada, Europe and Australia)	BMI (kg/m²)		Type I tumors	Stratified by study, age and race/ethnicity and adjusted for age at menarche, parity, OC use, menopausal status, menopausal hormone use and smoking status	P-heterogeneity (comparing categorical risk associations for type I versus type II tumors) < 0.0001
		<25	4602	1.00 (ref)		
		25 ≤ 30	3718	1.45 (1.37–1.53)		
		30 ≤ 35	2294	2.52 (2.35–2.69)		Similar risk associations were observed when restricting to postmenopausal women who never used menopausal hormones
		35 ≤ 40	1247	4.45 (4.05–4.89)		
		40+	992	7.14 (6.33–8.06)		
		[p-trend]		[<0.0001]		
		[per 2 kg/m²]	12,853	1.20 (1.19–1.21)		
		BMI (kg/m²)		Type II tumors		Separate risk estimates for cohort studies only were not provided
		<25	330	1.00 (ref)		
		25 ≤ 30	253	1.16 (0.98–1.38)		
		30 ≤ 35	159	1.73 (1.40–2.12)		
		35 ≤ 40	65	2.15 (1.60–2.88)		
		40+	47	3.11 (2.19–4.44)		
		[p-trend]		[<0.0001]		
		[per 2 kg/m²]	854	1.12 (1.09–1.14)		

[a]If the number of publications (rather than number of cases) is listed this is noted in the table

endometrial tumors. The stronger association of BMI with type I tumors was subsequently confirmed in a large study of 2825 endometrial cancer cases from a Gynecologic Oncology Group trial [18].

The objectives of this review are to summarize evidence from recent epidemiologic studies that have evaluated the association between obesity and endometrial cancer risk, to explore possible biological mechanisms that explain the link between obesity and endometrial carcinogenesis and to highlight areas for further research that are needed to improve strategies for the prevention of endometrial cancer in high risk women.

Body Mass Index in Relation to Endometrial Cancer Risk

The majority of studies that have focused on the association between obesity and endometrial cancer risk have utilized BMI as a measure of overweight (BMI ≥ 25 and <30 kg/m^2) and obesity (BMI ≥ 30 kg/m^2) as it is relatively straightforward to calculate requiring only estimates of weight and height. The body of work focusing on the association between BMI and endometrial cancer risk in prospective cohort studies was recently reported in a dose-response meta-analysis that summarized data for a large number of endometrial cancer cases (n = 22,320) from 30 studies [17] (Table 1.1). This study updated the earlier report published by the World Cancer Research Fund/American Institute for Cancer Research that concluded that there was convincing evidence to support the positive association between BMI and risk of endometrial cancer development [19]. Specifically, Aune et al. [17] observed a 1.54 times higher risk (95% CI: 1.47–1.61) to develop endometrial cancer with each 5 kg/m^2 increase in BMI. This meta-analysis included articles that were published up to February 2015 and at the time of writing this review we identified no additional cohort studies that had published on the association between BMI and endometrial cancer risk. The findings of Aune et al. [17] corroborated the results from two earlier meta-analyses that reported a 1.60 times higher risk for endometrial cancer with each five unit increase in BMI based on results from ≥ 19 prospective studies [8, 20]. These meta-analyses focused on the association between BMI and risk endometrial cancer overall. A recent pooled analysis further investigated the BMI-endometrial cancer association by comparing risk estimates between women diagnosed with type I and type II endometrial cancer (including n = 12,853 type I and n = 854 type II cases) and they observed that the risk of developing a type I tumor (per 2 kg/m^2 increase in BMI, odds ratio = 1.20 (95% CI: 1.19–1.21)) was stronger than the risk to develop a type II tumor (odds ratio = 1.12 (95% CI: 1.09–1.14)) (P-heterogeneity < 0.0001) [16].

A smaller number (n $\leq$ 9) of studies have evaluated BMI in younger women (at ages 18–25 years) and weight gain in relation to endometrial cancer risk (summarized in [17]). The dose-response meta-analysis reported a 1.45 times higher risk (95% CI: 1.28–1.64) of developing endometrial cancer for each 5 kg/m^2 increment increase in BMI among young women [17] (Table 1.1). When examining weight gain from the time of early adulthood to the study baseline, they observed a 1.16 times higher risk (95% CI: 1.12–1.20) to develop endometrial cancer for each 5 kg increase in weight. In the dose-response meta-analysis they observed high heterogeneity in most analyses of adiposity-related factors but they attributed this heterogeneity to differences in the strength of the association because almost all of the studies reported positive associations between adiposity measures and endometrial cancer risk.

Modification of the BMI-Endometrial Cancer Association by Menopausal Hormone Therapy Use

Menopausal hormone therapy (MHT) use, and use of the estrogen only MHT formulation in particular, is a key risk factor for endometrial cancer. Namely, use of estrogen only MHT versus never use was associated with an approximate twofold increased risk to develop postmenopausal endometrial cancer and a higher risk (approximately ninefold) was observed for women who reported long-term (≥10 years) estrogen only MHT use [21]. The inclusion of progestogens in combined estrogen plus progestogen MHT formulations may offset the proliferative effects of estrogen on the endometrium but it is uncertain whether it may do so completely [22, 23]. Interestingly, a recent report from the Women's Health Initiative randomized clinical trial observed that continuous combined estrogen plus progestin use in postmenopausal women lowered the risk of endometrial cancer by 35% [24].

It has been suggested that because postmenopausal MHT users are exposed to excess estrogen, this may obscure associations between endometrial cancer and body fatness that could act by modulating estrogen levels [20]. Consistent with this hypothesis, in the dose-response meta-analysis they observed that the increase in endometrial cancer risk with a higher BMI was stronger among women with naturally low estrogen levels (i.e., never-users of MHT) (summary relative risk (RR) per 5 kg/m^2 increase in BMI = 1.65 (95% CI: 1.33–2.05)) as compared with ever users of MHT (summary RR = 1.10 (95% CI: 1.06–1.14)) (P-heterogeneity = 0.005) [17]. In contrast, in the pooled analysis that examined endometrial cancer risk associations separately for type I and type II endometrial cancer, they observed similar associations for BMI when they restricted analyses to the subgroup of postmenopausal women who had never used MHT [16]. The dose-response meta-analysis also investigated whether the association with BMI differed according to menopausal status and there was a statistically significant 1.41-fold (95% CI: 1.37–1.45) and 1.54-fold (95% CI: 1.42–1.67) higher risk to develop endometrial cancer among both premenopausal and postmenopausal women, respectively [17].

Abdominal Obesity and Endometrial Cancer Risk

BMI is a measure of general obesity but it is limited in that it does not capture the body fat distribution. Other measures of abdominal obesity (commonly measured as waist circumference) may be better indicators of obesity-related metabolic stress [25]. The relevance of comparing different anthropometric measurements is that if some factors are more strongly related to endometrial cancer risk than others this could provide important insights regarding possible mechanisms liking obesity with endometrial cancer development. However, relatively few studies (n ≤ 5 identified in the dose-response meta-analysis) have investigated waist circumference and waist-hip ratio in relation to endometrial cancer risk [17]. Based on the available evidence, the findings are consistent with the conclusions based on BMI that there was an increased risk of developing endometrial cancer for women with a higher waist circumference (summary RR per 10 cm increment = 1.27 (95% CI: 1.17–1.39)) and waist-hip ratio (summary RR per 0.1 unit = 1.21 (95% CI: 1.13–1.29)). Aune et al. [17] concluded that all anthropometric measures were associated with increased risk of endometrial cancer; however, more studies are needed to investigate measures of abdominal obesity and in particular to try to clarify the possible independent associations of BMI (general adiposity) and waist circumference (abdominal obesity) with endometrial cancer risk.

Obesity-Related Pathologies and Endometrial Cancer

An additional link between obesity and endometrial cancer that has been explored is the development of metabolic syndrome defined using varying definitions such as BMI and/or waist circumference, hyperglycemia, higher blood pressure values and high triglyceride levels. As expected, a meta-analysis of metabolic syndrome and endometrial cancer risk including n = 6 studies (n = 2 prospective cohort studies) reported a significant positive association between metabolic syndrome and endometrial cancer (women with versus without metabolic syndrome, RR = 1.89 (95% CI: 1.34–2.67)) with high heterogeneity observed across the studies [26]. Notably, they observed that obesity/high waist circumference was more strongly related to endometrial cancer risk than any other metabolic syndrome component.

Several meta-analyses have reported that diabetes is a risk factor for endometrial cancer [27, 28] and risk estimates from the most recent report, based on n = 29 studies (including n = 17 prospective cohort studies), suggested that there was a 1.89-fold (95% CI: 1.46–2.45) increased risk of developing endometrial cancer in women with diabetes versus non-diabetics [29]. However, a recent investigation observed that out of eight cohort studies that had evaluated diabetes in relation to endometrial cancer incidence, only three studies had adjusted for BMI, hence it remains to be determined whether the diabetes-endometrial cancer association could be explained by obesity [30]. In the Women's Health Initiative study, Luo et al. [30] observed that the higher risk for endometrial cancer in women who had diabetes became non-significant after adjusting for BMI, hence concluding that the findings did not support an independent association between diabetes and risk of endometrial cancer.

A recent study used an alternative approach to assess whether hyperinsulinemia and type 2 diabetes were causally associated with endometrial cancer by using single nucleotide polymorphisms that were associated with type 2 diabetes, fasting glucose, fasting insulin, early insulin secretion (postchallenge insulin) and BMI as instrumental variables in Mendelian randomization analyses [31]. They observed that genetically predicted higher levels of fasting insulin, independent of BMI, were associated with a 2.3-fold higher risk (OR for each standard deviation increase = 2.34 (95% CI: 1.06–5.14)) of endometrial cancer. Similarly, there was an association between genetically predicted higher postchallenge insulin levels with a higher risk of endometrial cancer (OR for each standard deviation increase = 1.40 (95% CI: 1.12–1.76)). As expected, women with a genetically predicted higher BMI had an elevated endometrial cancer risk (OR for each genetically predicted standard deviation increase in BMI = 3.86 (95% CI: = 2.24–6.64)). In contrast, this study did not find evidence for an association between genetic risk of type 2 diabetes or fasting glucose with endometrial cancer risk.

Mechanisms Linking Obesity to Endometrial Carcinogenesis

Serologic Factors that may underlie the Obesity-Endometrial Cancer Association

Several serologic factors that are altered in obese individuals have also been shown to be associated with risk of developing endometrial cancer, including higher circulating levels of estrogen, insulin, leptin and inflammatory cytokines, and lower adiponectin levels [7] (Fig. 1.1). Obesity is associated with elevated endogenous estrogen levels in postmenopausal women, likely due to the enhanced peripheral conversion of androstenedione by adipocytes in obese individuals [5, 6, 32]. As outlined above it is thought that endometrial cancers develop under conditions of excess estrogen unopposed by progesterone [4]. Consistent with this hypothesis are observations that circulating estrogen levels are a significant positive risk factor for endometrial cancer (reviewed by [7]). In the largest study to date using data from the European Prospective Investigation into Cancer and Nutrition (EPIC), the ORs for endometrial cancer risk in postmenopausal women when comparing the highest versus lowest tertile were 2.66 (95% CI: 1.50–4.72, P-trend = 0.002) for estrone, 2.07 (95% CI: 1.20–3.60, P-trend = 0.001) for estradiol and 1.66 (95% CI 0.98–2.82, P-trend = 0.001) for free estradiol [33]. Conversely, in the same report there was a significant inverse association between sex hormone-binding globulin (SHBG) levels (OR for the highest versus lowest tertile = 0.57 (95% CI: 0.34–0.95,

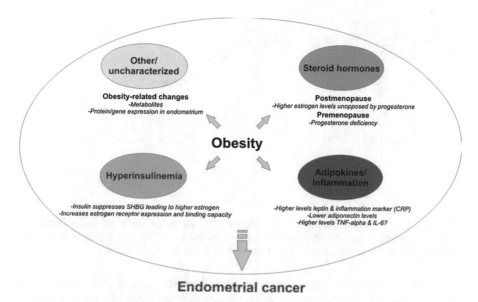

Fig. 1.1 Mechanisms linking obesity with endometrial cancer risk. *CRP* C-reactive protein, *IL-6* interleukin-6, *SHBG* sex hormone-binding globulin, *TNF-alpha* tumor necrosis factor-alpha

P-trend = 0.004)) and endometrial cancer risk which was anticipated as SHBG may decrease exposure to bioavailable estradiol levels. Although these data implicate estrogen in obesity-mediated endometrial carcinogenesis, the obesity-endometrial cancer relationship appears to be only partly explained by high estrogen levels as supported by the persistence of BMI as an important risk factor after adjusting for circulating estrogen levels [7, 34].

A related mechanism that may explain the association between obesity and endometrial cancer is hyperinsulinemia [35] (Fig. 1.2). Obesity is associated with high levels of insulin, which is a growth factor for a wide range of tissues, including endometrium. Insulin also suppresses levels of sex hormone binding globulin (SHBG), leading to higher levels of bioactive estrogen, and insulin increases estrogen receptor expression and binding capacity, raising the possibility that insulin and estrogen could act additively or even synergistically in endometrial carcinogenesis. Insulin and Insulin-like growth factor (IGF)-I share 40% amino acid sequence homology and can act as ligands for each other's receptors, albeit with low affinity. Binding of insulin or IGF-I to its own receptor can promote cell proliferation by activation of the same two downstream pathways: the Mitogen-Activated Protein Kinase and the phosphatidylinositol 3-kinase (PI3K) pathways. The IGFs differ from most other peptide hormones, such as insulin and growth hormone, in that they are maintained at continuously high levels throughout much of the body. Most IGF-I in circulation is produced by the liver and circulates bound to IGF-binding proteins (IGFBP) and approximately 75% of IGF-I is bound to IGFBP3. Approximately 1% of IGF-I circulates free (unbound) and the free fraction may be the most biologically active [36].

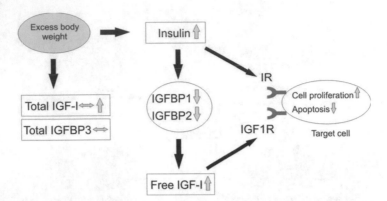

Fig. 1.2 Inter-relationships of obesity, insulin, the IGF axis, & their influence on cell growth & survival (adapted from [35]). *IGF* insulin-like growth factor, *IGFBP* insulin-like growth factor binding protein, *IGF1R* insulin-like growth factor-I receptor, *IR* insulin receptor

We previously investigated the association between circulating levels of estradiol, insulin, IGF-I and related serologic factors with endometrial cancer risk using biospecimens from postmenopausal women enrolled in the Women's Health Initiative [37]. We observed that baseline fasting insulin levels were positively associated with risk of the endometrioid histologic subtype endometrial cancer (hazard ratio (HR) for the highest versus lowest quartile = 2.33 (95% CI: 1.13–4.82)) among women not using MHT and after adjusting for estradiol levels, BMI and other risk factors [37]. In contrast, we observed that levels of free IGF-I (unbound to IGFBP) were inversely associated with endometrioid endometrial cancer risk (HR for the highest versus lowest quartile = 0.53 (95% CI: 0.31–0.90)) after adjusting for age, MHT use and estradiol [37]. The latter finding suggests a possible anti-tumorigenic role for IGF-I in endometrial cancer and similar observations have been reported in previous cross-sectional studies [37]. Most other prospective investigations reported similar positive associations between hyperinsulinaemia and endometrial cancer risk although these studies generally observed an attenuation of risk following adjustment for estradiol [38, 39]. In contrast to the insulin and free IGF-I results, other circulating insulin/IGF axis factors were not associated with endometrial cancer risk (total IGF-I, IGFBP3, IGF-I/IGFBP3 ratio investigated by Gunter et al. [37]; IGFBP1 and IGFBP2 measured by Cust et al. [38]; total IGF-I, IGBBP1, IGFBP2 and IGFBP3 investigated by Lukanova et al. [39]). These studies were limited by the number of endometrial cancer cases (the largest study evaluated n = 286 cases [38]), therefore it would be of interest to carry out a large pooled analysis of circulating insulin/IGF factors in relation to endometrial cancer risk. Consistent with these individual investigations, a meta-analysis of 25 studies (mostly retrospective case-control studies and including only two prospective cohort studies) reported a positive association between insulin resistance (measured as higher levels of insulin/C-peptide or homeostatic model assessment - insulin resistance values) and endometrial cancer risk [40].

Another mechanism that may link obesity to endometrial cancer development is the altered levels of hormones and cytokines (known as adipokines) that are produced in adipose tissue such as higher circulating levels of leptin and pro-inflammatory cytokines and lower levels of adiponectin (reviewed by [41]). There is evidence suggesting that dysregulated circulating adipokine levels are related to endometrial cancer risk and a recent meta-analysis reported a positive association with higher leptin levels (top versus lowest tertile, summary OR = 3.32 (95% CI: 1.98–5.56), n = 3 prospective studies) and an inverse association with adiponectin levels (top versus lowest tertile, summary OR = 0.65 (95% CI: 0.42–0.99), n = 5 prospective studies) [42]. Another recent meta-analysis using data from 12 cohort and case-control studies combined (a separate estimate for prospective cohort studies only was not provided) reported a 60% lower endometrial cancer risk (95% CI: 0.33–0.66) for subjects with the highest versus lowest adiponectin levels [43]. The positive association between circulating leptin levels and endometrial cancer risk is consistent with results from *in vitro* studies which showed that leptin promoted endometrial cancer cell growth and/or invasiveness [44, 45]. In contrast, adiponectin may have anti-inflammatory and insulin-sensitizing effects [46] which is consistent with the observation that lower levels of serologic adiponectin are associated with a higher risk of developing endometrial cancer.

Obesity is associated with changes in the physiological function of adipose tissue which may lead to chronic inflammation. Higher circulating levels of inflammatory markers have been reported in obese individuals including C-reactive protein (CRP) and proinflammatory cytokines such as tumor necrosis factor-alpha (TNF-α) and interleukin-6 (IL-6) which are secreted by dysfunctional adipose tissue (reviewed by [41]). In the largest prospective cohort study to date that evaluated inflammatory factors in n = 305 endometrial cancer cases from the EPIC study, there was an increased risk of endometrial cancer with higher levels of CRP (top versus bottom quartile, OR = 1.58 (95% CI: 1.03–2.41), P-trend = 0.02), IL-6 (top versus bottom quartile, OR = 1.66 (95% CI: 1.08–2.54), P-trend = 0.008) and the postulated chronic inflammatory factor, interleukin-1 receptor antagonist (top versus bottom quartile, OR = 1.82 (95% CI: 1.22–2.73), P-trend = 0.004) [47]. Notably, after adjustment for BMI the risk estimates were strongly reduced and became non-significant, therefore, the authors concluded that chronic inflammation could mediate the association between obesity and endometrial cancer. In a separate publication also using data from the EPIC study, a higher risk of endometrial cancer was observed with higher levels of TNF-α (OR = 1.73 (95% CI: 1.09–2.73), P-trend = 0.01) and there was a non-significant elevated risk with higher levels of TNF-α soluble receptors 1 and 2 (sTNFR1 and sTNFR2, OR = 1.68 (95% CI: 0.99–2.86), P-trend = 0.07 and OR = 1.53 (95%CI: 0.92–2.55), P-trend = 0.03, respectively) when accounting for BMI, parity, age at menopause and previous MHT use [48]. Wang et al. [49] also evaluated inflammatory markers in relation to endometrial cancer risk among postmenopausal women who were not using MHT in the Women's Health Initiative and they observed that CRP, but not IL-6 or TNF-α, was positively associated with endometrial cancer risk (quartile 4 versus quartile 1 of CRP, hazard ratio (HR) = 2.29 (95% CI: 1.13–4.65), P-trend = 0.01) after adjusting for age and BMI. However, with further adjustment for estradiol and insulin the association was attenuated and no longer significant therefore the authors concluded that the association between inflammation (indicated by high levels of CRP) and endometrial cancer risk may be partly explained by hyperinsulinemia and higher levels of estradiol. To our knowledge, inflammatory markers have only been evaluated in these two prospective studies in relation to endometrial cancer risk therefore additional studies are needed particularly to clarify the relationship between circulating IL-6 and TNF-α levels. Based on this limited evidence, there is modest support for the suggestion that inflammation (as indicated by higher CRP levels) is related to endometrial cancer risk, but rather than acting alone it appears that inflammation, together with other obesity-related factors including hyperinsulinemia and high estradiol levels, may contribute to endometrial cancer development.

Mechanistic Insights from Studies of Endometrial Tissues That May Explain the Obesity-Endometrial Cancer Association

It is of interest to identify molecular changes in the target tissue (endometrium) for endometrial cancer that may underlie the obesity-endometrial cancer risk association. Towards this goal we recently published a study that examined the impact of endometrial cancer risk factors, such as obesity (defined by BMI) and self-reported diabetes, in relation to the tissue expression of selected factors from the insulin/IGF and sex hormone axes in normal endometrial tissues from 107 women without cancer [50]. Specifically, we examined IGF ligands (IGF1, IGF2), IGFBP1 and IGFBP3, the tissue expression and activation of the insulin/IGF receptors (IR, IGF1R, phosphorylated (activated) IGF-I/insulin receptor (pIGF1R/pIR)), as well as the status of the hormone receptors (estrogen receptor, progesterone receptor) and expression of phosphatase and tensin homolog (PTEN). We evaluated these pathways because they would complement existing studies of circulating biomarkers and because of their important role in endometrial physiology [51, 52]. A key finding from this study was our observation of a higher frequency of positive immunohistochemical staining for pIGF1R/pIR in the endometrial tissues of postmenopausal diabetic versus non-diabetic women [50]. Interestingly, an earlier study reported up-regulation of pIGF1R/pIR in complex atypical endometrial hyperplasia, a putative precursor lesion for endometrial cancer, as well as in grade 1 endometrial cancers as compared with normal endometrium [53]. It will be of interest to examine the pIGF1R/pIR pathway in relation to obesity-mediated endometrial cancer development.

We did not observe differences in the insulin/IGF and sex hormone axes components according to BMI but we were unable to compare obese versus lean women due to the limited sample size and instead compared subgroups that were classified by splitting BMI levels at the median [50]. In our earlier study of PTEN loss using samples from the same normal endometrium study population there was no apparent difference in PTEN immunostaining patterns according to BMI or diabetes status [54]. Currently very few studies have investigated the relationship between risk factors and molecular profiling of normal endometrium, therefore further studies are needed to identify obesity-related molecular factors that may contribute to early events in the multistage process of endometrial carcinogenesis.

Conclusions and Future Directions

In this review we summarized several meta-analyses and a pooled analysis that have evaluated the association between obesity (assessed as BMI and other anthropometric measures) and endometrial cancer risk. Based on a recent dose-response meta-analysis that summarized data for the BMI-endometrial cancer risk association from 30 prospective cohort studies, there was a 1.54-fold higher risk of endometrial cancer for each 5 kg/m^2 incremental increase in BMI [17].

There is now convincing evidence that body fatness increases endometrial cancer risk [19] based mostly on the consistent positive associations with BMI that have been observed across different study populations. Given this well established obesity-endometrial cancer relationship, it is of great importance to identify potential mechanisms through which obesity may promote endometrial carcinogenesis. Several epidemiologic studies have investigated whether higher estrogen levels in obese postmenopausal women may explain the link between higher BMI and endometrial cancer risk. These studies concluded that the obesity-endometrial cancer relationship appears to be only partially explained by high estrogen levels based on observations that the association between BMI and endometrial cancer persisted after adjusting for circulating estrogen levels. Another serologic factor that may explain the obesity-endometrial cancer risk association is insulin based on evidence that insulin levels are positively associated with endometrial cancer risk in women with naturally low estrogen levels (non-users of MHT) [37] and a recent Mendelian Randomization study which observed that genetically predicted higher levels of fasting insulin, independent of BMI, were associated with a higher risk of endometrial cancer [31]. In our recent study of normal endometrium we observed a higher frequency of positive pIGF1R/pIR endometrial tissue immunohistochemical staining in diabetic versus non-diabetic postmenopausal women and we suggested that this could reflect the high levels of insulin in circulation among diabetic women [50]. Further studies are needed to investigate how hyperinsulinemia may lead to endometrial cancer development, and in particular it may be of interest to evaluate insulin-resistant women who have not yet developed diabetes and to account for the possible effects of diabetes treatment on the endometrium.

A current challenge in studying the link between obesity and endometrial cancer development is that only a small proportion of women who are obese or who exhibit high estrogen levels or hyperinsulinemia actually go on to develop endometrial cancer. Furthermore, there are women without these risk factors who develop endometrial cancer. Thus, the predictive values for estrogen and insulin

Fig. 1.3 Schematic demonstrating links between obesity and PI3K pathway (adapted from [59, 63]). *AKT* V-Akt Murine Thymoma Viral Oncogene Homolog, *IGF-I* insulin-like growth factor-I, *IL-6* interleukin-6, *mTORC* mechanistic target of rapamycin complex 1, *PDK* Phosphoinositide-dependent protein kinase, *PI3K* phosphatidylinositol 3-kinase, *PTEN* phosphatase and tensin homolog, *p85* PI3-Kinase Subunit p85, *TNF-alpha* tumor necrosis factor-alpha

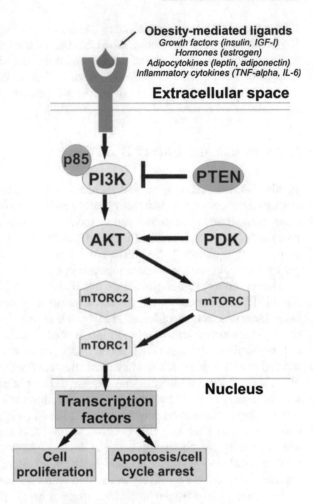

levels with respect to endometrial cancer are fairly low, even among obese women. It is likely that additional, currently unknown markers of endometrial cancer risk exist. Newer approaches to evaluating metabolic status, for example metabolomics, may offer powerful new insights into endometrial cancer development. A cross-sectional investigation of metabolite profiles in a population-based endometrial cancer case-control study (Polish Women's Health Study) reported that women with endometrial cancer had lower levels of C5-acylcarnitines, octenoylcarnitine and linoleic acid [55]. It is likely that future studies will apply metabolomics profiling to prospectively-collected biospecimens to identify biochemical intermediates that may help to explain the link between endometrial cancer and its risk factors, including BMI.

Mechanistic studies of normal endometrial tissues are complimentary to studies of serologic factors and could further contribute towards a comprehensive understanding of pathways that may be implicated in endometrial carcinogenesis. Aside from a few investigations [50, 54], very few studies that have examined tissue-level changes in response to risk factor exposures therefore this is an area that could be expanded upon in future research. For example, a key molecular pathway that is altered in endometrial cancer is the PI3K pathway and specifically more frequent mutations have been observed in the PI3K pathway than any other cancer that has been studied to date [56]. There is a large body of work focusing on the PI3K pathway in relation to endometrial cancer tumor aggressiveness [57, 58] and on targeting this pathway for the treatment of recurrent endometrial cancer using mammalian target of rapamycin (mTOR) and related inhibitors [59, 60] yet there is very limited knowledge regarding the role of the PI3K pathway in the early development of endometrial cancer. The PI3K pathway may have particular relevance to the obesity-endometrial cancer association because several factors that are altered in obese women, including higher circulating levels of estrogen, insulin, leptin, and inflammatory cytokines and lower adiponectin levels [7], are known to influence the PI3K pathway ([61, 62]; Figure 1; [45, 63–65]) (Fig. 1.3). In summary, the obesity-endometrial cancer relationship is an established association that requires further study to identify and evaluate molecular mechanisms that may explain this relationship. Such studies could assist in the development of improved strategies for endometrial cancer prevention that will become increasingly important given the current obesity epidemic and rising incidence of endometrial cancer.

References

1. American Cancer Society. Cancer facts and figures 2016: report. Atlanta: American Cancer Society; 2016. Accessed 28 Oct 2016
2. Ferlay J, Soerjomataram I, Ervik M, Dikshit R, Eser S, Mathers C, Rebelo M, Parkin DM, Forman D, Bray F. GLOBOCAN 2012 v1.0, Cancer Incidence and Mortality Worldwide: IARC CancerBase No. 11. International Agency for Research on Cancer. 2013. Lyon, France. Accessed 8 Apr 2015.
3. Cancer Research UK. CancerStats: Cancer statistics for the UK. N/A. 2016. Accessed 28 Oct 2016.
4. Key TJ, Pike MC. The dose-effect relationship between 'unopposed' oestrogens and endometrial mitotic rate: its central role in explaining and predicting endometrial cancer risk. Br J Cancer. 1988;57(2):205–12.
5. Longcope C, Pratt JH, Schneider SH, Fineberg SE. Aromatization of androgens by muscle and adipose tissue in vivo. J Clin Endocrinol Metab. 1978;46(1):146–52.
6. Perel E, Killinger DW. The interconversion and aromatization of androgens by human adipose tissue. J Steroid Biochem. 1979;10(6):623–7.
7. Kaaks R, Lukanova A, Kurzer MS. Obesity, endogenous hormones, and endometrial cancer risk: a synthetic review. Cancer Epidemiol Biomark Prev. 2002;11(12):1531–43.
8. Renehan AG, Tyson M, Egger M, Heller RF, Zwahlen M. Body-mass index and incidence of cancer: a systematic review and meta-analysis of prospective observational studies. Lancet. 2008;371(9612):569–78. doi:10.1016/S0140-6736(08)60269-X. pii:S0140-6736(08)60269-X.
9. Bhaskaran K, Douglas I, Forbes H, dos-Santos-Silva I, Leon DA, Smeeth L. Body-mass index and risk of 22 specific cancers: a population-based cohort study of 5.24 million UK adults. Lancet. 2014;384(9945):755–65. doi:10.1016/S0140-6736(14)60892-8. pii:S0140-6736(14)60892-8.

10. Bokhman JV. Two pathogenetic types of endometrial carcinoma. Gynecol Oncol. 1983;15(1):10–7.
11. Sherman ME. Theories of endometrial carcinogenesis: a multidisciplinary approach. Mod Pathol. 2000;13(3):295–308.
12. Sherman ME, Sturgeon S, Brinton L, Kurman RJ. Endometrial cancer chemoprevention: implications of diverse pathways of carcinogenesis. J Cell Biochem Suppl. 1995b;23:160–4.
13. Sherman ME, Bur ME, Kurman RJ. p53 in endometrial cancer and its putative precursors: evidence for diverse pathways of tumorigenesis. Hum Pathol. 1995a;26(11):1268–74.
14. Hamilton CA, Cheung MK, Osann K, Chen L, Teng NN, Longacre TA, Powell MA, Hendrickson MR, Kapp DS, Chan JK. Uterine papillary serous and clear cell carcinomas predict for poorer survival compared to grade 3 endometrioid corpus cancers. Br J Cancer. 2006;94(5):642–6.
15. Hendrickson M, Ross J, Eifel P, Martinez A, Kempson R. Uterine papillary serous carcinoma: a highly malignant form of endometrial adenocarcinoma. Am J Surg Pathol. 1982;6(2):93–108.
16. Setiawan VW, Yang HP, Pike MC, McCann SE, Yu H, Xiang YB, Wolk A, Wentzensen N, Weiss NS, Webb PM, van den Brandt PA, van de Vijver K, Thompson PJ, Strom BL, Spurdle AB, Soslow RA, Shu XO, Schairer C, Sacerdote C, Rohan TE, Robien K, Risch HA, Ricceri F, Rebbeck TR, Rastogi R, Prescott J, Polidoro S, Park Y, Olson SH, Moysich KB, Miller AB, ML MC, Matsuno RK, Magliocco AM, Lurie G, Lu L, Lissowska J, Liang X, Lacey JV Jr, Kolonel LN, Henderson BE, Hankinson SE, Hakansson N, Goodman MT, Gaudet MM, Garcia-Closas M, Friedenreich CM, Freudenheim JL, Doherty J, De Vivo I, Courneya KS, Cook LS, Chen C, Cerhan JR, Cai H, Brinton LA, Bernstein L, Anderson KE, Anton-Culver H, Schouten LJ, Horn-Ross PL. Type I and II endometrial cancers: have they different risk factors? J Clin Oncol. 2013;31(20):2607–18. doi:10.1200/JCO.2012.48.2596. pii:JCO.2012.48.2596.
17. Aune D, Navarro Rosenblatt DA, Chan DS, Vingeliene S, Abar L, Vieira AR, Greenwood DC, Bandera EV, Norat T. Anthropometric factors and endometrial cancer risk: a systematic review and dose-response meta-analysis of prospective studies. Ann Oncol. 2015;26(8):1635–48. doi:10.1093/annonc/mdv142. pii:mdv142.
18. Brinton LA, Felix AS, McMeekin DS, Creasman WT, Sherman ME, Mutch D, Cohn DE, Walker JL, Moore RG, Downs LS, Soslow RA, Zaino R. Etiologic heterogeneity in endometrial cancer: evidence from a Gynecologic Oncology Group trial. Gynecol Oncol. 2013;129(2):277–84. doi:10.1016/j.ygyno.2013.02.023. pii:S0090-8258(13)00094-2.
19. World Cancer Research Fund/American Institute for Cancer Research. Continuous Update Project Report. Food, Nutrition, Physical Activity, and the Prevention of Endometrial Cancer. N/A. 2013. Accessed 28 May 2015.
20. Crosbie EJ, Zwahlen M, Kitchener HC, Egger M, Renehan AG. Body mass index, hormone replacement therapy, and endometrial cancer risk: a meta-analysis. Cancer Epidemiol Biomark Prev. 2010;19(12):3119–30. doi:10.1158/1055-9965.EPI-10-0832. pii:1055-9965. EPI-10-0832.
21. Grady D, Gebretsadik T, Kerlikowske K, Ernster V, Petitti D. Hormone replacement therapy and endometrial cancer risk: a meta-analysis. Obstet Gynecol. 1995;85(2):304–13. doi:10.1016/0029-7844(94)00383-O. pii:0029-7844(94)00383-O.
22. Allen NE, Tsilidis KK, Key TJ, Dossus L, Kaaks R, Lund E, Bakken K, Gavrilyuk O, Overvad K, Tjonneland A, Olsen A, Fournier A, Fabre A, Clavel-Chapelon F, Chabbert-Buffet N, Sacerdote C, Krogh V, Bendinelli B, Tumino R, Panico S, Bergmann M, Schuetze M, van Duijnhoven FJ, Bueno-de-Mesquita HB, Onland-Moret NC, van Gils CH, Amiano P, Barricarte A, Chirlaque MD, Molina-Montes ME, Redondo ML, Duell EJ, Khaw KT, Wareham N, Rinaldi S, Fedirko V, Mouw T, Michaud DS, Riboli E. Menopausal hormone therapy and risk of endometrial carcinoma among postmenopausal women in the European Prospective Investigation Into Cancer and Nutrition. Am J Epidemiol. 2010;172(12):1394–403. doi:10.1093/aje/kwq300. pii:kwq300.
23. Pike MC, Peters RK, Cozen W, Probst-Hensch NM, Felix JC, Wan PC, Mack TM. Estrogen-progestin replacement therapy and endometrial cancer. J Natl Cancer Inst. 1997;89(15):1110–6.

24. Chlebowski RT, Anderson GL, Sarto GE, Haque R, Runowicz CD, Aragaki AK, Thomson CA, Howard BV, Wactawski-Wende J, Chen C, Rohan TE, Simon MS, Reed SD, Manson JE. Continuous combined estrogen plus progestin and endometrial cancer: the Women's health initiative randomized trial. J Natl Cancer Inst. 2016;108(3):pii:djv350. doi:10.1093/jnci/djv350.

25. Burkhauser RV, Cawley J. Beyond BMI: the value of more accurate measures of fatness and obesity in social science research. J Health Econ. 2008;27(2):519–29. doi:10.1016/j.jhealeco.2007.05.005. pii:S0167-6296(07)00113-0.

26. Esposito K, Chiodini P, Capuano A, Bellastella G, Maiorino MI, Giugliano D. Metabolic syndrome and endometrial cancer: a meta-analysis. Endocrine. 2014;45(1):28–36. doi:10.1007/s12020-013-9973-3.

27. Friberg E, Orsini N, Mantzoros CS, Wolk A. Diabetes mellitus and risk of endometrial cancer: a meta-analysis. Diabetologia. 2007;50(7):1365–74. doi:10.1007/s00125-007-0681-5.

28. Zhang ZH, Su PY, Hao JH, Sun YH. The role of preexisting diabetes mellitus on incidence and mortality of endometrial cancer: a meta-analysis of prospective cohort studies. Int J Gynecol Cancer. 2013;23(2):294–303. doi:10.1097/IGC.0b013e31827b8430.

29. Liao C, Zhang D, Mungo C, Andrew TD, Zeidan AM. Is diabetes mellitus associated with increased incidence and disease-specific mortality in endometrial cancer? A systematic review and meta-analysis of cohort studies. Gynecol Oncol. 2014;135(1):163–71. doi:10.1016/j.ygyno.2014.07.095. pii:S0090-8258(14)01218-9.

30. Luo J, Beresford S, Chen C, Chlebowski R, Garcia L, Kuller L, Regier M, Wactawski-Wende J, Margolis KL. Association between diabetes, diabetes treatment and risk of developing endometrial cancer. Br J Cancer. 2014;111(7):1432–9. doi:10.1038/bjc.2014.407. pii:bjc2014407.

31. Nead KT, Sharp SJ, Thompson DJ, Painter JN, Savage DB, Semple RK, Barker A, Perry JR, Attia J, Dunning AM, Easton DF, Holliday E, Lotta LA, O'Mara T, McEvoy M, Pharoah PD, Scott RJ, Spurdle AB, Langenberg C, Warcham NJ, Scott RA. Evidence of a causal association between insulinemia and endometrial cancer: a mendelian randomization analysis. J Natl Cancer Inst. 2015;107(9):pii:djv178. doi:10.1093/jnci/djv178.

32. Siiteri PK. Adipose tissue as a source of hormones. Am J Clin Nutr. 1987;45(1 Suppl):277–82.

33. Allen NE, Key TJ, Dossus L, Rinaldi S, Cust A, Lukanova A, Peeters PH, Onland-Moret NC, Lahmann PH, Berrino F, Panico S, Larranaga N, Pera G, Tormo MJ, Sanchez MJ, Ramon QJ, Ardanaz E, Tjonneland A, Olsen A, Chang-Claude J, Linseisen J, Schulz M, Boeing H, Lundin E, Palli D, Overvad K, Clavel-Chapelon F, Boutron-Ruault MC, Bingham S, Khaw KT, Bueno-de-Mesquita HB, Trichopoulou A, Trichopoulos D, Naska A, Tumino R, Riboli E, Kaaks R. Endogenous sex hormones and endometrial cancer risk in women in the European Prospective Investigation into Cancer and Nutrition (EPIC). Endocr Relat Cancer. 2008;15(2):485–97. doi:10.1677/ERC-07-0064. pii:15/2/485.

34. Potischman N, Gail MH, Troisi R, Wacholder S, Hoover RN. Measurement error does not explain the persistence of a body mass index association with endometrial cancer after adjustment for endogenous hormones. Epidemiology. 1999;10(1):76–9. pii:00001648-199901000-00011.

35. Renehan AG, Frystyk J, Flyvbjerg A. Obesity and cancer risk: the role of the insulin-IGF axis. Trends Endocrinol Metab. 2006;17(8):328–36. doi:10.1016/j.tem.2006.08.006. pii:S1043-2760(06)00157-3.

36. Juul A, Holm K, Kastrup KW, Pedersen SA, Michaelsen KF, Scheike T, Rasmussen S, Muller J, Skakkebaek NE. Free insulin-like growth factor I serum levels in 1430 healthy children and adults, and its diagnostic value in patients suspected of growth hormone deficiency. J Clin Endocrinol Metab. 1997;82(8):2497–502. doi:10.1210/jcem.82.8.4137.

37. Gunter MJ, Hoover DR, Yu H, Wassertheil-Smoller S, Manson JE, Li J, Harris TG, Rohan TE, Xue X, Ho GY, Einstein MH, Kaplan RC, Burk RD, Wylie-Rosett J, Pollak MN, Anderson G, Howard BV, Strickler HD. A prospective evaluation of insulin and insulin-like growth factor-I as risk factors for endometrial cancer. Cancer Epidemiol Biomark Prev. 2008;17(4):921–9. doi:10.1158/1055-9965.EPI-07-2686. pii:17/4/921.

38. Cust AE, Allen NE, Rinaldi S, Dossus L, Friedenreich C, Olsen A, Tjonneland A, Overvad K, Clavel-Chapelon F, Boutron-Ruault MC, Linseisen J, Chang-Claude J, Boeing H, Schulz M, Benetou V, Trichopoulou A, Trichopoulos D, Palli D, Berrino F, Tumino R, Mattiello A,

Vineis P, Quiros JR, Agudo A, Sanchez MJ, Larranaga N, Navarro C, Ardanaz E, Bueno-de-Mesquita HB, Peeters PH, van Gils CH, Bingham S, Khaw KT, Key T, Slimani N, Riboli E, Kaaks R. Serum levels of C-peptide, IGFBP-1 and IGFBP-2 and endometrial cancer risk; results from the European prospective investigation into cancer and nutrition. Int J Cancer. 2007;120(12):2656–64. doi:10.1002/ijc.22578.

39. Lukanova A, Zeleniuch-Jacquotte A, Lundin E, Micheli A, Arslan AA, Rinaldi S, Muti P, Lenner P, Koenig KL, Biessy C, Krogh V, Riboli E, Shore RE, Stattin P, Berrino F, Hallmans G, Toniolo P, Kaaks R. Prediagnostic levels of C-peptide, IGF-I, IGFBP-1, −2 and −3 and risk of endometrial cancer. Int J Cancer. 2004;108(2):262–8. doi:10.1002/ijc.11544.

40. Hernandez AV, Pasupuleti V, Benites-Zapata VA, Thota P, Deshpande A, Perez-Lopez FR. Insulin resistance and endometrial cancer risk: a systematic review and meta-analysis. Eur J Cancer. 2015;51(18):2747–58. doi:10.1016/j.ejca.2015.08.031. pii:S0959-8049(15)00851-5.

41. van Kruijsdijk RC, van der Wall E, Visseren FL. Obesity and cancer: the role of dysfunctional adipose tissue. Cancer Epidemiol Biomark Prev. 2009;18(10):2569–78. doi:10.1158/1055-9965.EPI-09-0372. pii:1055-9965.EPI-09-0372.

42. Gong TT, Wu QJ, Wang YL, Ma XX. Circulating adiponectin, leptin and adiponectin-leptin ratio and endometrial cancer risk: evidence from a meta-analysis of epidemiologic studies. Int J Cancer. 2015;137(8):1967–78. doi:10.1002/ijc.29561.

43. Zheng Q, Wu H, Cao J. Circulating adiponectin and risk of endometrial cancer. PLoS One. 2015;10(6):e0129824. doi:10.1371/journal.pone.0129824. pii:PONE-D-14-53656.

44. Catalano S, Giordano C, Rizza P, Gu G, Barone I, Bonofiglio D, Giordano F, Malivindi R, Gaccione D, Lanzino M, De AF, Ando S. Evidence that leptin through STAT and CREB signaling enhances cyclin D1 expression and promotes human endometrial cancer proliferation. J Cell Physiol. 2009;218(3):490–500. doi:10.1002/jcp.21622.

45. Sharma D, Saxena NK, Vertino PM, Anania FA. Leptin promotes the proliferative response and invasiveness in human endometrial cancer cells by activating multiple signal-transduction pathways. Endocr Relat Cancer. 2006;13(2):629–40. doi:10.1677/erc.1.01169. pii:13/2/629.

46. Kelesidis I, Kelesidis T, Mantzoros CS. Adiponectin and cancer: a systematic review. Br J Cancer. 2006;94(9):1221–5. doi:10.1038/sj.bjc.6603051. pii:6603051.

47. Dossus L, Rinaldi S, Becker S, Lukanova A, Tjonneland A, Olsen A, Stegger J, Overvad K, Chabbert-Buffet N, Jimenez-Corona A, Clavel-Chapelon F, Rohrmann S, Teucher B, Boeing H, Schutze M, Trichopoulou A, Benetou V, Lagiou P, Palli D, Berrino F, Panico S, Tumino R, Sacerdote C, Redondo ML, Travier N, Sanchez MJ, Altzibar JM, Chirlaque MD, Ardanaz E, Bueno-de-Mesquita HB, van Duijnhoven FJ, Onland-Moret NC, Peeters PH, Hallmans G, Lundin E, Khaw KT, Wareham N, Allen N, Key TJ, Slimani N, Hainaut P, Romaguera D, Norat T, Riboli E, Kaaks R. Obesity, inflammatory markers, and endometrial cancer risk: a prospective case-control study. Endocr Relat Cancer. 2010;17(4):1007–19. doi:10.1677/ERC-10-0053. pii:ERC-10-0053.

48. Dossus L, Becker S, Rinaldi S, Lukanova A, Tjonneland A, Olsen A, Overvad K, Chabbert-Buffet N, Boutron-Ruault MC, Clavel-Chapelon F, Teucher B, Chang-Claude J, Pischon T, Boeing H, Trichopoulou A, Benetou V, Valanou E, Palli D, Sieri S, Tumino R, Sacerdote C, Galasso R, Redondo ML, Bonet CB, Molina-Montes E, Altzibar JM, Chirlaque MD, Ardanaz E, Bueno-de-Mesquita HB, van Duijnhoven FJ, Peeters PH, Onland-Moret NC, Lundin E, Idahl A, Khaw KT, Wareham N, Allen N, Romieu I, Fedirko V, Hainaut P, Romaguera D, Norat T, Riboli E, Kaaks R. Tumor necrosis factor (TNF)-alpha, soluble TNF receptors and endometrial cancer risk: the EPIC study. Int J Cancer. 2011;129(8):2032–7. doi:10.1002/ijc.25840.

49. Wang T, Rohan TE, Gunter MJ, Xue X, Wactawski-Wende J, Rajpathak SN, Cushman M, Strickler HD, Kaplan RC, Wassertheil-Smoller S, Scherer PE, Ho GY. A prospective study of inflammation markers and endometrial cancer risk in postmenopausal hormone nonusers. Cancer Epidemiol Biomark Prev. 2011;20(5):971–7. doi:10.1158/1055-9965.EPI-10-1222. pii:1055-9965.EPI-10-1222.

50. Merritt MA, Strickler HD, Einstein MH, Yang HP, Sherman ME, Wentzensen N, Brouwer-Visser J, Cossio MJ, Whitney KD, Yu H, Gunter MJ, Huang GS. Insulin/IGF and sex hormone axes in human endometrium and associations with endometrial cancer risk factors.

Cancer Causes Control. 2016;27(6):737–48. doi:10.1007/s10552-016-0751-4. pii:10.1007/s10552-016-0751-4.

51. Rutanen EM. Insulin-like growth factors in endometrial function. Gynecol Endocrinol. 1998;12(6):399–406.

52. Zhu L, Pollard JW. Estradiol-17beta regulates mouse uterine epithelial cell proliferation through insulin-like growth factor 1 signaling. Proc Natl Acad Sci U S A. 2007;104(40):15847–51. doi:10.1073/pnas.0705749104. pii:0705749104.

53. McCampbell AS, Broaddus RR, Loose DS, Davies PJ. Overexpression of the insulin-like growth factor I receptor and activation of the AKT pathway in hyperplastic endometrium. Clin Cancer Res. 2006;12(21):6373–8. doi:10.1158/1078-0432.CCR-06-0912. pii:12/21/6373.

54. Yang HP, Meeker A, Guido R, Gunter MJ, Huang GS, Luhn P, d'Ambrosio L, Wentzensen N, Sherman ME. PTEN expression in benign human endometrial tissue and cancer in relation to endometrial cancer risk factors. Cancer Causes Control. 2015;26(12):1729–36. doi:10.1007/s10552-015-0666-5. pii:10.1007/s10552-015-0666-5.

55. Gaudet MM, Falk RT, Stevens RD, Gunter MJ, Bain JR, Pfeiffer RM, Potischman N, Lissowska J, Peplonska B, Brinton LA, Garcia-Closas M, Newgard CB, Sherman ME. Analysis of serum metabolic profiles in women with endometrial cancer and controls in a population-based case-control study. J Clin Endocrinol Metab. 2012;97(9):3216–23. doi:10.1210/jc.2012-1490. pii:jc.2012-1490.

56. Cancer Genome Atlas Research Network. Integrated genomic analyses of ovarian carcinoma. Nature. 2011;474(7353):609–15. doi:10.1038/nature10166.

57. Salvesen HB, Carter SL, Mannelqvist M, Dutt A, Getz G, Stefansson IM, Raeder MB, Sos ML, Engelsen IB, Trovik J, Wik E, Greulich H, Bo TH, Jonassen I, Thomas RK, Zander T, Garraway LA, Oyan AM, Sellers WR, Kalland KH, Meyerson M, Akslen LA, Beroukhim R. Integrated genomic profiling of endometrial carcinoma associates aggressive tumors with indicators of PI3 kinase activation. Proc Natl Acad Sci U S A. 2009;106(12):4834–9. doi:10.1073/pnas.0806514106. pii:0806514106.

58. Wik E, Trovik J, Kusonmano K, Birkeland E, Raeder MB, Pashtan I, Hoivik EA, Krakstad C, Werner HM, Holst F, Mjos S, Halle MK, Mannelqvist M, Mauland KK, Oyan AM, Stefansson IM, Petersen K, Simon R, Cherniack AD, Meyerson M, Kalland KH, Akslen LA, Salvesen HB. Endometrial Carcinoma Recurrence Score (ECARS) validates to identify aggressive disease and associates with markers of epithelial-mesenchymal transition and PI3K alterations. Gynecol Oncol. 2014;134(3):599–606. doi:10.1016/j.ygyno.2014.06.026. pii:S0090-8258(14)01067-1.

59. Dedes KJ, Wetterskog D, Ashworth A, Kaye SB, Reis-Filho JS. Emerging therapeutic targets in endometrial cancer. Nat Rev Clin Oncol. 2011;8(5):261–71. doi:10.1038/nrclinonc.2010.216. pii:nrclinonc.2010.216.

60. Salvesen HB, Haldorsen IS, Trovik J. Markers for individualised therapy in endometrial carcinoma. Lancet Oncol. 2012;13(8):e353–61. doi:10.1016/S1470-2045(12)70213-9. pii:S1470-2045(12)70213-9.

61. Pereira RI, Draznin B. Inhibition of the phosphatidylinositol 3′-kinase signaling pathway leads to decreased insulin-stimulated adiponectin secretion from 3T3-L1 adipocytes. Metabolism. 2005;54(12):1636–43. doi:10.1016/j.metabol.2005.07.002. pii:S0026-0495(05)00263-5.

62. Schmandt RE, Iglesias DA, Co NN, Lu TH. Understanding obesity and endometrial cancer risk: opportunities for prevention. Am J Obstet Gynecol. 2011;205(6):518–25.

63. Huang XF, Chen JZ. Obesity, the PI3K/Akt signal pathway and colon cancer. Obes Rev. 2009;10(6):610–6. doi:10.1111/j.1467-789X.2009.00607.x. pii:OBR607.

64. Miller TW, Balko JM, Arteaga CL. Phosphatidylinositol 3-kinase and antiestrogen resistance in breast cancer. J Clin Oncol. 2011;29(33):4452–61. doi:10.1200/JCO.2010.34.4879. pii:JCO.2010.34.4879.

65. Slomovitz BM, Coleman RL. The PI3K/AKT/mTOR pathway as a therapeutic target in endometrial cancer. Clin Cancer Res. 2012;18(21):5856–64. doi:10.1158/1078-0432.CCR-12-0662. pii:1078-0432.CCR-12-0662.

Chapter 2
Epidemiologic Relationship Between Obesity and Ovarian Cancer

Carmen Jochem, Inga Schlecht, and Michael Leitzmann

Abstract Ovarian cancer is the seventh most common cancer in women worldwide. Several systematic reviews and meta-analyses have shown a positive association between obesity and ovarian cancer, and the American Institute for Cancer Research and World Cancer Research Fund recently concluded that body fatness (marked by body mass index) is a probable risk factor for ovarian cancer. The positive relation of body fatness to ovarian cancer appears to be more evident among non-users of hormone therapy. Furthermore, compared to normal weight, obesity is associated with poorer ovarian cancer survival. Possible biological mechanisms linking obesity with ovarian cancer risk and progression include insulin resistance and hyperinsulinaemia, increased levels of circulating growth factors, chronic inflammation, and altered levels of sex hormones. Thus, obesity, as a modifiable risk factor, should be targeted for preventing ovarian cancer and for improving ovarian cancer survival.

Keywords Ovarian cancer age standardized incidence rate • Ovarian cancer risk factor • Obesity • Ovarian cancer mortality • Insulin resistance

Introduction

The ovaries – as reproductive glands – are the sites of ovum production and they are also the main source of the sex hormones oestrogen and progesterone in premenopausal women. Ovarian cancer can originate from the three types of cells that make up the ovaries: epithelial cells, which cover the outer surface of the ovary; hormone producing stromal cells (structural tissue cells); and egg producing germ cells. Up to 95% of ovarian tumors are epithelial cell tumors.

C. Jochem • I. Schlecht • M. Leitzmann (✉)
Department of Epidemiology and Preventive Medicine, University of Regensburg,
Franz-Josef-Strauss-Allee 11, Regensburg 93053, Germany
e-mail: Carmen.Jochem@klinik.uni-regensburg.de; Inga.Schlecht@klinik.uni-regensburg.de;
Michael.Leitzmann@klinik.uni-regensburg.de

© Springer International Publishing AG 2018
N.A. Berger et al. (eds.), *Focus on Gynecologic Malignancies*, Energy Balance and Cancer 13, DOI 10.1007/978-3-319-63483-8_2

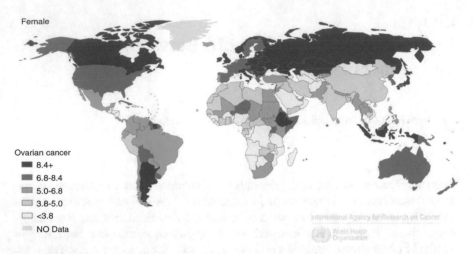

Fig. 2.1 Estimated age-standardized incidence rates of ovarian cancer worldwide in 2012 (reproduced with permission from the International Agency for Research on Cancer [29])

Ovarian cancer is the seventh most common cancer in women worldwide [1]. In 2012, approximately 239,000 cases of ovarian cancer were recorded, accounting for 3.6% of all new cancer cases in women [1]. Almost half of all new ovarian cancer cases were reported in Asia (N = 112,000).

The age-standardized incidence rate of ovarian cancer is 6.1 per 100,000. Incidence rates are lower in less developed regions of the world (ASR 4.9 per 100,000) than more developed regions of the world (ASR 9.1 per 100,000) and they range from 3.6 per 100,000 in Western Africa to ≥11 per 100,000 women in Central, Eastern, and Northern Europe (Fig. 2.1) [1]. The estimated cumulative risk of developing ovarian cancer before the age of 75 years ranges from 0.5% in less developed regions of the world to 1% in more developed regions, and it reaches 1.3% in Central and Eastern Europe [1].

Ovarian cancer is the eighth most common cause of death from cancer in women, with an estimated number of 152,000 deaths worldwide in 2012 (4.3% of deaths from cancer in women) [1]. Similar to its incidence rates, estimated age-standardized mortality rates (ASR) of ovarian cancer are lower in less developed regions of the world (ASR 3.1 per 100,000) and higher in more developed regions (ASR 5.0 per 100,000), such as North America (ASR 5.0), Northern Europe (ASR 5.9), Central and Eastern Europe (ASR 6.0), and Melanesia (ASR 6.5) [1].

According to the Global Burden of Disease Study, prevalent ovarian cancer cases contributed to an estimated 135,000 years lived with disability (YLDs) in 2013 – a figure that is comparable to the YLDs due to kidney cancer and malignant skin melanoma [2]. Thus, ovarian cancer is a relevant public health issue and it is crucial to gain a deeper understanding of its major risk factors – particularly those that are preventable, such as obesity.

Ovarian Cancer Characteristics and Risk Factors

Ovarian cancer frequently has no clinical symptoms in its early stages. Therefore, the disease is generally advanced when it is diagnosed. The 5-year survival rate ranges from approximately 30–50% [3].

Ovarian cancer is a heterogeneous disease with distinct histologic subtypes and thus, it is characterized by differences in epidemiologic and genetic risk factors, clinical presentation, response to treatment, and prognosis [4]. Five different tumor types account for 98% of ovarian cancers: high-grade serous carcinoma (70%), endometrioid carcinoma (10%), clear-cell carcinoma (19%), mucinous carcinoma (5%), and low-grade serous carcinoma (3%) [4].

Although ovarian cancer risk factors differ between distinct tumor histologic types, there are a number of established risk factors for total ovarian cancer, including age, reproductive history, modifiable lifestyle factors, family history, and genetic mutations.

Several factors concerning the reproductive history and life events during a woman's lifetime may influence the risk of developing ovarian cancer. Whereas oral contraceptives seem to have a beneficial effect on the risk of developing ovarian cancer [5], intrauterine device use may pose a potential risk factor for ovarian cancer [6]. Early menarche and late natural menopause, and consecutively a higher number of menstrual cycles during a woman's lifetime, increase the risk of ovarian cancer. In line with this, late menarche, breast feeding (lactation), early menopause, and number of pregnancies are beneficial factors that decrease the risk of developing ovarian cancer [5, 7]. It has been shown that the use of hormone therapy (HT) increases the risk of ovarian cancer [8, 9].

Polycystic ovarian syndrome is a potential risk factor for developing ovarian cancer [10]. However, the available evidence is not yet clear [11]. Furthermore, endometriosis is a risk factor for certain but not all histologic types of ovarian cancer [12]. Findings from a meta-analysis show positive associations between self-reported endometriosis and risks of clear-cell, low-grade serous, and endometrioid invasive ovarian cancers [12].

Smoking – as a modifiable lifestyle factor – is a risk factor for mucinous ovarian cancer, but not for other types of ovarian cancers [13]. Other lifestyle factors including obesity have been evaluated and the American Institute for Cancer Research and World Cancer Research Fund recently concluded that there is probable evidence for a positive association between obesity and ovarian cancer [14]. By comparison, the relations with other lifestyle factors, such as physical activity or dietary factors and ovarian cancer remain unclear [14].

Hereditary ovarian cancer makes up about 5–10% of all cases of ovarian cancer. The majority of hereditary ovarian cancers are based on mutations in the *BRCA1* and *BRCA2* genes [15]. In contrast to the lifetime risk of developing ovarian cancer in the general population (approximately 1%), women with a *BRCA1* mutation have a lifetime risk of approximately 40% [16]. Mean cumulative ovarian cancer risk for *BRCA2* mutation carriers is somewhat lower, at approximately 20% at age 70 [16].

Another type of hereditary ovarian cancer is based on mutations in genes such as *MSH2* or *MLH1,* which represent DNA mismatch repair genes that are linked to hereditary non-polyposis colorectal cancer (HNPCC; also called Lynch syndrome), an autosomal dominant disorder that predisposes to colorectal, endometrial, and ovarian cancers, among others [15]. In women with Lynch syndrome, lifetime risk of ovarian cancer is between 3 and 14% [17]. Overall, at least 16 genes have been associated with ovarian cancer [15] – and it is likely that advances in genomic technologies will detect more genes associated with ovarian cancer in the future.

Association Between Obesity and Ovarian Cancer Incidence and Mortality

Numerous observational studies have investigated the association between obesity and the risk of ovarian cancer. However, results have not been entirely consistent. The current section aims at providing an overview of the existing evidence by summarizing the main findings from published meta-analyses, reviews, and observational studies.

Research on the relation between obesity and ovarian cancer risk has increased substantially in the past decade. In 2007, the World Cancer Research Fund/American Institute for Cancer Research stated that the evidence relating body fatness, abdominal fatness and weight change to ovarian cancer risk was inconclusive [18]. Since then, several systematic reviews and meta-analyses have been conducted, reflecting the increased number of available epidemiologic studies on adiposity and ovarian cancer.

The Continuous Update Project "Ovarian Cancer 2014 Report" published by the World Cancer Research Fund and the American Institute for Cancer Research concluded that greater body fatness (marked by body mass index (BMI)) is a probable cause of ovarian cancer [14]. The systematic literature review underlying that report compared the highest versus lowest BMI levels and it included 26 prospective studies on ovarian cancer incidence and mortality [14]. The dose-response meta-analysis of that report included a total of 15,899 cases from 25 prospective studies (22 risk estimates) and it showed a statistically significant increased ovarian cancer risk of 6% per 5 BMI units (relative risk (RR) = 1.06; 95% confidence interval (CI): 1.02–1.11) (Fig. 2.2). However, there was evidence of substantial heterogeneity between studies (I^2 = 55%). Results from additional analyses identified several possible sources of heterogeneity, such as tumor type, use of HT, and menopausal status. With respect to tumor type, the positive association between BMI and risk for ovarian cancer was slightly more pronounced for borderline serous, invasive endometrioid, and invasive mucinous tumors, with pooled RRs per 5 BMI units of 1.24 (95% CI: 1.18–1.30), 1.17 (95% CI: 1.11–1.23), and 1.19 (95% CI: 1.06–1.32), respectively [14]. By comparison, there was no association with serous invasive cancer (pooled OR per 5 BMI units: 0.98; 95% CI: 0.94–1.02).

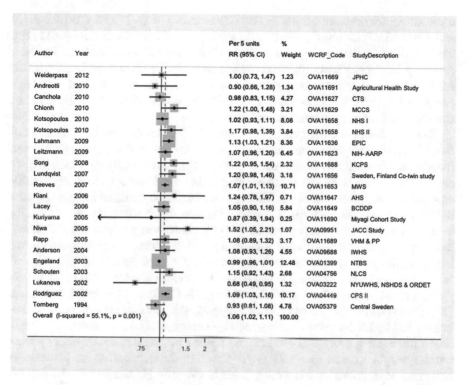

Author	Year		Per 5 units RR (95% CI)	% Weight	WCRF_Code	StudyDescription
Weiderpass	2012		1.00 (0.73, 1.47)	1.23	OVA11669	JPHC
Andreotti	2010		0.90 (0.66, 1.28)	1.34	OVA11691	Agricultural Health Study
Canchola	2010		0.98 (0.83, 1.15)	4.27	OVA11627	CTS
Chionh	2010		1.22 (1.00, 1.48)	3.21	OVA11629	MCCS
Kotsopoulos	2010		1.02 (0.93, 1.11)	8.08	OVA11658	NHS I
Kotsopoulos	2010		1.17 (0.98, 1.39)	3.84	OVA11658	NHS II
Lahmann	2009		1.13 (1.03, 1.21)	8.36	OVA11636	EPIC
Leitzmann	2009		1.07 (0.96, 1.20)	6.45	OVA11623	NIH- AARP
Song	2008		1.22 (0.95, 1.54)	2.32	OVA11688	KCPS
Lundqvist	2007		1.20 (0.98, 1.46)	3.18	OVA11656	Sweden, Finland Co-twin study
Reeves	2007		1.07 (1.01, 1.13)	10.71	OVA11653	MWS
Kiani	2006		1.24 (0.78, 1.97)	0.71	OVA11647	AHS
Lacey	2006		1.05 (0.90, 1.16)	5.84	OVA11649	BCDDP
Kuriyama	2005		0.87 (0.39, 1.94)	0.25	OVA11690	Miyagi Cohort Study
Niwa	2005		1.52 (1.05, 2.21)	1.07	OVA09951	JACC Study
Rapp	2005		1.08 (0.89, 1.32)	3.17	OVA11689	VHM & PP
Anderson	2004		1.08 (0.93, 1.26)	4.55	OVA09688	IWHS
Engeland	2003		0.99 (0.96, 1.01)	12.48	OVA01399	NTBS
Schouten	2003		1.15 (0.92, 1.43)	2.68	OVA04756	NLCS
Lukanova	2002		0.68 (0.49, 0.95)	1.32	OVA03222	NYUWHS, NSHDS & ORDET
Rodriguez	2002		1.09 (1.03, 1.16)	10.17	OVA04449	CPS II
Tomberg	1994		0.93 (0.81, 1.08)	4.78	OVA05379	Central Sweden
Overall (I-squared = 55.1%, p = 0.001)			1.06 (1.02, 1.11)	100.00		

Fig. 2.2 Dose-response meta-analysis of BMI and ovarian cancer (conducted by and reproduced with permission from the World Cancer Research Fund/American Institute for Cancer Research [14])

In addition to BMI, the Continuous Update Project summarized the findings on weight, waist circumference, and waist-to-hip ratio in relation to ovarian cancer risk. With respect to weight, a dose-response meta-analysis of three cohort studies revealed a summary RR of 1.05 (95% CI: 1.02–1.07) per 5 kg increase in weight. A dose-response meta-analysis of four studies on the association between waist cir-cumference and ovarian cancer risk showed a statistically non-significant positive association, with a RR of 1.03 (95% CI: 0.97–1.10 per 10 cm). Furthermore, four studies were included in a dose-response meta-analysis for waist-to-hip ratio and ovarian cancer and no association was observed (RR = 0.99; 95% CI: 0.92–1.06 per 10 cm).

The Continuous Update Project concluded that there was evidence of positive association between obesity (as assessed by BMI) and ovarian cancer risk, with the exception of serous invasive cancer. By comparison, the evidence for abdominal fatness (as assessed by waist circumference and waist-to-hip ratio) was judged lim-ited and inconclusive [14].

A recently published meta-analysis included 13 case-control and 13 cohort stud-ies with a total of 12,963 ovarian cancer cases and 2,164,977 participants [19]. As compared with normal weight (BMI = 18.5–24.9 kg/m²), that meta-analysis showed a pooled RR for overweight (BMI = 25.0–29.9 kg/m^2) of 1.07 (95% CI: 1.02–1.12) and a pooled RR for obesity (BMI $\geq$ 30 kg/m^2) of 1.28 (95% CI: 1.16–1.41) [19]. The positive association held true for both Caucasian and Asian studies. However, subgroup analyses showed that overweight and obesity were associated with an increased risk of ovarian cancer in premenopausal women only (RR for over-weight = 1.31; 95% CI: 1.04–1.65; RR for obesity = 1.50; 95% CI: 1.12–2.00), but showed no relation in postmenopausal women [19].

The Collaborative Group on Epidemiological Studies of Ovarian Cancer con-ducted an individual participant meta-analysis on the association between body size (height and BMI) and risk of ovarian cancer [13]. The investigators included 47 studies and a total of 25,157 ovarian cancer cases and found a statistically signifi-cant positive association between BMI and ovarian cancer risk that did not substan-tially vary by age, year of birth, ethnicity, education, age at menarche, parity, family history of ovarian or breast cancer, use of oral contraceptives, menopausal status, hysterectomy, smoking, or alcohol consumption. However, there was significant heterogeneity between ever-users and never-users of HT. Specifically, a 5 kg/m^2 increase in BMI was associated with a RR of 1.10 (95% CI: 1.07–1.13) in HT never-users, whereas it was related to a RR of 0.95 (95% CI: 0.92–0.99) in HT ever-users [13]. Data showing that the association between BMI and ovarian cancer incidence is modified by HT had first been reported by Leitzmann and colleagues [20]. They found that among never users of HT, the risk of ovarian cancer for obese versus normal weight women was 1.83 (95% CI: 1.18–2.84), whereas no association between BMI and ovarian cancer was noted among ever HT users (RR = 0.96; 95% CI: 0.65–1.43; P for interaction = 0.02).

Dixon and colleagues pooled data from 39 studies of the International Ovarian Cancer Association Consortium in a Mendelian randomization study, including a total of 14,047 ovarian cancer cases, to investigate the association between BMI and subtypes of ovarian cancer [21]. Mendelian randomization uses genetic markers (instrumental variables) as proxies for risk factors. In that study, a weighted genetic risk score for BMI was constructed by summing alleles associated with higher BMI across a predefined number of single nucleotide polymorphisms that had previously been associated with BMI. The researchers found that genetically predicted increas-ing BMI (per 5 kg/m^2) was associated with an increased risk of non-high grade serous ovarian cancer (pooled OR = 1.29; 95% CI: 1.03–1.61) but was unrelated to the more common high grade serous ovarian cancer (pooled OR = 1.06; 95% CI: 0.88–1.27).

Compared to BMI as a metric of adiposity, adult weight gain better reflects the dynamic pattern of weight trajectories throughout adult life. Whereas BMI captures both fat mass and lean body mass, adult weight gain primarily captures increasing fat mass. Keum and colleagues conducted a dose-response meta-analysis of pro-spective observational studies to investigate the association between adult weight gain and adiposity-related cancers [22]. The dose-response meta-analysis was based on two eligible prospective studies among postmenopausal women. Findings showed that each 5 kg increase in adult weight gain was associated with a 13%

increase in risk of developing ovarian cancer (RR = 1.13; 95% CI: 1.03–1.23) in postmenopausal women with no/low HT use [22].

Summarizing the results from meta-analyses and reviews, it can be concluded that there is a positive relationship between BMI and risk of developing ovarian cancer. An increase of 5 BMI units is associated with a 6% increased risk of ovarian cancer. However, the strength of the association varies according to menopausal status, HT use, and tumor histologic type.

Association Between Obesity and Ovarian Cancer Survival

Obesity may not only be associated with an increased risk of developing ovarian cancer, but may also produce poor survival among women with ovarian cancer. As individual studies on the association between obesity and ovarian cancer survival have yielded conflicting results, the following section summarizes the main findings from published meta-analyses.

Bae et al. conducted a meta-analysis on obesity five years before diagnosis, obesity at young age, and obesity at diagnosis in relation to ovarian cancer survival [23]. The pooled results from three cohort studies that investigated the relationship between obesity in adolescence and ovarian cancer survival yielded a summary hazard ratio (HR) of 1.67 (95% CI: 1.29–2.16). Three cohort studies on obesity 5 years before ovarian cancer diagnosis and ovarian cancer survival showed a weaker relation (HR = 1.35; 95% CI: 1.03–1.76), as did studies examining the association between obesity at diagnosis and ovarian cancer survival (HR = 1.11; 95% CI: 0.97–1.27).

A meta-analysis by Protani and colleagues included 14 cohort studies and showed that ovarian cancer survival was poorer in obese women compared to non-obese women (HR = 1.17; 95% CI: 1.03–1.34) [24]. The pooled risk estimates did not vary between studies that measured pre-diagnosis BMI (HR = 1.13; 95% CI: 0.95–1.35), BMI at the time of diagnosis (HR = 1.13; 95% CI: 0.81–1.57), or BMI at the time of chemotherapy (HR = 1.13; 95% CI: 0.92–1.39), although all risk estimates were statistically non-significant.

Nagle and colleagues used data from 21 case-control studies, including 12,390 women with ovarian cancer from the Ovarian Cancer Association Consortium to investigate the association between pre-diagnosis BMI and progression-free survival, ovarian cancer-specific survival, and overall survival [25]. Multivariate analyses showed that overweight and obese women experienced worse survival than women with normal weight, although associations were not statistically significant. Furthermore, each 5-unit increase in BMI was related to a borderline significant 3% increased risk of death (95% CI: 1.00–1.07). Results stratified by tumor histologic type revealed a borderline significant positive association for survival among women with high-grade serous cancer, with a pooled HR of 1.04 (95% CI: 1.00–1.09) for each 5-unit increase in BMI. Positive but statistically non-significant associations were noted for survival among women with low-grade serous and endometrioid cancers. No associations were noted for mucinous and clear cell tumors [25]. Compared to women with normal weight, obese women showed poorer progression-free and overall survival, with HRs of 1.10 (95% CI: 0.99–1.23) and 1.12 (95% CI: 1.01–1.26), respectively.

Taken together, the evidence regarding the relationship between obesity and ovarian cancer survival is less clear than that between obesity and ovarian cancer incidence, but results from epidemiologic studies suggest that obesity is associated with poor ovarian cancer survival.

In addition to ovarian cancer survival, several studies investigated the relation between adiposity and surgical morbidity and clinical outcomes in ovarian cancer patients. A meta-analysis of five studies showed that compared to non-obese ovarian cancer patients, obese patients had an increased incidence of wound complications (odds ratio (OR) = 4.81; 95% CI: 2.40–9.62) [26]. However, there were no significant associations between BMI and febrile complications, ileus, or venous thromboembolism. In addition, there were no significant relations between BMI and intra-operative outcomes, such as cytoreduction status, estimated blood loss, or operation time. While obese patients showed a statistically significantly longer hospital stay than non-obese patients, there were no differences between obese and non-obese patients regarding 30-day mortality or transfusion rates [26].

Potential Biological Mechanisms

Obesity has been associated with increased risk and poor survival regarding cancers at multiple body sites, including several gynecological malignancies [27]. Possible mechanisms linking obesity with ovarian cancer risk and progression include insulin resistance and hyperinsulinaemia, increased levels of circulating growth factors, chronic inflammation, and altered levels of sex hormones [28].

Circulating levels of insulin and leptin are elevated in obese people and may promote the growth of cancer cells. In addition, obesity-related insulin resistance leads to compensatory increased insulin production and thus to hyperinsulinemia, which, in turn, may increase the risk of cancer. Furthermore, sex hormones, including estrogens, androgens, and progesterone, are likely to play a mechanistic role in ovarian cancer development. Additionally, obesity is related to a chronic state of low-grade inflammation. Compared to people with normal weight, levels of pro-inflammatory factors, such as tumor necrosis factors (TNF-) alpha, interleukin 6, and C-reactive protein are increased in obese people. Chronic inflammation can promote cancer development.

Chapter 6 of this book provides detailed information on the underlying biologic mechanisms linking obesity with ovarian cancer.

Conclusions

As outlined in this chapter, BMI is associated with an increased risk of developing ovarian cancer. The positive relation of body fatness to ovarian cancer is more evident among HT non-users than HT users. Furthermore, obesity appears to be associated with poor survival among ovarian cancer patients. Additional studies are needed to strengthen the evidence and to further investigate the underlying biological mechanisms.

References

1. Ferlay J, Soerjomataram I, Dikshit R, Eser S, Mathers C, Rebelo M, et al. Cancer incidence and mortality worldwide: sources, methods and major patterns in GLOBOCAN 2012. Int J Cancer. 2015;136(5):E359–86.
2. Global Burden of Disease Study 2013 Collaborators. Global, regional, and national incidence, prevalence, and years lived with disability for 301 acute and chronic diseases and injuries in 188 countries, 1990–2013: a systematic analysis for the Global Burden of Disease Study 2013. Lancet (London, England). 2015;386(9995):743–800.
3. De Angelis R, Sant M, Coleman MP, Francisci S, Baili P, Pierannunzio D, et al. Cancer survival in Europe 1999-2007 by country and age: results of EUROCARE--5-a population-based study. Lancet Oncol. 2014;15(1):23–34.
4. Prat J. Ovarian carcinomas: five distinct diseases with different origins, genetic alterations, and clinicopathological features. Virchows Arch. 2012;460(3):237–49.
5. Beral V, Doll R, Hermon C, Peto R, Reeves G. Ovarian cancer and oral contraceptives: collaborative reanalysis of data from 45 epidemiological studies including 23,257 women with ovarian cancer and 87,303 controls. Lancet (London, England). 2008;371(9609):303–14.
6. Tworoger SS, Fairfield KM, Colditz GA, Rosner BA, Hankinson SE. Association of oral contraceptive use, other contraceptive methods, and infertility with ovarian cancer risk. Am J Epidemiol. 2007;166(8):894–901.
7. Jordan SJ, Cushing-Haugen KL, Wicklund KG, Doherty JA, Rossing MA. Breast-feeding and risk of epithelial ovarian cancer. Cancer Causes Control. 2012;23(6):919–27.
8. Rodriguez C, Patel AV, Calle EE, Jacob EJ, Thun MJ. Estrogen replacement therapy and ovarian cancer mortality in a large prospective study of US women. JAMA. 2001;285(11):1460–5.
9. Beral V, Gaitskell K, Hermon C, Moser K, Reeves G, Peto R. Menopausal hormone use and ovarian cancer risk: individual participant meta-analysis of 52 epidemiological studies. Lancet (London, England). 2015;385(9980):1835–42.
10. Chittenden BG, Fullerton G, Maheshwari A, Bhattacharya S. Polycystic ovary syndrome and the risk of gynaecological cancer: a systematic review. Reprod Biomed Online. 2009;19(3):398–405.
11. Barry JA, Azizia MM, Hardiman PJ. Risk of endometrial, ovarian and breast cancer in women with polycystic ovary syndrome: a systematic review and meta-analysis. Hum Reprod Update. 2014;20(5):748–58.
12. Pearce CL, Templeman C, Rossing MA, Lee A, Near AM, Webb PM, et al. Association between endometriosis and risk of histological subtypes of ovarian cancer: a pooled analysis of case-control studies. Lancet Oncol. 2012;13(4):385–94.
13. Collaborative Group on Epidemiological Studies of Ovarian C. Ovarian cancer and body size: individual participant meta-analysis including 25,157 women with ovarian cancer from 47 Epidemiological Studies. PLoS Med. 2012;9(4):e1001200.

14. World Cancer Research Fund and American Institute for Cancer Research. Continuous update project: ovarian cancer 2014 report: food, nutrition, physical activity, and the prevention of ovarian cancer. 2014.

15. Pennington KP, Swisher EM. Hereditary ovarian cancer: beyond the usual suspects. Gynecol Oncol. 2012;124(2):347–53.

16. Chen S, Parmigiani G. Meta-analysis of BRCA1 and BRCA2 penetrance. J Clin Oncol. 2007;25(11):1329–33.

17. Koornstra JJ, Mourits MJ, Sijmons RH, Leliveld AM, Hollema H, Kleibeuker JH. Management of extracolonic tumours in patients with Lynch syndrome. Lancet Oncol. 2009;10(4):400–8.

18. World Cancer Research Fund & American Institute for Cancer Research. Food, nutrition, physical activity, and the prevention of cancer: a global perspective. Washington DC: AICR; 2007.

19. Liu Z, Zhang TT, Zhao JJ, Qi SF, Du P, Liu DW, et al. The association between overweight, obesity and ovarian cancer: a meta-analysis. Jpn J Clin Oncol. 2015;45(12):1107–15.

20. Leitzmann MF, Koebnick C, Danforth KN, Brinton LA, Moore SC, Hollenbeck AR, et al. Body mass index and risk of ovarian cancer. Cancer. 2009;115(4):812–22.

21. Dixon SC, Nagle CM, Thrift AP, Pharoah PD, Pearce CL, Zheng W, et al. Adult body mass index and risk of ovarian cancer by subtype: a Mendelian randomization study. Int J Epidemiol. 2016;45(3):884–95.

22. Keum N, Greenwood DC, Lee DH, Kim R, Aune D, Ju W, et al. Adult weight gain and adiposity-related cancers: a dose-response meta-analysis of prospective observational studies. J Natl Cancer Inst. 2015;107(2)

23. Bae HS, Kim HJ, Hong JH, Lee JK, Lee NW, Song JY. Obesity and epithelial ovarian cancer survival: a systematic review and meta-analysis. J Ovarian Res. 2014;7:41.

24. Protani MM, Nagle CM, Webb PM. Obesity and ovarian cancer survival: a systematic review and meta-analysis. Cancer Prev Res (Phila). 2012;5(7):901–10.

25. Nagle CM, Dixon SC, Jensen A, Kjaer SK, Modugno F, de Fazio A, et al. Obesity and survival among women with ovarian cancer: results from the Ovarian Cancer Association Consortium. Br J Cancer. 2015;113(5):817–26.

26. Smits A, Lopes A, Das N, Kumar A, Cliby W, Smits E, et al. Surgical morbidity and clinical outcomes in ovarian cancer - the role of obesity. BJOG. 2016;123(2):300–8.

27. Bhaskaran K, Douglas I, Forbes H, dos-Santos-Silva I, Leon DA, Smeeth L. Body-mass index and risk of 22 specific cancers: a population-based cohort study of 5.24 million UK adults. Lancet (London, England). 2014;384(9945):755–65.

28. Allott EH, Hursting SD. Obesity and cancer: mechanistic insights from transdisciplinary studies. Endocr Relat Cancer. 2015;22(6):R365–86.

29. International Agency for Research on Cancer. GLOBOCAN 2012: Estimated cancer incidence, mortality and prevalence worldwide in 2012 2012. http://globocan.iarc.fr/Pages/Map.aspx. Accessed 13 Sept 2016.

Chapter 3
Public Knowledge of Obesity and Gynecologic Cancer Risk

Shannon Armbruster and Pamela T. Soliman

Abstract In the United States, obesity continues to be a significant health issue, with strong evidence supporting the association between excess body weight and several health conditions, including gynecologic cancer. As obesity is a modifiable condition, it is important to determine the public perception of the gynecologic cancer risks associated obesity. Studies conducted in various populations of women consistently show a gap in knowledge, thus providing a rationale for increasing the education of women on these important health issues. The data support including information on the concepts of body mass index (BMI) and obesity, as well as the increased risk of gynecologic cancers related to excess adiposity.

Keywords Obesity endometrial cancer awareness • Patient awareness • Physician awareness

Obesity and Health

Across the United States, increases in body weight have resulted in a true epidemic, with 70.7% of adults being classified as overweight or obese [1, 2]. The increase in prevalence of obesity most frequently impacts women and minority groups [3, 4]. From 1984 to 2014, the number of obese females increased by 21.6% [4]. Black women, compared to White and Hispanic women, and those with less than 12 years of education are the most likely to become obese or severely obese [2]. Obesity is a well-established risk factor for hypertension, hyperinsulinemia, type 2 diabetes mellitus, hyperlipidemia, cardiovascular disease, sleep apnea, and osteoarthritis [5]. Furthermore, excess adiposity has been shown to increase the incidence of certain cancers. According to the National

S. Armbruster • P.T. Soliman (✉)
The University of Texas MD Anderson Cancer Center,
1155 Herman Pressler, Room Number: CPB6.3244, Unit Number: 1362,
Houston, TX 77030, USA
e-mail: SDArmbruster@mdanderson.org; psoliman@mdanderson.org

© Springer International Publishing AG 2018
N.A. Berger et al. (eds.), *Focus on Gynecologic Malignancies*, Energy Balance and Cancer 13, DOI 10.1007/978-3-319-63483-8_3

Cancer Institute, eight obesity-related cancers have been identified, including esophageal, pancreatic, colon/rectum, post-menopausal breast, renal, thyroid, gallbladder, and endometrial cancer [6]. Earlier chapters reported the strong evidence supporting the relationship between obesity and endometrial cancer as well as the inconsistent data for the relationship between obesity and ovarian cancer. Investigation into the impact of obesity on cervical adenocarcinoma suggests a possible, but not certain link [7]. For endometrial cancer survivors, increased body weight not only increases the likelihood of developing the disease, but also increases mortality rates (RR 6.25, 95% CI 3.75–10.42) [8]. When considering endometrial cancer survivors, African American women with endometrial cancer have a significantly higher mortality rate when compared to Caucasian women [9]. Given that obesity is a modifiable disease, determining public knowledge of the relationship between obesity and gynecologic cancer is important and can serve to identify groups who should be targeted by educational programs and interventions.

Methodology

Several studies have investigated public knowledge of the correlation between increased body weight and endometrial cancer. Most of these studies used written questionnaires to obtain quantitative data, while the use of focus groups to obtain qualitative data occurred less frequently. The majority of researchers developed their own questionnaires based on literature reporting the risk factors relating to obesity [10–15]. A limited number of studies used select questions from the validated questionnaire Behavioral Risk Factor Surveillance System provided by the Center for Disease Control and Prevention [16] as well as from the Harvard Forms on Health survey [17–20]. Research investigating public perception of the correlation between obesity and ovarian or cervical cancer is lacking and thus will not be discussed in this chapter.

Obesity and Endometrial Cancer Awareness

The majority of women, in all but one study, were unaware of the link between obesity and endometrial cancer, with anywhere from 18 to 66% of women correctly identifying the correlation [10–14, 18–20]. These results were determined from individuals with different demographic, anthropometric, and medical histories and thus information obtained should be considered in the context in which the data was collected. A brief description of the referenced studies can be found in Table 3.1. As most women are not aware of the association between obesity and endometrial cancer, an opportunity exists to provide education for all groups of women.

Table 3.1 Referenced studies relating to obesity and endometrial cancer.

Reference	Location; Sample size; Gender	Location of patient recruitment; Gender	Race/ethnicity	Weight status based on BMI (% of n) or mean
Ackermann et al. [10]	Dusseldorf, Germany; n = 2108	Gynecologic outpatient clinics; Female	Not included	Not included
George et al. [11]	New South Wales, Australia; n = 329	Gynecologic outpatient clinics; Female	Not included	Not included
Cardozo et al. [12]	Chicago, IL; n = 207	Community fair; Female	African American 99.0 Hispanic 0.5 Asian 0.5 Caucasian/ Other 0	Mean = 31.2 ± 6.7 kg/m²
Cardozo et al. [13]	Chicago, IL; n = 150	Infertility patients at academic medical center; Female	Caucasian 54.7 African American 26.7 Hispanic 6.7 Asian 8.7 Other 3.3	Underweight: 2.7[a] Normal weight: 54.0 Overweight: 19.3 Obese Class I: 10.7 Obese Class II: 7.3 Obese Class III: 6.0
Henretta et al. [14]	Charlottesville, VA; n = 93	Bariatric surgery clinic appointment; Female	African-American 17.2 Caucasian 77.4 Other/ multiracial 2.2 No response 3.2	Obese: 14.0[b] Morbidly Obese: 51.6 Super Obese: 33.3
Cooper et al. [15]	Miami, FL; New York City, NY; Los Angelis, CA; Chicago, IL n = 132	Participant databases from focus group facilities; Female	Caucasian 40.2 African American 32.6 Hispanic 18.9 Asian 8.3	Not included
Beavis et al. [18]	Los Angelis, CA; n = 163	Gynecology, infertility, and gynecologic oncology clinics; Female	Hispanic 66.9 Caucasian 17.2 African American 6.1 Asian 4.9 Native American 0.6 No response 4.3	Mean = 31.4 ± 7.8 kg/m²
Soliman et al. [19]	Houston, Texas; n = 1545	Local events, health care waiting rooms, online; Female	Caucasian (50%) African American (27%) Hispanic (15%) Asian (6%) Other (1%) Unknown (1%)	Normal: 28.2[c] Overweight: 23.6 Obese: 44.6 Missing: 3.5

(continued)

Table 3.1 (continued)

Reference	Location; Sample size; Gender	Location of patient recruitment; Gender	Race/ethnicity	Weight status based on BMI (% of n) or mean
Clark et al. [20]	Chapel Hill, NC n = 108	Chart review of gynecologic oncology patients; Female	Caucasian 84 African American 12 Hispanic 1 Asian 1 Other 1	Mean = 29.8 kg/m²
Post et al. [23]	West Virginia and New Jersey; n = 515	Health care waiting rooms; Male (44%) and Female (56%)	Not included	Underweight: 2.0[c] Normal: 27.9 Overweight: 31.3 Obese: 38.7

[a]BMI Categories: Underweight (BMI <18.5 kg/m²), Normal range (BMI 18.5–24.9 kg/m²), Overweight (BMI 25.0–29.9 kg/m²), Obese class I (BMI 30.0–34.9 kg/m²), Obese class II (BMI 35.0–39.9 kg/m²), Obese class III (BMI >40.0 kg/m²).
[b]BMI Categories: Obese (BMI 30–39.9 kg/m²), Morbidly Obese (BMI 40–49.9 kg/m²), Super Obese (BMI ≥50 mg/kg²).
[c]BMI Categories: Underweight (BMI <18.5 kg/m²), Normal (BMI 18.5–24.9 kg/m²), Overweight (BMI 25.0–29.9 kg/m²), Obese (BMI ≥ 30.0 kg/m²).

Awareness of Risk Factors for Endometrial Cancer

Women's knowledge of risk factors for endometrial cancer is inconsistent and often incomplete. Cooper et al. utilized focus groups to elicit patient-reported risk factors for gynecologic cancer. During these sessions, women were unable to identify any risk factors specifically related to endometrial cancer [15]. Studies utilizing questionnaires that inquired about a listed risk factor have yielded better, but not overwhelming results. Two studies were conducted in outpatient gynecologic clinics and reported that the minority of women were aware of the correlation of obesity to endometrial cancer [10, 11]. The first study, from Germany, reported that women most commonly (93%) associated genetic factors with endometrial cancer, while significantly fewer (36%) related "obesity, diabetes, and hypertension" to endometrial cancer [10]. Similarly, women from an Australian study most frequently cited genetic factors, followed by history of breast cancer, and less frequently "obesity, high, blood pressure, and diabetes" as factors associated with endometrial cancer [11]. The results of these studies show that although most women accurately identify the link between genetics and personal history of breast cancer to endometrial cancer, they are far less aware of relationship to obesity, which is the most common risk factor.

Awareness of Obesity and Related Comorbidities

Several studies have compared the percentages of women acknowledging the relationship between obesity and other obesity-related health conditions to those recognizing the risk of endometrial cancer related to excess adiposity. These studies help to determine if the problem is a general lack of knowledge surrounding obesity or a concentrated knowledge deficit of the association of obesity with endometrial cancer.

The knowledge of the relationship of obesity to comorbid conditions, excluding cancer, has been compared to awareness of the obesity-related endometrial cancer risk. A survey conducted in gynecologic, infertility, and gynecologic oncology clinics by Beavis et al. revealed that hypertension and heart disease were correlated with obesity by 67% of women, in comparison to endometrial cancer that was related to obesity by only 37.4% of respondents [18]. Similarly, diabetes, hypertension, and cardiovascular disease were all correlated with obesity by the majority of responders (79%, 74%, and 73%, respectively) in a study of urban African American women [12]. These findings are in sharp contrast to the 18.1% of responders who identified that increased body weight was related to endometrial cancer risk [12]. Overall, women relate medical comorbidities to obesity more frequently than they do to endometrial cancer, indicating a knowledge deficit related to the awareness of the elevated endometrial cancer risk due to obesity.

Analogous to the awareness of obesity-related comorbidities compared to endometrial cancer risk, women also more frequently acknowledge the correlation of obesity to breast or colon cancer than the relationship of obesity to endometrial cancer. Soliman et al. queried 1545 women, most of whom where were Caucasian (50%, n = 772), followed by African American (25%, n = 411), and Hispanic (15%, n = 232). Overall, only 42% of women (n = 625) knew that obesity was a risk factor for endometrial cancer, in contrast to over 50% of respondents who identified the association of obesity to colon and breast cancer [19]. Cardozo et al. reported similar findings from a study of infertility patients, showing women were more likely to identify obesity-related breast cancer risk (38.7%) compared to endometrial cancer risk (20.7%) [13].

The highest recognition of risk for endometrial cancer was seen in a study of obese women who were presenting for bariatric surgery. Sixty-six percent of women correctly identified obesity as a risk factor for endometrial cancer, however 45% of these obese women who retained their uterus reported that it was not likely/possible for them to develop uterine cancer [14]. Along similar lines, only 50% of women responded that obesity "increased /increased a lot" their risk of endometrial cancer [14]. This percentage is similar to those perceiving an "increase/increase of a lot" of the risk of breast and colon cancer due to obesity (48% and 47% respectively) [14]. This study supports the idea that simply acknowledging a correlation does not equate to perceiving a personal risk. Therefore, an approach that makes the data personal could be beneficial when educating overweight or obese women. Taken together, these studies demonstrate a wide-reaching knowledge gap relating to endometrial cancer that in many cases is greater than that of other obesity-related cancers and requires attention.

Health History and Sociodemographic Variables affecting Obesity and Cancer Awareness

Lack of knowledge of the relationship of obesity to breast and colon cancers has been reported based on certain demographic characteristics, including age, income, educational level, and race [19, 21, 22]. Investigation into potentially relevant variables relating to endometrial cancer knowledge has been undertaken to see if there is a subpopulation of women who has the greatest knowledge deficit.

Race, Age, Education Level, and Socioeconomic Status

The data supporting differences in knowledge of obesity and endometrial cancer based on race and educational attainment are inconsistent. Soliman et al. reported that African American women were more likely to be unaware of the correlation, while Asian women more frequently acknowledged the relationship [19]. Other studies report no difference in knowledge based on race [13, 18]. Similar to race, studies correlating educational attainment to knowledge level are inconsistent. Cardozo et al. reported that having less than a 4 year college education was associated with lack of knowledge [12]. However, the majority of studies report that education level, age, household income, or insurance level have no bearing on the knowledge of association between obesity and endometrial cancer [10, 11, 13, 18, 19]. These data support wide-reaching educational programs that are not confined to certain socio-demographic populations.

Obesity stratification

Several studies have investigated the knowledge of the association of obesity to endometrial cancer based on the BMI of the respondent, to determine if one BMI category is more educated than the others. These studies have yielded mixed results. Cardozo et al. reported an association of body weight to lack of knowledge, finding obese women more frequently unaware of the relationship [12]. However, two other studies report that there was no association of knowledge of endometrial cancer risk associated with obesity when comparing weight groups [18, 19]. Taken together, these data provide evidence to provide education to all women, especially those that are overweight and obese because they are at higher risk for comorbidities.

Cancer survivors

Survivors of obesity-related cancers should have a high understanding of the relationship of their adiposity to their disease. Unfortunately, the literature does not support this concept. A study of 108 endometrial cancer survivors reported that only

46% of respondents were aware of the connection between obesity and endometrial cancer [20]. A second study of endometrial cancer survivors demonstrated that their recognition of obesity as a risk factor for endometrial cancer was higher after diagnosis of endometrial hyperplasia or cancer (54%) compared to women without a cancer diagnosis (32%) [18]. It is encouraging that approximately half of survivors are aware of the etiology of their disease, however there is room for improvement. Education should include the survivor population who is at risk for recurrence, a second obesity related cancer, or other comorbidities. Additionally, information must be extended beyond the survivor population to provide incentive for women to maintain a healthy weight or lose excess body mass to avoid obesity-relate health conditions such as endometrial cancer.

Obesity Awareness

In order to enhance knowledge of the relationship between obesity and endometrial cancer, education must reach all women, especially those that are overweight and obese. For this education to resonate with women, they need to have a basic understanding of obesity and accurately perceive their weight class. Thus, several researchers have sought to describe women's ability to accomplish these tasks. Post et al. reported that patients seen in primary care practices frequently relate the concept of BMI to obesity, however less than 20% of respondents could identify BMI levels or their meaning [23]. These findings were similar to a study of urban African American women revealing that merely 21.8% knew the normal BMI range and only 8.4% knew their BMI within 1 kg/m^2 [12]. In comparison, 47.3% of infertility patients could identify the normal BMI range, while only 11% could correctly report their BMI within 1 kg/m^2 [13]. BMI awareness was higher in a study of gynecologic oncology patients, who correctly identified their BMI category 85% of the time, including 45 of 47 women who knew they were obese [20]. Regardless of the group investigated, these studies indicate that knowledge and awareness of obesity are lacking, especially in the general population. Interestingly, obese females who presented for bariatric surgery were better able to accurately identify their BMI group as weight increased, with correct identification occurring in 23% of obese, 77% of morbidly obese, and 85% of super obese women [14]. This study suggests that information about BMI class is beneficial to all women with a BMI $\geq$ 30 mg/kg^2, but should be sure to target women in the obese range.

A cross-sectional study querying women who presented to general gynecologic oncology, infertility, or gynecologic oncology clinics highlights the impact of provider intervention [18]. Fifty-five percent of overweight or obese respondents reported being told they were overweight or obese by their physician and 83.6% of those women correctly identified themselves as overweight or obese [18]. Although this was a cross-sectional study, the data is hypothesis generating, pointing to a plausible increase in knowledge due to provider education. Taken together, these studies bring to light the need for basic obesity counseling and the potential impact medical providers can have on self-awareness of BMI. Education programs should not assume that women are familiar with BMI categories, or their own BMI. Education should begin with an assessment of a woman's current knowledge of basic BMI concepts before proceeding to co-morbidity specific information.

Increasing Awareness on the National Level

The United States government and large national organizations have noted the deficiency in recognition of the relationship between obesity and endometrial cancer. In 2007, Congress passed the Gynecologic Cancer Education and Awareness Act that sanctioned the creation of a national program to promote symptoms, signs, risk factors and prevention of gynecologic cancers [24]. In 2014, the American Society of Clinical Oncology (ASCO) published their Statement Priorities and Activities Focused on Obesity and Cancer that included an objective and clinical goal intended to increase patient knowledge about the relationship between obesity and cancer risk [25]. Despite these mandates, in 2016, the Womb Cancer Alliance published their top ten unanswered questions relating to endometrial cancer, which included a task to increase public awareness about endometrial cancer [26], indicating that more education is still needed.

Increasing Awareness in the Clinical Setting

In alignment with national efforts, women desire more information about endometrial cancer. Survey data confirm that the vast majority of women, 94–96%, desire information about the risk factors for endometrial cancer [10, 11]. Who should discuss these risk factors and lifestyle changes with gynecologic cancer survivors is debatable. One study examined the rates of counseling between primary care physicians (PCP) and gynecologic oncologists (GO). The study reported 52% of survivors received PCP counseling, compared to 35% of survivors being counseled by their GO. When comparing PCPs to GOs, PCPs were more likely to specifically give diet (47% versus 25%, respectively) and physical activity (62% versus 37%, respectively) recommendations [20]. Interestingly, of those counseled by a PCP, 56% of survivors attempted weight loss, while 100% of those counseled by GOs attempted weight reduction. Eighty-eight percent (28/32) however, were counseled by both their GO and PCP [20]. Regardless of who counseled the women, those that received any weight loss counseling attempted to lose weight more often than those who did not [20]. This data encourages a multi-disciplinary approach, including both PCPs and GOs to educate as many women as possible.

Future Direction

Understanding the need for education is the first step toward addressing the problem. The next steps involve development of educational programs and the utilization of existing resources such as the ASCO Obesity Toolkit [27]. These interventions should be tested for efficacy relating to the actual content delivery as well as recipient comprehension of the material. Now that the knowledge deficit has been identified, the challenge for the medical community is to improve awareness of the risk for endometrial cancer related to obesity, as well as increase women's accountability for their health.

References

1. U.S. Department of Health and Human Services. Health, United States, 2015. 2015.
2. Ljungvall A, Zimmerman FJ. Bigger bodies: long-term trends and disparities in obesity and body-mass index among U.S. adults, 1960-2008. Soc Sci Med. 2012;75(1):109–19.
3. Ogden CL, Carroll MD, Fryar CD, Flegal KM. Prevalence of obesity among adults and youth: United States, 2011–2014. NCHS Data Brief. 2015(219):1–8.
4. An R, Xiang X. Age–period–cohort analyses of obesity prevalence in US adults. Public Health. 2016;141:163–9.
5. Kopelman PG. Obesity as a medical problem. Nature. 2000;404(6778):635–43.
6. National Cancer Institute. Obesity and cancer risk. https.//www.cancer.gov/about-cancer/causes-prevention/risk/obesity/obesity-fact-sheet. Accessed 2 Jan 2017.
7. Modesitt SC, Van Nagell Jr JR. The impact of obesity on the incidence and treatment of gynecologic cancers: A review. Obstet Gynecol Surv. 2005;60(10):683–92.
8. Calle EE, Rodriguez C, Walker-Thurmond K, Thun MJ. Overweight, obesity, and mortality from cancer in a prospectively studied cohort of U.S. Adults. N Engl J Med. 2003;348(17):1625–38.
9. Siegel RL, Miller KD, Jemal A. Cancer statistics, 2016. CA Cancer J Clin. 2016;66(1):7–30.
10. Ackermann S, Renner SP, Fasching PA, Poehls U, Bender HG, Beckmann MW. Awareness of general and personal risk factors for uterine cancer among healthy women. Eur J Cancer Prev. 2005;14(6):519–24.
11. George M, Asab NA, Varughese E, Irwin M, Oldmeadow C, Hollebone K, et al. Risk awareness on uterine cancer among Australian women. Asian Pac J Cancer Prev. 2014;15(23):10251–4.
12. Cardozo ER, Dune TJ, Neff LM, Brocks ME, Ekpo GE, Barnes RB, et al. Knowledge of obesity and its impact on reproductive health outcomes among urban women. J Community Health. 2013;38(2):261–7.
13. Cardozo ER, Neff LM, Brocks ME, Ekpo GE, Dune TJ, Barnes RB, et al. Infertility patients' knowledge of the effects of obesity on reproductive health outcomes. Am J Obstet Gynecol. 2012;207(6):509.e1–e10.
14. Henretta MS, Copeland AR, Kelley SL, Hallowell PT, Modesitt SC. Perceptions of obesity and cancer risk in female bariatric surgery candidates: Highlighting the need for physician action for unsuspectingly obese and high risk patients. Gynecol Oncol. 2014;133(1):73–7.
15. Cooper CP, Polonec L, Gelb CA. Women's knowledge and awareness of gynecologic cancer: A multisite qualitative study in the United States. J Women's Health. 2011;20(4):517–24.
16. Behavioral Risk Factor Surveillance System. https://www.cdc.gov/BRFSS/. Accessed 12 Dec 2016.
17. Obesity as a Public Health Issue: a look at solutions. In: Lake S Perry and Associates, editor. 20082003.

18. Beavis AL, Cheema S, Holschneider CH, Duffy EL, Amneus MW. Almost half of women with endometrial cancer or hyperplasia do not know that obesity affects their cancer risk. Gynecol Oncol Rep. 2015;13:71–5.
19. Soliman PT, Bassett RL, Wilson EB, Boyd-Rogers S, Schmeler KM, Milam MR, et al. Limited public knowledge of obesity and endometrial cancer risk: what women know. Obstet Gynecol. 2008;112(4):835–42.
20. Clark LH, Ko EM, Kernodle A, Harris A, Moore DT, Gehrig PA, et al. Endometrial cancer survivors' perceptions of provider obesity counseling and attempted behavior change: are we seizing the moment? Int J Gynecol Cancer. 2016;26(2):318–24.
21. Leite-Pereira F, Medeiros R, Dinis-Ribeiro M. Overweight and obese patients do not seem to adequately recognize their own risk for colorectal cancer. J Cancer Educ. 2011;26(4):767–73.
22. Consedine NS, Magai C, Spiller R, Neugut AI, Conway F. Breast cancer knowledge and beliefs in subpopulations of African American and Caribbean women. Am J Health Behav. 2004;28(3):260–71.
23. Post RE, Mendiratta M, Haggerty T, Bozek A, Doyle G, Xiang J, et al. Patient understanding of body mass index (BMI) in primary care practices: a two-state practice-based research (PBR) collaboration. J Am Board Fam Med. 2015;28(4):475–80.
24. Cancer Education and Awareness Act, S. HR 1245(2005).
25. Ligibel JA, Alfano CM, Courneya KS, Demark-Wahnefried W, Burger RA, Chlebowski RT, et al. American Society of Clinical Oncology Position Statement on Obesity and Cancer. J Clin Oncol. 2014;32(31):3568–74.
26. Wan YL, Beverley-Stevenson R, Carlisle D, Clarke S, Edmondson RJ, Glover S, et al. Working together to shape the endometrial cancer research agenda: the top ten unanswered research questions. Gynecol Oncol. 2016;143(2):287–93.
27. Ligibel JA, Wollins D. American society of clinical oncology obesity initiative: Rationale, progress, and future directions. J Clin Oncol. 2016;34(35):4256–60.

Chapter 4
Role of Estrogen and Progesterone in Obesity Associated Gynecologic Cancers

For Publication in Energy Balance and Gynecologic Cancers

Louise A. Brinton and Britton Trabert

Abstract Obesity is an established endometrial cancer risk factor, and may, to a lesser extent, also increase ovarian cancer. Given that the primary source of post-menopausal estrogens is through peripheral conversion of precursors in adipose tissue and that endometrial cancer arises from an imbalance of estrogen to progesterone levels, much attention has focused on these two hormones.

Indirect evidence for an important role of these hormones derives from studies of menopausal hormones and oral contraceptives, whose use is, respectively, directly and inversely associated with both endometrial and ovarian cancer risks. Endometrial cancer risks are particularly enhanced if unopposed estrogens are prescribed, especially among thin women.

Studies have demonstrated a link between high endogenous estrogen levels and increased endometrial cancer risk, with most metabolites showing evidence of uterotropic activity. Estrogens are less strongly related to ovarian cancer, although may predispose some to non-serous cancers, which are also enhanced among obese women.

Difficulties in measuring progesterone levels have hampered our understanding of their effects, although improved assays have recently been developed. To fully understand the role of estrogens and progestogens, additional attention should focus on other hormones (e.g., androgens), insulin, growth factors, and such obesity-related biomarkers as adiponectin.

While cervical and vulvar cancers do not show strong relations of risk with obesity, it is possible that hormonal changes associated with obesity may enhance the effects of the human papillomaviruses, important causes of both of these tumors.

L.A. Brinton, Ph.D. (✉) • B. Trabert, Ph.D.
Division of Cancer Epidemiology and Genetics, National Cancer Institute,
9609 Medical Center Drive, Rm SG/6E422, Bethesda, MD 20892-9774, USA
e-mail: brintonl@mail.nih.gov; trabertbl@mail.nih.gov

© Springer International Publishing AG 2018
N.A. Berger et al. (eds.), *Focus on Gynecologic Malignancies*, Energy Balance and Cancer 13, DOI 10.1007/978-3-319-63483-8_4

With obesity rates rapidly increasing, further clarification of the biologic under-pinnings of gynecologic cancers are needed to inform future prevention efforts.

Keywords Oral contraceptives • Menopausal hormones • Androgens • Insulin • Adiponectin • Estrogen • Progesterone • Uterine cancer • Endometrial cancer • Luteinizing hormone • Follicle stimulating hormone • Polycystic ovary syndrome • Selective estrogen receptor modulator • Hydroxyestrone

Introduction

Over the last couple of decades, there has been increasing recognition of the impor-tance of obesity in the etiology of a variety of cancers, including several gyneco-logic cancers. One of the cancers recognized as being most strongly influenced by obesity is that of uterine cancer, with other gynecologic cancers also being affected, although to lesser extents. Obesity has been extensively investigated as it influences not only cancer risk and survival, but also other established risk factors. Although a variety of biologic mechanisms have been postulated as explanatory to the effects of obesity on risk, the most accepted mechanism has been alterations in the production and metabolism of estrogens and progesterones. Below, we review the epidemiol-ogy of gynecologic cancers as it relates to obesity and associated endogenous hor-monal changes.

Uterine Cancers

Uterine corpus cancer (hereafter referred to as uterine cancer) is the most common invasive gynecologic cancer and the fourth most frequently diagnosed cancer among American women today, with one in 40 women developing the disease during their lives [1]. The vast majority of uterine cancers are endometrial cancers, prompting most epidemiologic studies to focus on these malignancies. Numerous epidemio-logic studies have identified a variety of risk factors for endometrial cancers. Obesity is one of the strongest risk factors for the disease apart from age and exogenous menopausal hormone use (Table 4.1). Additional risk factors include infertility or nulliparity, early menarche and/or late menopause, and several diseases, including diabetes. In contrast, oral contraceptive use, physical activity, and smoking appear to decrease risk.

Obesity has been estimated to account for up to 25% of endometrial cancers [2]. Studies indicate that for every 5 kg. increase in weight that women have an associ-ated relative risk (and 95% confidence interval, CI) of 1.59 (1.50–1.68) [3]. Women who are clinically obese (body mass indices, or BMIs exceeding 40) are at excep-tionally high risks, on the order of fivefold elevations compared to women with

Table 4.1 Risk factors for endometrial cancer

Factors influencing risk	Estimated relative risk[a]
Long-term use of menopausal estrogens	10.0–20.0
Stein-Leventhal disease or estrogen-producing tumors	<5.0
Residency in North America, northern Europe	3.0–18.0
High cumulative doses of tamoxifen	3.0–7.0
Obesity	2.0–5.0
Older age	2.0–3.0
Late age at natural menopause	2.0–3.0
History of infertility	2.0–3.0
White race	2
Nulliparity	2
Higher levels of education or income	1.5–2.0
Early age at menarche	1.5–2.0
Menstrual irregularities	1.5
Histories of diabetes, hypertension, gallbladder disease, or thyroid disease	1.3–3.0
Use of oral contraceptives	0.3–0.5
Cigarette smoking	0.5
Moderate-to-vigorous physical activity	0.5–0.8

[a]Relative risks depend on the study and referent group employed

BMIs in the normal range (<25) [4]. Obesity appears to affect both premenopausal and postmenopausal endometrial cancer risk.

Adding to the evidence of a causal association between increased BMI and elevations in the risk of endometrial cancer is the demonstration that women undergoing bariatric surgery experience reductions in endometrial cancer incidence [5]. Similarly, women who report intentional weight loss and who maintain this loss are not at increased risk compared to women who maintain heavier weights [6]; in addition, women who lose weight demonstrate lower levels of a variety of inflammatory and hormonal biomarkers believed to be involved in endometrial carcinogenesis [7].

Although initial studies hypothesized that adolescent and long-standing obesity may be more important than adult weight, recent studies support that contemporary weight and weight gain during adulthood are the most important predictors of endometrial cancer risk [8]. As detailed below, relationships with obesity appear stronger among women not currently exposed to exogenous hormones.

Recent interest has focused on determining whether the distribution of body fat predicts endometrial cancer risk. A number of studies have shown that central obesity may have an effect independent of overall body size [9], although not all studies confirm this relationship [10].

Physical activity has also been recognized as being inversely associated with endometrial cancer risk [11]. The reductions in risk appear to be restricted to overweight and obese women [12]. The extent to which physical activity induced changes in endogenous hormones and other biologic markers are involved has been the topic of a number of investigations, without definitive conclusions.

Biologic Underpinning of Obesity as an Etiologic Factor

Endometrial cancer arises in the context of prolonged estrogen stimulation unopposed by sufficient progesterone levels [13]. Imbalances in these hormones lead to increases in mitotic activity of endometrial cells with increased opportunities for DNA replication errors and subsequent neoplastic transformation. The natural history of endometrial cancer has been well investigated, with an established intermediate marker of risk being endometrial hyperplasia, particularly atypical hyperplasia. Altered circulatory hormone levels are reported in endometrial hyperplasia patients, particularly in those with metabolic syndrome, with findings of elevated levels of estrogen, testosterone, insulin, leptin, and luteinizing hormone (LH), and of LH/follicle stimulating hormone (FSH) ratios. Increased estrogen bioavailability in hyperplastic endometrium, as a consequence of increased local aromatase expression and activity, has also been postulated to affect risk [14].

Obesity is believed to play a central role in the natural history of endometrial pathologies, including endometrial hyperplasias, most likely because estrogens are formed in peripheral fat tissue from the conversion of precursor elements, including androgens [15]. Estrogen (estradiol) production is thought to primarily be an endocrine product of the ovary, but many additional tissues have the ability to synthesize estrogens from androgen precursors. Most notably, aromatase activity in adipose tissue accounts for extraglandular formation of endogenous estrogens, which increases as a function of body weight, particularly in postmenopausal women.

The relation of obesity to endometrial pathology has been shown to be enhanced in women with conditions associated with specific alterations in hormone levels, such as polycystic ovary syndrome (PCOS), a condition characterized by clinical features of obesity and diabetes as well as primary hormonal aberrations of unopposed estrogens, insulin resistance, and hyperandrogenism. Notably women with PCOS are at between a two and threefold increased risk of developing endometrial cancer [16, 17], translating into a lifetime risk of 9% (as compared to the background risk of 3% in the general population) [18]. Diabetics are also at an increased risk of developing endometrial cancers, with some evidence that this relation may be independent of increased levels of obesity among such patients. Further support for the relationship derives from findings that users of the antidiabetic medication metformin experience substantial reductions in endometrial cancer risk [19].

There is an increasing epidemic of obesity and diabetes in the United States (as well as an increasing proportion of older adults) and, as such, we can expect that obesity-related cancer diagnoses will rise. Specifically, the incidence of endometrial cancer is estimated to increase by 55% between 2010 and 2030 [20], although there is uncertainty in this estimate given possible influences of changing hysterectomy patterns.

Exogenous Hormones

In clarifying the roles of estrogens and progestogens in the etiology of endometrial cancer, much has been learned from studies of exogenous hormones, with many studies linking oral contraceptives to decreases in risk and most menopausal hormone therapies to increases in risk.

Oral Contraceptives. The use of combination oral contraceptives has been shown to be associated with marked reductions in the risk of endometrial cancer, with the greatest decreases seen among long-term users. In a recent pooled analysis, 5 years of use was associated with a relative risk (RR) of 0.76 (95% CI 0.73–0.78) [21]. This reduction in risk persisted for more than 30 years, with no apparent difference in risk across calendar time periods, despite use of higher estrogen dose pills in earlier years. The similar protective effect observed in high and low dose estrogen-containing pills [22] suggests that reductions in risk may be driven by lifetime progestin exposures. In support of this, one study found that higher progestin potency oral contraceptives were required to reduce risk in obese women, a relation that was not observed among thinner women [22].

Of particular interest in this regard are studies of systemic high doses of progestins, such as depot medroxyprogesterone acetate (DMPA), which induce a hypoestrogenic state with profound ovarian suppression. To date there are no definitive studies evaluating the long-term effects on cancer risk of DMPA, possibly reflecting its recent marketing (1992). Progestin-containing intra-uterine devices (IUDs) are also of interest. Although studies have confirmed reductions in endometrial cancer risk associated with use of earlier IUDs [23], the relations have not specifically been related to progestin-containing devices, again most likely reflecting an inability to evaluate long-term effects.

Menopausal Hormones. It is well established that unopposed estrogens are associated with a 2- to 12-fold elevation in endometrial cancer risk [24]. In most investigations, the increased risk does not become apparent until the drugs have been used for at least 2–3 years, and longer use of estrogens is generally associated with higher risk. The highest RRs have been observed with higher drug dosages and after 10 years of use (up to 20-fold), although it is unclear whether risk increases after 15 years. Most but not all studies have found that cessation of use is associated with a relatively rapid decrease in risk, although a number of studies have found significantly elevated risks persisting for 10 or more years after last usage.

The large body of evidence linking estrogen use to increases in the risk of endometrial cancers has led to estrogens being prescribed in conjunction with progestins among women who have not had a hysterectomy since progestins cause regression of endometrial hyperplasia, the presumed precursor of endometrial cancers. In the Women's Health Initiative (WHI) clinical trial, after 5.6 years' median intervention and 13 years of follow-up, women assigned daily to 0.625 mg of conjugated equine estrogen plus 2.5 mg of medroxyprogesterone acetate had a hazard ratio (HR) of 0.65 (95% confidence interval, CI 0.48–0.89) compared to those assigned to placebo [25]. Similar results derive from a number of observational studies, including the Million Women Study in the United Kingdom, where women whose last usage of hormones comprised continuous combined therapy had a RR of 0.71 (95% CI 0.56–0.90) compared to never users [24].

Although studies indicate that the excess risk of endometrial cancer associated with estrogens can be significantly reduced if progestins are given for at least 10 days each month [26], some studies have shown that subjects prescribed progestins for less than 10 days per month (sequential users) experience some increase in risk, with only a slight risk reduction compared to estrogen-only users [27]. The sharp contrast between the effects of <10 and ≥10 days of progestin use has led to the suggestion that the extent of uterine sloughing or of "terminal" differentiation at the completion of the progestin phase may play a critical role in determining risk. It remains questionable whether 10 days of progestin administration per month is sufficient for complete protection, particularly for long-term users. Few studies have had large numbers of long-term sequential users, but there is some evidence that this pattern of usage may result in persistent elevations in risk [28].

The type of progestin prescribed may also be a factor affecting endometrial cancer risk. Notably, there are some data to support higher risks when micronized progesterones are prescribed [29]. Tibolone, a synthetic steroid drug with estrogenic, progestogenic, and weak androgenic actions, has also been shown to be significantly related to elevated endometrial cancer risks [24, 30].

Most data regarding effects of hormones derive from studies of users of pills. Unresolved is whether the use of estrogen patches, creams, or injections can affect risk; given relationships of risk with even low dose estrogen pills, it is plausible that other routes of administration confer some increases in risk.

Studies have shown that the effects of hormonal therapy (both unopposed estrogens as well as combination therapy) may vary by user characteristics, most notably by a woman's body mass. Investigations have shown that the adverse effects of unopposed estrogens are greatest in non-obese women and that the beneficial effects of combined therapy (particularly continuous combined therapy) are greatest in obese women (Fig. 4.1) [27].

Tamoxifen. An adverse effect of estrogens derives further support from studies that have linked use of tamoxifen, a selective estrogen receptor modulator (SERM), to increases in endometrial cancer risk. A number of clinical trials have demonstrated an increased risk of uterine cancer among tamoxifen-treated breast cancer patients, with a recent meta-analysis showing a HR of 2.18 (95% CI 1.39–3.42) [31], consistent with tamoxifen's estrogenic effects on the endometrium. Elevated risks have been observed primarily within relatively short periods after exposure and among women receiving high cumulative doses of therapy. Certain uterine cancer histologies that are normally associated with a poor prognosis, such as serous cancers, may be especially elevated [32].

While some of the newer SERMs, such as Raloxifene, Bazedoxifene and Ospemifene, appear to have neutral effects on the endometrium [33], Lasofoxifene may increase endometrial thickness, although studies have not yet confirmed a higher risk of hyperplasia or endometrial cancer after 5 years of follow-up [34].

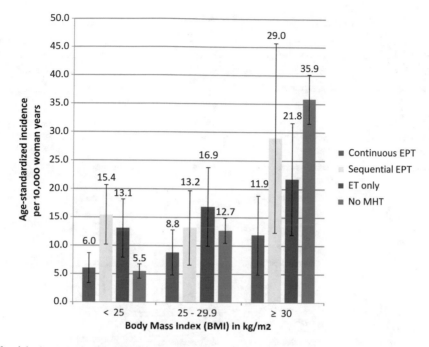

Fig. 4.1 Age-standardized incidence of endometrial cancer by menopausal hormone therapy use and body mass index (BMI) groups (in kg/m²), NIH-AARP Diet and Health Study, 1995–2006. Error bars indicate 95% confidence intervals on the age-standardized incidence. From [27]

Endogenous Hormones and Other Biomarkers

Evidence for direct effects of endogenous hormones on endometrial cancer risk derives from studies that have measured estrogens, progesterone and androgens in relation to risk. Results of these studies are detailed below.

Estrogens. Despite the acceptance of the hormonal etiology of endometrial cancers [35], relatively few studies have explored the etiologic role of endogenous hormones [36]. The studies have generally been based on limited numbers of cases and radioimmunological assays, which have recognized limitations, particularly for measuring low concentrations of hormones in postmenopausal women. The studies conducted to date, however, have all shown increased risks of endometrial cancers associated with high levels of estradiol. This has included studies of 124 postmenopausal cancers from three cohort studies in which a fourfold increased risk was found for the highest vs. lowest quartile of estradiol [37]; 247 menopausal cancers from the European Investigation of Cancer (EPIC) in which a twofold increased risk was found for the highest versus lowest tertile of estradiol [38]; and 250 cancers from the Women's Health Initiative Observational Study (WHI-OS) in which a 3.6-fold increased risk was found for the highest versus lowest tertile of estradiol [39].

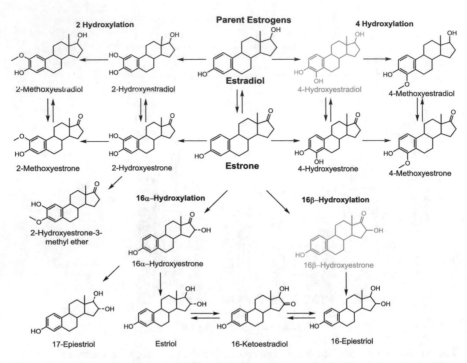

Fig. 4.2 Formation of 2-, 4-, and 16-hydroxylation pathway estrogen metabolites from parent estrogens. The serum estrogen metabolite assay measures 15 of the 17 metabolites pictured, 4-Hydroxyestradiol and 16β-Hydroxyestrone (in light gray) are not measured with the mass spectrometry assay due to very low abundance in circulation

The use of mass spectrometry to measure endogenous hormones has recently opened up new research avenues [40]. In addition to improving sensitivity, accuracy, and reproducibility, mass spectrometry assays have enabled concurrent measurements of parent estrogens as well as estrogen metabolites, which purportedly have divergent effects on cancer development. The metabolism of estradiol or estrone with irreversible hydroxylation at the C-2, C-4, or C-16 positions of the steroid ring results in metabolites with varying mitogenic and genotoxic properties (Fig. 4.2).

Two major hypotheses about estrogen metabolites have emerged from experimental research, namely that (i) 16α-hydroxyestrone ($16\alpha OHE_1$) is carcinogenic because it can bind covalently to the estrogen receptor with strong mitogenic effects, and (ii) the 2- and 4-hydroxylation catechol estrogen metabolites (2-hydroxyestrone, 2-hydroxyestradiol, 4-hydroxyestrone, 4-hydroxyestradiol) are carcinogenic because they can be oxidized into mutagenic quinones that form DNA adducts and lead to oxidative DNA damage [40].

Estrogen metabolites have been most extensively evaluated with respect to breast cancer risk, with some support for mutagenic effects of estrogen metabolites. Notably, two studies have noted decreased risks of postmenopausal breast cancer associated with elevated ratios of 2-pathway metabolites relative to parent estrogens [41, 42], and one study has found increased risks for higher levels of catechols to methylated catechols [42]. However, for endometrial cancer, which is known to be influenced by epithelial cell proliferation (particularly in the absence of progesterone), estrogen metabolites that are mitogenic have been proposed as possibly most etiologically relevant.

To date, only a limited number of studies have explored the role of estrogen metabolites in endometrial carcinogenesis. One prospective study, involving 124 cases, evaluated circulating 2-OHE$_1$ and 16αOHE$_1$ levels using an enzyme immunoassay and found some increases with high levels of both metabolites, but this relation did not persist after adjustment for estrone or estradiol levels [43]. In another cohort study (66 cases), estradiol was significantly associated with risk, but there was no further discrimination of risk according to levels of metabolites or their ratios [44]. Two endometrial cancer case-control studies have also evaluated estrogen metabolites, with suggestive relationships for certain metabolites, although interpretation of the results was limited by small numbers and assessment of hormone levels after disease onset [45, 46].

In the latest study, estrone, estradiol, and 13 estrogen metabolites were measured among 313 incident endometrial cancer cases and 354 matching controls within the WHI-OS [47]. Parent estrogens (estrone and estradiol) were positively related to risk, with the highest risk observed for unconjugated estradiol (OR 5th vs. 1st quintile = 6.19, 95% CI 2.95–13.03). Nearly all metabolites were significantly associated with elevated risks, with some attenuation after adjustment for unconjugated estradiol (residual risks of two to threefold) for most metabolites. Thus, the study provided little support for the hypothesis that endometrial cancer is especially affected by metabolites that have unique mitogenic or mutagenic properties. Instead, similar to experimental data that have failed to support unique antineoplastic activity of 2-hydroxy metabolites in endometrial cancer [48, 49], these epidemiologic results are consistent with the notion that all three estrogen pathways (2, 4, and 16) have uterotropic activity that results in endometrial proliferation [50] and endometrial tumor progression [51].

Estrogens and Endometrial Cancer Heterogeneity. It is increasingly being recognized that endometrial cancer is a heterogeneous disease, defined by at least two different entities that show different etiologies, clinical manifestations and prognoses. Type I tumors, the predominant form that corresponds histologically to endometrioid adenocarcinomas, are believed to arise from atypical endometrial hyperplasia, whereas type II tumors encompass most non-endometrioid cancers and most likely develop as a result of malignant changes in the endometrial surface epithelium. Type I tumors have been shown in epidemiologic studies to demonstrate stronger relations with a variety of hormonally-related risk factors, including obesity, parity, and cigarette smoking [32, 52, 53]. A recent Danish investigation demonstrated that menopausal hormone relations were restricted to Type I tumors [54]. Thus, it has been speculated that endogenous hormones might show similar differences in risk relations. Indeed, one small study has demonstrated higher ovarian vein levels of estradiol in type I as compared to II patients [55]. Further, in the latest epidemiologic investigation, the investigation within the WHI-OS that was previously discussed, unconjugated estradiol was more strongly related to risk of type I than II tumors [47], consistent with a central role for estrogens in influencing the progression of endometrial hyperplasias to these malignancies [56].

Interrelationship of Obesity and Endogenous Estrogens on Endometrial Cancer. Given the recognition that estrogens are produced from conversion of androgen precursors in adipose tissue, attention has focused on the interrelationships of obesity and estrogens on endometrial cancer risk. Several studies have assessed the effects of obesity on endometrial cancer risk after adjustment for estrogen levels and found persistent risks, suggesting that there may be other mediating factors [38, 47]. Androgens have been suggested to also be etiologically involved, with several studies showing positive associations of endometrial cancer risk with serum androstenedione and testosterone levels [38]. This may reflect a role of chronic anovulation and progesterone deficiency in premenopausal women, whereas after the menopause aromatase and local conversion of estrone from androstenedione appear to be more etiologically relevant.

Progestogens. Somewhat enigmatic given the strong relationships that have been established between endometrial cancer and high levels of endogenous estrogens is the observation that oral contraceptives are associated with profound reductions in risk. The fact that these compounds also contain progestogens suggests that attention should also focus on risk relations with endogenous progestogens, particularly given additional observations that administration of exogenous progestins given in the context of menopausal hormone therapy can significantly attenuate the effects of exogenous estrogens on endometrial cancer risk. Further support for assessing the role of endogenous progestogens on endometrial cancer risk derive from numerous observations that endometrial hyperplasia can be ameliorated by administration of either oral progestins or progestin-containing intrauterine devices in both pre- and post-menopausal women [57].

Despite the compelling evidence to support an evaluation of progesterone levels on endometrial cancer risk, epidemiologic investigations of the effects of endogenous levels have not yet been undertaken. This may reflect that assays to measure progesterone have in the past been associated with considerable measurement limitations, namely insufficient sensitivity to detect low levels of circulating progesterone in postmenopausal women. Of note is a newly developed assay that measures progesterone precursors, progesterone and progesterone metabolites [58], which has great potential for clarifying the effects of different endogenous levels on endometrial cancer risk.

Other Biomarkers. The notion that the effects of obesity on endometrial cancer risk cannot be entirely explained by endogenous estrogen levels has prompted an interest in other biomarkers, including obesity-related biomarkers such as adiponectin, which has been shown to be inversely related to risk [59]. Inflammation, which has also been recognized as being associated with obesity, has also been recognized as a risk factor for endometrial cancer [60]. While several studies have focused on effects on endometrial cancer risk of surrogate markers, such as non-steroidal anti-inflammatory drug use [61], recent research has benefitted from advances in measuring specific inflammatory markers [62]. A role for hyperinsulinemia has also been supported by findings that high levels of either insulin or C-peptide relate to

Table 4.2 Risk factors for ovarian cancer

Factors influencing risk	Estimated relative risk[a]
Long-term use of menopausal estrogens	3.0–5.0
Female relative with ovarian cancer	3.0–4.0
Older age	3.0
Residency in North America, northern Europe	2.0–5.0
History of infertility	2.0–5.0
Nulligravity	2.0–3.0
Higher levels of education or income	1.5–2.0
Late age at natural menopause	1.5–2.0
Perineal talc exposure	1.5–2.0
White race	1.5
Early age at menarche	1.5
Use of oral contraceptives	0.3–0.5
History of hysterectomy or tubal ligation	0.5–0.7

[a]Relative risks depend on the study and referent group employed

elevated endometrial cancer risks [63, 64]. Finally, insulin like growth factors have been examined in a number of investigations [39], albeit without conclusive results as to whether their effects on endometrial cancer risk are independent of those associated with obesity itself or of obesity-related conditions (e.g., diabetes).

Ovarian Cancer

Ovarian cancer accounts for 1.3% of all incident cancers in U.S. women, with approximately 1 in 70 American women developing ovarian cancer during their lives [1]. Similar to endometrial cancer, most attention regarding risk factors for ovarian cancer has focused on a variety of menstrual and reproductive factors, with increased risks having been related to early ages at menarche, nulligravidity or nulliparity, and late ages at menopause (Table 4.2). Obesity has not generally been viewed as a major risk factor for ovarian cancer, although its importance in the etiology of the disease has recently received increased scrutiny. Most individual studies fail to show an association, but pooling projects and meta-analyses that have enhanced power for detecting associations are beginning to indicate increased risks associated with higher BMIs. In the latest meta-analysis [65], however, there was significant heterogeneity in relations of BMI to ovarian cancer risk that varied according to the history of menopausal hormone therapy usage, with stronger relations observed for non-hormone users. Notably, the RR per 5 kg/m^2 increase in BMI was 1.10 (95% CI 1.07–1.13) in never users and 0.95 (0.92–0.99) in ever users [2].

Some investigations have also shown stronger anthropometric relationships among other subgroups, including those who have never had children, premenopausal women, postmenopausal women, women without a family history of ovarian cancer, and physically inactive women. Further, some studies have suggested that obesity is a risk factor only for certain types of tumors, with most evidence pointing to increased risks for borderline serous and invasive endometrioid and mucinous tumors [66, 67].

Exogenous Hormones

Similar to endometrial cancer, much has been learned regarding the etiology of ovarian cancers by studying relations with exogenous hormones. Oral contraceptive use is associated with profound reductions in risk, whereas menopausal hormone use has been related to risk increases, although not to the extent as seen for endometrial cancers.

Oral Contraceptives. Oral contraceptive use has been consistently associated with reduced risks of ovarian cancer. The overall estimated protection is approximately 40% for ever use and increases to more than 50% with 5 years of use or longer. A pooled analysis of 45 studies confirmed that the reduction in risk persists for 30 years beyond last use [68]. The lower-dose formulations now in use seem to reduce risk at least as effectively as higher dose predecessors and androgenicity of the progestins used does not appear to differentiate risks.

Menopausal Hormones. Unopposed estrogen menopausal hormone therapy has consistently been associated with an increased risk of ovarian cancer. Associations between estrogen plus progestin use and ovarian cancer risk have been less consistent. In the WHI clinical trial, women exposed to estrogen plus progestin therapy had an increased, albeit non-significant, risk of ovarian cancer compared to those receiving a placebo (RR 2.42; 95% CI: 0.64–9.12) [69]. A pooled analysis of 52 epidemiologic studies reported similar increased risks of ovarian cancer for both estrogen-only and estrogen plus progestin use [68]. The Danish Sex Hormone Register study reported increased risk for both sequential and continuous estrogen plus progestin use [30], suggesting that progestins do not mitigate the increased risk associated with unopposed estrogens.

Fertility Medications. The risk of ovarian cancer among women who are prescribed fertility medications is of particular interest given that these drugs stimulate ovulation, which is a recognized risk factor for ovarian cancer. Usage also raises estradiol levels [70]. Although several early studies indicated large increases in risk associated with the usage of ovulation-stimulating drugs, more recent studies have been more reassuring [71]. There are a few reports that drug usage may preferentially increase the risk of cancers among women who remain nulliparous after treatment [71], which could reflect effects of indications for usage rather than that of the drugs themselves since such conditions as endometriosis and anovulation can impart independent effects on risk. In addition, several studies have noted increased risks of low-malignant potential or borderline ovarian tumors among women receiving either ovulation-stimulating drugs or *in vitro* fertilization (IVF) [72]. Whether this is due to a drug effect or increased surveillance is as yet unresolved.

Endogenous Hormones

Studies evaluating circulating estrogens and ovarian cancer risk have been quite limited. Three studies [44, 73, 74], including one project that pooled data from three cohorts [74], failed to find relationships with either prediagnostic circulating estrone or estradiol levels, but all were limited by relatively small samples sizes (respective samples sizes of 31, 132 and 67 ovarian cancer cases) and most relied on radioimmunoassays to evaluate relations. The most recent investigation, which involved 169 cases within the WHI-OS and measured estrogen metabolites via mass spectrometry [75], observed no overall relationships, but did detect significant associations of parent estrogens with non-serous cancers. This result was consistent with a study of early pregnancy hormones that found null relations for estradiol related to serous cancers, but some evidence of elevated risks for non-serous cancers [76]. However, the relevance of estrogen levels measured during pregnancy to levels measured during the postmenopausal period remains unclear.

Similar to endometrial cancer, more recent studies have focused on estrogen metabolism. One study involving 67 ovarian cancer cases [44] found no distinctive relations according to any estrogen metabolites (similar to their findings for parent estrogens), but was unable to assess relations with specific ovarian cancer subtypes. The other study previously discussed in terms of parent estrogens [75], did not note strong associations with any metabolites for all cancer, but found that many of the 2-, 4-, and 16-pathway metabolites were positively associated with non-serous cancers.

Stronger relations with non-serous tumors have also been seen for BMI [67, 77, 78], which is not surprising given that circulating estrogens derive from adipose tissue. However, in one study that attempted to disentangle the effects of endogenous estrogens from those associated with BMI, the two measures appeared quite independent from each other [75], supporting the notion that other factors (e.g., other hormones, inflammatory factors) might contribute—both to BMI and to other hormonally-related risk factors, whose correlation with endogenous hormones has not been well explored.

The role of androgens in the etiology of ovarian cancer has also received attention. Although a number of studies have not found levels to be strongly related to risk [66, 74, 79], one study found some suggestion that free testosterone might play a role in early onset ovarian cancers [80]. In addition, a study evaluating early pregnancy hormone levels and cancer development later in life reported increased risks of invasive tumors with higher testosterone and androstenedione levels, while progesterone, 17-hydroxyprogesterone, and sex hormone binding globulin (SHBG) were not substantially related to risk [76]. Further interest has focused on gonadotropin levels, including FSH, which have been reported in one study to be inversely related to risk [81]. Thus, there remains interest in further exploring the role of endogenous hormones in the etiology of ovarian cancers, especially given that hormones may interact with immunologic factors, which have been suggested to play an important role in ovarian carcinogenesis [82]. There has also been some interest in a putative role of insulin-like growth factors (IGFs), although studies to date have provided inconclusive results regarding their effects on ovarian cancer risk [83].

Our knowledge of the etiology of ovarian cancer is rapidly changing, with recent recognition that many ovarian tumors, notably serous cancers, most likely arise in the fallopian tube. It is likely that hormones and other biomarkers have distinctive effects on the origins of different types of ovarian cancers, which undoubtedly will be the focus of much future research [84, 85].

Cervical Cancer

Cervical cancer, a disease that is well-established as resulting from infection with the human papillomaviruses (HPV), shows tremendous variation in incidence and mortality worldwide, primarily as a result of differential prevalence of PaP smear screening and vaccination services. In the U.S., invasive cancers are quite rare (estimate that 12,990 will be diagnosed annually), resulting in a focus on the identification of risk factors for precursor conditions, including various types of cervical intraepithelial neoplasias (CIN) [1]. There is little evidence for a link of obesity with overall disease risk, but some studies show higher risks of cervical adenocarcinomas (which account for only about 10% of all cervical cancers) among obese women [86]. This is consistent with the well-established role of obesity in endometrial adenocarcinomas.

Exogenous Hormones

Oral contraceptives. Use of oral hormonal contraceptives could plausibly potentiate the carcinogenicity of HPV infection, because transcriptional regulatory regions of HPV DNA contain hormone-recognition elements and hormones have been shown *in vitro* to enhance and transform the effects of viral DNA [87]. A pooled analysis of multiple case-control studies found an elevated risk of invasive cervical cancer among HPV-positive women who used oral contraceptives for more than 5 years, an increased risk that persisted after careful adjustment for sexual and reproductive factors, duration of HPV infection, and screening history [88]. Short durations of use or use more than 5 years prior to cancer onset were not associated with elevated risk. The latest investigation within the EPIC Study found increased risks related to long-term (≥15 years) oral contraceptive use for both CIN3/carcinoma *in situ* (CIS) and invasive cancer (respective RRs versus non-users of 1.6 and 1.8).

Other hormonal contraceptives. The effect of other long-acting steroid preparations, notably DMPA, has also been of concern with respect to cervical abnormalities. Although these agents are widely used in many countries, studies evaluating their effects are limited. Further, assessment of relations may be problematic given that longer term DMPA appears to be associated with the detection of oncogenic HPVs [89].

IUD use, which is also a common contraception option in developing countries, has been evaluated in a few studies, including a pooled analysis of ten case–control studies of cervical cancer and 16 HPV prevalence surveys from four continents. This showed a decreased risk of cervical cancer, regardless of duration of use (few months to up to 9 years) and after adjustment for screening status [90]. A reduced risk associated with IUD usage was also recently noted in the EPIC Study [91], although neither this investigation or the pooling project was able to assess effects of specific types of IUDs, including hormone-containing ones. The evidence contradicts a widely held assumption that IUDs may increase the risk of cervical cancer, and might suggest their role as protective cofactors in cervical carcinogenesis, similar to the role they play in reducing endometrial cancer risk. While the precise mechanisms are subject to future investigations, it has been suggested that local cellular immunity may be triggered during the process of IUD insertion or by the device itself.

Menopausal Hormones. The role of menopausal hormone therapy and its interrelationship with overweight/obesity as determinants of either cervical cancer risk or of circulating estrogen levels in postmenopausal women is not well understood [92]. The latest analysis, within EPIC, noted a significantly reduced risk of invasive cervical cancer associated with menopausal hormone therapy use [91]. The extent to which this finding reflects a screening bias has yet to be determined.

Endogenous Hormones

The relationship between endogenous hormones and cervical cancer risk is unclear and is a topic of ongoing investigation [93]. Some results point to the role of circulating levels of testosterone and estradiol in modulating cervical cancer risk in premenopausal women [94]. Mechanistic evidence to confirm these associations and exploration of signaling pathways suggests hormone-receptor modulation in cervical cancer likely differs from other estrogen-dependent cancers (such as endometrial cancer) [95].

Vulvar Cancer

Vulvar cancer is a rare malignancy, accounting for only about 4% of cancers of the female reproductive organs and 0.6% of all cancers among American women. In the U.S., women have a 1 in 333 chance of developing vulvar cancer at some point during their lives [1], with it primarily being a disease of older women. The risk of developing invasive vulvar cancer is increased among women with a history of cervical carcinoma *in situ* [96], consistent with the recognition that both diseases are etiologically linked to HPV infection.

Although early studies were contradictory as to whether or not obesity was a risk factor for the disease, the latest investigation within a large cohort showed a RR of 1.71 (95% CI 1.44–2.04) for women who had BMIs of 30 or greater compared to those with BMIs under 25 [96]. This has prompted further interest in the etiologic role of a variety of hormonal factors in the etiology of the disease, including effects of exogenous and endogenous hormones.

Exogenous and Endogenous Hormones in the Etiology of Vulvar Cancer

Several studies have noted higher risks of both invasive and in situ vulvar cancers among oral contraceptive users [97], although the extent to which this association is confounded by HPV infection status remains unknown given that these studies were conducted prior to routine HPV testing. The rarity of this tumor has hampered efforts to understand the etiologic role of exogenous and endogenous hormones, but this would appear to be a worthwhile endeavor given the recent recognition of the role of obesity in its etiology.

Summary and Conclusions

The vast majority of gynecologic cancers, and in particular endometrial cancer, are more common in obese women, with much of the association presumably due to effects of endogenous estrogens. Given increasing rates of obesity, concern has been expressed regarding possible increases in incidence. Incidence projections for endometrial cancer, as well as other cancers, are difficult, however, given changing time trends in hysterectomies/oophorectomies and usage of menopausal hormones, which may have lesser effects in obese women.

We have learned much in the last decade regarding the effects of endogenous hormones, specifically estrogens, on the risks of various gynecologic cancers, but it is apparent that these relations are complex—not only because of relatively low levels of risk, but also because of intervening effects of other endogenous hormones and other biomarkers (androgens, IGFs, etc.), most of which have not been adequately investigated. The etiologic heterogeneity of gynecologic cancers is also increasingly being recognized, with different patterns of risk being noted with both obesity and hormones (both exogenous and endogenous)—particularly for endometrial and ovarian cancers.

References

1. American Cancer Society: Cancer Facts & Figures 2015, 2015.
2. Schmandt RE, Iglesias DA, Co NN, et al. Understanding obesity and endometrial cancer risk: opportunities for prevention. Am J Obstet Gynecol. 2011;205:518–25.
3. Renehan AG, Tyson M, Egger M, et al. Body-mass index and incidence of cancer: a systematic review and meta-analysis of prospective observational studies. Lancet. 2008;371:569–78.
4. Sponholtz TR, Palmer JR, Rosenberg L, et al. Body size, metabolic factors, and risk of endometrial cancer in black women. Am J Epidemiol. 2016;183:259–68.
5. Upala S, Anawin S. Bariatric surgery and risk of postoperative endometrial cancer: a systematic review and meta-analysis. Surg Obes Relat Dis. 2015;11:949–55.
6. Nagle CM, Marquart L, Bain CJ, et al. Impact of weight change and weight cycling on risk of different subtypes of endometrial cancer. Eur J Cancer. 2013;49:2717–26.
7. Linkov F, Maxwell GL, Felix AS, et al. Longitudinal evaluation of cancer-associated biomarkers before and after weight loss in RENEW study participants: implications for cancer risk reduction. Gynecol Oncol. 2012;125:114–9.
8. Dougan MM, Hankinson SE, Vivo ID, et al. Prospective study of body size throughout the life-course and the incidence of endometrial cancer among premenopausal and postmenopausal women. Int J Cancer. 2015;137:625–37.
9. Friedenreich C, Cust A, Lahmann PH, et al. Anthropometric factors and risk of endometrial cancer: the European prospective investigation into cancer and nutrition. Cancer Causes Control. 2007;18:399–413.
10. Ju W, Kim HJ, Hankinson SE, et al. Prospective study of body fat distribution and the risk of endometrial cancer. Cancer Epidemiol. 2015;39:567–70.
11. Schmid D, Behrens G, Keimling M, et al. A systematic review and meta-analysis of physical activity and endometrial cancer risk. Eur J Epidemiol. 2015;30:397–412.
12. Moore SC, Lee IM, Weiderpass E, et al. Association of Leisure-Time Physical Activity with Risk of 26 types of cancer in 1.44 million adults. JAMA Intern Med. 2016;176:816–25.
13. Key TJ, Pike MC. The dose-effect relationship between 'unopposed' oestrogens and endometrial mitotic rate: its central role in explaining and predicting endometrial cancer risk. Br J Cancer. 1988;57:205–12.
14. Zhao S, Chlebowski RT, Anderson GL, et al. Sex hormone associations with breast cancer risk and the mediation of randomized trial postmenopausal hormone therapy effects. Breast Cancer Res. 2014;16:R30.
15. Siiteri PK. Adipose tissue as a source of hormones. Am J Clin Nutr. 1987;45:277–82.
16. Fearnley EJ, Marquart L, Spurdle AB, et al. Polycystic ovary syndrome increases the risk of endometrial cancer in women aged less than 50 years: an Australian case-control study. Cancer Causes Control. 2010;21:2303–8.
17. Gottschau M, Kjaer SK, Jensen A, et al. Risk of cancer among women with polycystic ovary syndrome: a Danish cohort study. Gynecol Oncol. 2015;136:99–103.
18. Haoula Z, Salman M, Atiomo W. Evaluating the association between endometrial cancer and polycystic ovary syndrome. Hum Reprod. 2012;27:1327–31.
19. Pandey A, Forte V, Abdallah M, et al. Diabetes mellitus and the risk of cancer. Minerva Endocrinol. 2011;36:187–209.
20. Sheikh MA, Althouse AD, Freese KE, et al. USA endometrial cancer projections to 2030: should we be concerned? Future Oncol. 2014;10:2561–8.
21. Collaborative Group on Epidemiological Studies on Endometrial C. Endometrial cancer and oral contraceptives: an individual participant meta-analysis of 27 276 women with endometrial cancer from 36 epidemiological studies. Lancet Oncol. 2015;16:1061–70.
22. Maxwell GL, Schildkraut JM, Calingaert B, et al. Progestin and estrogen potency of combination oral contraceptives and endometrial cancer risk. Gynecol Oncol. 2006;103:535–40.

23. Felix AS, Gaudet MM, La Vecchia C, et al. Intrauterine devices and endometrial cancer risk: a pooled analysis of the epidemiology of endometrial cancer consortium. Int J Cancer. 2015;136:E410–22.
24. Beral V, Bull D, Reeves G, et al. Endometrial cancer and hormone-replacement therapy in the million women study. Lancet. 2005;365:1543–51.
25. Chlebowski RT, Anderson GL, Sarto GE, et al. Continuous combined estrogen plus progestin and endometrial cancer: the Women's Health Initiative randomized trial. J Natl Cancer Inst. 2016;108
26. Razavi P, Pike MC, Horn-Ross PL, et al. Long-term postmenopausal hormone therapy and endometrial cancer. Cancer Epidemiol Biomark Prev. 2010;19:475–83.
27. Trabert B, Wentzensen N, Yang HP, et al. Is estrogen plus progestin menopausal hormone therapy safe with respect to endometrial cancer risk? Int J Cancer. 2013;132:417–26.
28. Yang TY, Cairns BJ, Allen N, et al. Postmenopausal endometrial cancer risk and body size in early life and middle age: prospective cohort study. Br J Cancer. 2012;107:169–75.
29. Sjogren LL, Morch LS, Lokkegaard E. Hormone replacement therapy and the risk of endometrial cancer: a systematic review. Maturitas. 2016;91:25–35.
30. Morch LS, Lokkegaard E, Andreasen AH, et al. Hormone therapy and ovarian cancer. JAMA. 2009;302:298–305.
31. Cuzick J, Sestak I, Bonanni B, et al. Selective oestrogen receptor modulators in prevention of breast cancer: an updated meta-analysis of individual participant data. Lancet. 2013;381:1827–34.
32. Brinton LA, Felix AS, McMeekin DS, et al. Etiologic heterogeneity in endometrial cancer: evidence from a gynecologic oncology group trial. Gynecol Oncol. 2013;129:277–84.
33. Kamal A, Tempest N, Parkes C, et al. Hormones and endometrial carcinogenesis. Horm Mol Biol Clin Investig. 2016;25:129–48.
34. Gennari L. Lasofoxifene, a new selective estrogen receptor modulator for the treatment of osteoporosis and vaginal atrophy. Expert Opin Pharmacother. 2009;10:2209–20.
35. Kaaks R, Lukanova A, Kurzer MS. Obesity, endogenous hormones, and endometrial cancer risk: a synthetic review. Cancer Epidemiol Biomark Prev. 2002;11:1531–43.
36. Brown SB, Hankinson SE. Endogenous estrogens and the risk of breast, endometrial, and ovarian cancers. Steroids. 2015;99:8–10.
37. Lukanova A, Lundin E, Micheli A, et al. Circulating levels of sex steroid hormones and risk of endometrial cancer in postmenopausal women. Int J Cancer. 2004;108:425–32.
38. Allen NE, Key TJ, Dossus L, et al. Endogenous sex hormones and endometrial cancer risk in women in the European prospective investigation into cancer and nutrition (EPIC). Endocr Relat Cancer. 2008;15:485–97.
39. Gunter MJ, Hoover DR, Yu H, et al. A prospective evaluation of insulin and insulin-like growth factor-I as risk factors for endometrial cancer. Cancer Epidemiol Biomark Prev. 2008;17:921–9.
40. Ziegler RG, Fuhrman BJ, Moore SC, et al. Epidemiologic studies of estrogen metabolism and breast cancer. Steroids. 2015;99:67–75.
41. Dallal CM, Tice JA, Buist DS, et al. Estrogen metabolism and breast cancer risk among postmenopausal women: a case-cohort study within B~FIT. Carcinogenesis. 2014;35:346–55.
42. Fuhrman BJ, Schairer C, Gail MH, et al. Estrogen metabolism and risk of breast cancer in postmenopausal women. J Natl Cancer Inst. 2012;104:326–39.
43. Zeleniuch-Jacquotte A, Shore RE, Afanasyeva Y, et al. Postmenopausal circulating levels of 2- and 16alpha-hydroxyestrone and risk of endometrial cancer. Br J Cancer. 2011;105:1458–64.
44. Dallal CM, Lacey JV Jr, Pfeiffer RM, et al. Estrogen metabolism and risk of postmenopausal endometrial and ovarian cancer: the B approximately FIT cohort. Horm Cancer. 2016;7:49–64.
45. Audet-Walsh E, Lepine J, Gregoire J, et al. Profiling of endogenous estrogens, their precursors, and metabolites in endometrial cancer patients: association with risk and relationship to clinical characteristics. J Clin Endocrinol Metab. 2011;96:E330–9.
46. Zhao H, Jiang Y, Liu Y, et al. Endogenous estrogen metabolites as biomarkers for endometrial cancer via a novel method of liquid chromatography-mass spectrometry with hollow fiber liquid-phase microextraction. Horm Metab Res. 2015;47:158–64.

47. Brinton LA, Trabert B, Anderson GL, et al. Serum Estrogens and Estrogen Metabolites and Endometrial Cancer Risk among Postmenopausal Women. Cancer Epidemiol Biomark Prev. 2016;25:1081–9.
48. Newbold RR, Liehr JG. Induction of uterine adenocarcinoma in CD-1 mice by catechol estrogens. Cancer Res. 2000;60:235–7.
49. Reddy VV, Hanjani P, Rajan R. Synthesis of catechol estrogens by human uterus and leiomyoma. Steroids. 1981;37:195–203.
50. Zhu BT, Conney AH. Functional role of estrogen metabolism in target cells: review and perspectives. Carcinogenesis. 1998;19:1–27.
51. Takahashi M, Shimomoto T, Miyajima K, et al. Effects of estrogens and metabolites on endometrial carcinogenesis in young adult mice initiated with N-ethyl-N'-nitro-N-nitrosoguanidine. Cancer Lett. 2004;211:1–9.
52. Setiawan VW, Yang HP, Pike MC, et al. Type I and II endometrial cancers: have they different risk factors? J Clin Oncol. 2013;31:2607–18.
53. Yang HP, Wentzensen N, Trabert B, et al. Endometrial cancer risk factors by 2 main histologic subtypes: the NIH-AARP diet and health study. Am J Epidemiol. 2013;177:142–51.
54. Morch LS, Kjaer SK, Keiding N, et al. The influence of hormone therapies on type I and II endometrial cancer: a nationwide cohort study. Int J Cancer. 2016;138:1506–15.
55. Ashihara K, Tanaka T, Maruoka R, et al. Postmenopausal patients with endometrial cancer of type 1 have elevated serum estradiol levels in the ovarian vein. Int J Gynecol Cancer. 2014;24:1455–60.
56. Sherman ME. Theories of endometrial carcinogenesis: a multidisciplinary approach. Mod Pathol. 2000;13:295–308.
57. Armstrong AJ, Hurd WW, Elguero S, et al. Diagnosis and management of endometrial hyperplasia. J Minim Invasive Gynecol. 2012;19:562–71.
58. Trabert B, Falk RT, Stanczyk FZ, et al. Reproducibility of an assay to measure serum progesterone metabolites that may be related to breast cancer risk using liquid chromatography tandem mass spectrometry. Horm Mol Biol Clin Investig. 2015;23:79–84.
59. Zheng Q, Wu H, Cao J. Circulating adiponectin and risk of endometrial cancer. PLoS One. 2015;10:e0129824.
60. Dossus L, Lukanova A, Rinaldi S, et al. Hormonal, metabolic, and inflammatory profiles and endometrial cancer risk within the EPIC cohort--a factor analysis. Am J Epidemiol. 2013;177:787–99.
61. Brons N, Baandrup L, Dehlendorff C, et al. Use of nonsteroidal anti-inflammatory drugs and risk of endometrial cancer: a nationwide case-control study. Cancer Causes Control. 2015;26:973–81.
62. Friedenreich CM, Langley AR, Speidel TP, et al. Case-control study of inflammatory markers and the risk of endometrial cancer. Eur J Cancer Prev. 2013;22:374–9.
63. Cust AE, Allen NE, Rinaldi S, et al. Serum levels of C-peptide, IGFBP-1 and IGFBP-2 and endometrial cancer risk: results from the European prospective investigation into cancer and nutrition. Int J Cancer. 2007;120:2656–64.
64. Hernandez AV, Pasupuleti V, Benites-Zapata VA, et al. Insulin resistance and endometrial cancer risk: a systematic review and meta-analysis. Eur J Cancer. 2015;51:2747–58.
65. Collaborative Group on Epidemiological Studies of Ovarian C. Ovarian cancer and body size: individual participant meta-analysis including 25,157 women with ovarian cancer from 47 epidemiological studies. PLoS Med. 2012;9:e1001200.
66. Olsen CM, Nagle CM, Whiteman DC, et al. Obesity and risk of ovarian cancer subtypes: evidence from the ovarian cancer association consortium. Endocr Relat Cancer. 2013;20:251–62.
67. Yang HP, Trabert B, Murphy MA, et al. Ovarian cancer risk factors by histologic subtypes in the NIH-AARP diet and health study. Int J Cancer. 2012;131:938–48.
68. Collaborative Group on Epidemiological Studies of Ovarian C, Beral V, Doll R, et al. Ovarian cancer and oral contraceptives: collaborative reanalysis of data from 45 epidemiological studies including 23,257 women with ovarian cancer and 87,303 controls. Lancet. 2008;371:303–14.

69. Anderson GL, Judd HL, Kaunitz AM, et al. Effects of estrogen plus progestin on gynecologic cancers and associated diagnostic procedures: the Women's Health Initiative randomized trial. JAMA. 2003;290:1739–48.
70. Sovino H, Sir-Petermann T, Devoto L. Clomiphene citrate and ovulation induction. Reprod Biomed Online. 2002;4:303–10.
71. Brinton LA, Sahasrabuddhe VV, Scoccia B. Fertility drugs and the risk of breast and gynecologic cancers. Semin Reprod Med. 2012;30:131–45.
72. van Leeuwen FE, Klip H, Mooij TM, et al. Risk of borderline and invasive ovarian tumours after ovarian stimulation for in vitro fertilization in a large Dutch cohort. Hum Reprod. 2011;26:3456–65.
73. Helzlsouer KJ, Alberg AJ, Gordon GB, et al. Serum gonadotropins and steroid hormones and the development of ovarian cancer. JAMA. 1995;274:1926–30.
74. Lukanova A, Lundin E, Akhmedkhanov A, et al. Circulating levels of sex steroid hormones and risk of ovarian cancer. Int J Cancer. 2003;104:636–42.
75. Trabert B, Brinton LA, Anderson GL, et al. Circulating estrogens and postmenopausal ovarian cancer risk in the Women's Health Initiative observational study. Cancer Epidemiol Biomark Prev. 2016;25(4):648–56.
76. Schock H, Surcel HM, Zeleniuch-Jacquotte A, et al. Early pregnancy sex steroids and maternal risk of epithelial ovarian cancer. Endocr Relat Cancer. 2014;21:831–44.
77. Fortner RT, Ose J, Merritt MA, et al. Reproductive and hormone-related risk factors for epithelial ovarian cancer by histologic pathways, invasiveness and histologic subtypes: results from the EPIC cohort. Int J Cancer. 2015;137:1196–208.
78. Gates MA, Rosner BA, Hecht JL, et al. Risk factors for epithelial ovarian cancer by histologic subtype. Am J Epidemiol. 2010;171:45–53.
79. Ose J, Fortner RT, Rinaldi S, et al. Endogenous androgens and risk of epithelial invasive ovarian cancer by tumor characteristics in the European prospective investigation into cancer and nutrition. Int J Cancer. 2015;136:399–410.
80. Rinaldi S, Dossus L, Lukanova A, et al. Endogenous androgens and risk of epithelial ovarian cancer: results from the European prospective investigation into cancer and nutrition (EPIC). Cancer Epidemiol Biomark Prev. 2007;16:23–9.
81. McSorley MA, Alberg AJ, Allen DS, et al. Prediagnostic circulating follicle stimulating hormone concentrations and ovarian cancer risk. Int J Cancer. 2009;125:674–9.
82. Ness RB, Cottreau C. Possible role of ovarian epithelial inflammation in ovarian cancer. J Natl Cancer Inst. 1999;91:1459–67.
83. Ose J, Fortner RT, Schock H, et al. Insulin-like growth factor I and risk of epithelial invasive ovarian cancer by tumour characteristics: results from the EPIC cohort. Br J Cancer. 2015;112:162–6.
84. Cardenas C, Alvero AB, Yun BS, et al. Redefining the origin and evolution of ovarian cancer: a hormonal connection. Endocr Relat Cancer. 2016;23:R411–22.
85. Gharwan H, Bunch KP, Annunziata CM. The role of reproductive hormones in epithelial ovarian carcinogenesis. Endocr Relat Cancer. 2015;22:R339–63.
86. Lacey JV Jr, Swanson CA, Brinton LA, et al. Obesity as a potential risk factor for adenocarcinomas and squamous cell carcinomas of the uterine cervix. Cancer. 2003;98:814–21.
87. de Villiers EM. Relationship between steroid hormone contraceptives and HPV, cervical intraepithelial neoplasia and cervical carcinoma. Int J Cancer. 2003;103:705–8.
88. International Collaboration of Epidemiological Studies of Cervical C. Cervical carcinoma and reproductive factors: collaborative reanalysis of individual data on 16,563 women with cervical carcinoma and 33,542 women without cervical carcinoma from 25 epidemiological studies. Int J Cancer. 2006;119:1108–24.
89. Harris TG, Miller L, Kulasingam SL, et al. Depot-medroxyprogesterone acetate and combined oral contraceptive use and cervical neoplasia among women with oncogenic human papillomavirus infection. Am J Obstet Gynecol. 2009;200:489 e1–8.

90. Arbyn M, Castellsague X, de Sanjose S, et al. Worldwide burden of cervical cancer in 2008. Ann Oncol. 2011;22:2675–86.
91. Roura E, Travier N, Waterboer T, et al. The influence of hormonal factors on the risk of developing cervical cancer and pre-cancer: results from the EPIC cohort. PLoS One. 2016;11:e0147029.
92. Roberts JN, Kines RC, Katki HA, et al. Effect of pap smear collection and carrageenan on cervicovaginal human papillomavirus-16 infection in a rhesus macaque model. J Natl Cancer Inst. 2011;103:737–43.
93. Poorolajal J, Jenabi E. The association between BMI and cervical cancer risk: a meta-analysis. Eur J Cancer Prev. 2016;25:232–8.
94. Rinaldi S, Plummer M, Biessy C, et al. Endogenous sex steroids and risk of cervical carcinoma: results from the EPIC study. Cancer Epidemiol Biomark Prev. 2011;20:2532–40.
95. den Boon JA, Pyeon D, Wang SS, et al. Molecular transitions from papillomavirus infection to cervical precancer and cancer: role of stromal estrogen receptor signaling. Proc Natl Acad Sci U S A. 2015;112:E3255–64.
96. Coffey K, Gaitskell K, Beral V, et al. Past cervical intraepithelial neoplasia grade 3, obesity, and earlier menopause are associated with an increased risk of vulval cancer in postmenopausal women. Br J Cancer. 2016;115:599–606.
97. Newcomb PA, Weiss NS, Daling JR. Incidence of vulvar carcinoma in relation to menstrual, reproductive, and medical factors. J Natl Cancer Inst. 1984;73:391–6.

Chapter 5
Obesity and Endometrial Cancer Precursors

Jaclyn Watkins

Abstract The menstrual cycle is composed of two phases – proliferative and secretory. During the proliferative phase, estrogen stimulates the endometrium leading to growth of both the stromal and epithelial compartments. During this period of abundant mitotic activity, mutations inevitably arise within the epithelial compartment. It is typically the rise of progesterone during the secretory cycle that selects against further proliferation of these mutant cells. However, in patients with excess estrogen (e.g., obesity), these mutant populations have a selective advantage, leading to further proliferation and increased mutation rates. The result is a progression of "latent precancers" to endometrial intraepithelial neoplasia (EIN) – a precursor of endometrial endometrioid-type adenocarcinoma.

Keywords Endometrial intra epithelial neoplasia • Phosphatase and tensin homolog (PTEN) • Paired box gene 2 (PAX2) • Endometroid Cancer – Latent Precursors

Endometrial Cancer and Obesity

Chronic excess estrogen, whether endogenous or exogenous, is a well-known risk factor for the development of endometrial cancer and its precursor, endometrial intraepithelial neoplasia (EIN). In postmenopausal patients, estrogen predominantly derives from the presence of aromatase within adipose tissue. Aromatase is an enzyme responsible for the conversion of androgens to estrone and estradiol. Levels of aromatase are known to increase with age and, given its location within adipose tissue, with increasing BMI. The result is a direct relationship between BMI and circulating estrogen [1, 2].

However in obese patients, aromatase levels, and the subsequent increase in circulating estrogen, provide only a partial explanation for observed elevated risk of endometrial carcinoma and EIN. Another key component is a relative lack of progesterone [2]. Progesterone is known to inhibit endometrial proliferation and induce

J. Watkins, M.D., M.S. (✉)
Department of Pathology, Microbiology, and Immunology, Vanderbilt University Medical Center, 1161 21st Avenue South, C-3321 MCN, Nashville, TN 37212, USA
e-mail: jaclyn.c.watkins@vanderbilt.edu

© Springer International Publishing AG 2018
N.A. Berger et al. (eds.), *Focus on Gynecologic Malignancies*, Energy Balance and Cancer 13, DOI 10.1007/978-3-319-63483-8_5

endometrial differentiation - functions that decrease the probability of mutations accruing within the endometrial epithelial compartment [3]. Therefore, it is the balance between progesterone and estrogen that is critical in the progression of latent precancers to EIN and carcinoma [2].

PTEN and Endometrial Precancers

Mutations in PTEN, a tumor suppressor gene involved in the mediation of cell division and apoptosis [4], are amongst the most common genetic changes in endometrioid-type endometrial cancer. In fact, up to 83% of endometrioid-type endometrial adenocarcinoma demonstrate biallelic somatic inactivation of PTEN [5].

The role of PTEN mutations in endometrial carcinogenesis has been proven in both mouse models [6] and in humans [5]. Further, germline mutations in PTEN, as occurs in Cowden's Syndrome, are known to increase the risk of developing cancers of multiple sites including the thyroid, breast, and endometrium [7–9]. However, PTEN mutations in isolation do not definitively lead to endometrial cancer [5]; rather, PTEN inactivation is an early event that sets the stage for cancer [10].

PTEN inactivation within the endometrial epithelial compartment is a common event. In fact, somatic PTEN inactivation has been documented in a small subset of histologically normal endometrial glands in up to 43% of normally cycling premenopausal women [10]. Despite the large number of women with PTEN-deficient glands, only 2% of such glands will persist as a unique clone [11] and lifetime risk of endometrial cancer only approaches 2.5% [12, 13]. For this reason, such histologically normal PTEN deficient glands are referred to as "latent precancers," a term which implies that additional mutations are required to produce neoplasia [11]. Such findings are subclinical – meaning they are below the threshold that pathologists would consider clinically relevant – as the frequency of such clones progressing to cancer is low.

Latent precancers are histologically defined by the absence of PTEN expression by immunohistochemistry [10]. The glands do not display cytologic or architectural atypia. They are typically few in number and are generally scattered or clustered within a background of normal endometrium [10]. They generally display proliferative features, namely mitoses [10]. Over 75% of such PTEN negative clones are retained through multiple menstrual cycles, with some clones persisting upwards of 1 year. [10, 14].

Over time, PTEN-negative latent precancers that are not shed during the normal endometrial cycle may become persistently proliferative [10]. At first, the expansion is due to increased gland size [10]. Eventually, however, the population of PTEN-mutant glands becomes increasingly dense, taking on features that approach EIN. [10].

Endometrial Intraepithelial Neoplasia: The Endometrial Endometrioid Adenocarcinoma Precursor

Endometrioid-type endometrial adenocarcinoma is the most common endometrial malignancy, accounting for 70–80% of sporadic endometrial cancer cases [15]. This particular subtype is often indolent, arising from premalignant glandular lesions that result from prolonged estrogen stimulation [15]. Historically, these premalignant lesions fell at one end of a spectrum of endometrial changes known as "endometrial hyperplasia" [15].

Endometrial hyperplasia, as was delineated in the 1994 World Health Organization schema, was a catch-all term for both clonal premalignant lesions and benign field effect changes of the endometrium that occurred in hyperestrogenic states. However, the WHO system, which divided hyperplasia in four categories, showed poor reproducibility among pathologists [16–18].

Since the 1994 categorization, the mechanisms underlying endometrial hyperplasia have become more fully understood. Today, true "hyperplasia" of the endometrium is thought to be the result of unopposed estrogenic stimulation [15]. Histormophologically speaking, such hyperplasias are diffuse entities, representing a field effect in the endometrium. While it had been assumed that such hyperplastic lesions might ultimately evolve into cancer, it has since been realized that endometrioid adenocarcinoma results from the malignant transformation of a single gland, which in turn grows into a localized premalignant lesion [15]. Such localized lesions, which typically arise 3–4 years prior to the development of overt carcinoma, [19] are histomorphologically discrete from the background endometrium and are now designated endometrial intraepithelial neoplasia (EIN) [15].

EIN, a monoclonal proliferation of endometrial glands that displays both architectural and cytologic changes, has distinct histomorphologic features that allow pathologists to diagnose it on H&E alone (Fig. 5.1) [20]. First, an EIN lesion must measure at least 1 mm in greatest dimension within a single tissue fragment [15].

Fig. 5.1 An endometrial biopsy demonstrating a benign proliferative population of glands (*left*) and endometrial intraepithelial neoplasia (EIN) (*right*). Note that the EIN population demonstrates the three necessary histopathologic features to render a diagnosis – size >1 mm, gland density greater than stromal density, and a cytomorphologic shift in the glandular epithelium

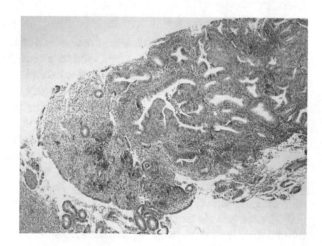

This particular cutoff is critical as it is the minimum size that reproducibly alters clinical outcomes (i.e., increased risk of carcinoma) [20]. Secondly, greater than 50% of the lesion should be composed of glands (i.e., glandular epithelium plus lumens) [15]. This gives the lesion a characteristically crowded appearance in which the surrounding stroma is relatively reduced. Lastly, the diagnosis of EIN requires a shift in the cytomorphologic features of the lesion relative to background endometrial glands. This shift does not necessarily mean that the glands harbor atypical features (e.g., round nuclei, prominent nucleoli, loss of polarity), though one or more of these features are often present [15]. EIN lesions do not share a common altered cytology; therefore, the shift in cytomorphology must be determined on a case-by-case basis. [15] EIN is commonly a localized process, often occurring in a background of estrogenic effect; however, it may also grow to occupy the entire endometrial compartment, giving rise to what is known as "extensive EIN" [15].

EIN has been associated with a high likelihood of progression to adenocarcinoma. In fact, 1/3–1/2 of women who are diagnosed with EIN will be diagnosed with adenocarcinoma within 1 year [20, 21]. If a patient remains cancer free in the first year after diagnosis, she holds a 45-fold increased risk of progression to endometrial cancer thereafter, with the average interval to progression being 4 years [20]. In comparison, atypical hyperplasia, as defined by the former WHO criteria, confers only a 14-fold increased risk of cancer [22].

PTEN inactivation has been documented in up to 63% of EIN lesions [10] and 83% of endometrial adenocarcinomas [5]. However, it is thought that an accumulation of multiple genetic "hits" is necessary to turn latent precancers into EIN [19]. These "hits" often include mutations in KRAS [23], CTNNB1 [24], PIK3CA [24], PAX2 [25], and mismatch repair genes [23, 24]. Microsatellite instability has also been documented in 20–25% of EIN lesions [26].

PAX2 Expression in Latent Precancers and Endometrial Cancer

In addition to PTEN inactivation, loss of expression of PAX2, a gene involved in the embryonic development of the kidneys, ureters, uterus, fallopian tubes, vas deferens and epididymis, is common in latent precancers and endometrial cancer [27]. The endometrium persistently expresses PAX2 throughout the life course [28], indicating that PAX2 likely plays a critical role in endometrial proliferation and renewal [25]. In fact, there is some data to suggest that loss of constitutive expression of PAX2 in the endometrium is associated with both endometrial and cervical malignant transformation [29]. One such study, which examined the expression of PAX2 through quantitative RNA, demonstrated that benign endometrium displays the highest levels of PAX2 expression [30]. The level of PAX2 expression drops twofold with the initiation of tamoxifen therapy and fivefold in endometrial cancers [30]. Therefore, it is likely that PAX2 functions as a tumor suppressor gene within the endometrium, likely working in parallel with PTEN [25].

PAX2 expression is lost in 77% of endometrial adenocarcinomas [25]. It is also evident, at least focally, in 36% of normal endometrial samples. [25] Interestingly, PAX2 loss in the normal endometrium tends to occur in glands separate from those that are PTEN null. [25] However as neoplasia arises, first as EIN and then as adenocarcinoma, the likelihood of overlap increases with 31% of EIN and 55% of carcinomas displaying coincident loss in an overlapping clonal distribution (Fig. 5.2). [25].

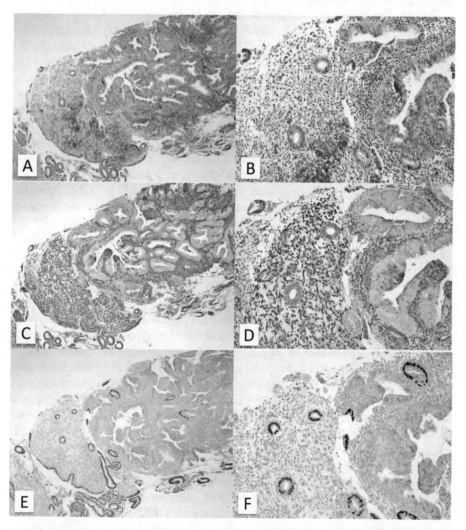

Fig. 5.2 Endometrial intraepithelial neoplasia (EIN) as displayed in the right side of image (**a**, low power) and (**b**, high power) frequently displays a loss of PTEN expression by immunohistochemistry (low power, **c**; high power, **d**) due to biallelic somatic inactivation. Such a pattern of staining is also seen in latent precancers. Background endometrial glands (left portion of image, **c**, **d**) show intact expression by immunohistochemistry. EIN, unlike most latent precancers, may also show concurrent loss of PAX2 expression with background benign endometrial glands demonstrating intact staining (low power, **e**; high power **f**)

PTEN-Negative Latent Precursors and Nongenetic Risk Modifiers

Nongenetic risk modifiers (e.g., hormones) alter the likelihood of latent precancers progressing to malignancy by functioning as selection factors, either for or against, the outgrowth of PTEN-negative clones [14].

To fully understand how nongenetic risk modifiers alter the progression of latent precancers, it is first necessary to address normal PTEN expression throughout the menstrual cycle. Within the uterus, PTEN expression is primarily located in the endometrial functionalis, in both the stromal and glandular compartments [31]. Beginning with the estrogen-driven proliferative phase of the menstrual cycle, PTEN expression increases in the epithelial and stromal compartments [31]. With the beginning of the progesterone dominant secretory phase, PTEN expression decreases in the epithelial compartment, but increases in the stromal compartment, especially as the stroma becomes decidualized [31]. This transition of expression (i.e., expression of PTEN within the epithelium during the proliferative phase and a reduction of epithelial expression during the secretory phase) likely represents a functional need for PTEN expression during the high mitotic period of epithelial proliferation. [31] Expression is less necessary during the progesterone-dominant periods as proliferation ceases and differentiation begins [31].

Nongenetic Risk Modifiers and Selection of Latent Precancers

It has been hypothesized that the transition from precancer to overt malignancy is the result of positive selection of mutant clones (i.e., latent precancers) by hormonal mechanisms. A high burden of somatic mutations occur with each menstrual cycle [10]. However, it is only the subsequent hormonal selection of these mutated clones, or latent precancers, that leads to the expansion of genetically defective cells [32].

One of the most well-known cancer-causing nongenetic modifiers is unopposed estrogen. Unopposed estrogen exposure, which commonly occurs in obese patients, increases endometrial cancer risk up to tenfold [33]. This risk-elevating exposure is not thought to increase the number of latent precursors; rather, it is thought to promote the progression of existing latent precursors through an increase in glandular proliferation or mutation rate [14]. PTEN-defective latent endometrial precancers maintain high levels of nuclear estrogen and progesterone receptors [10]. Furthermore, physiologic expression of PTEN is highest during the proliferative phase of the menstrual cycle, which is stimulated by estrogen [31]. Therefore, when excess estrogen is present, PTEN clones are likely to have a selective advantage. The result is clonal expansion of the mutated population and an increased likelihood of the accumulation of additional mutations [15]. PTEN-mutant populations in the presence of high estrogen levels therefore have a high risk of becoming carcinoma. [31].

Nongenetic Risk Modifiers and Involution of Latent Precancers

One of the most cancer-protective modifiers is progesterone (or progestin if exogenous). Progesterone has been shown to selectively ablate PTEN mutant latent precancers within the background endometrium [3]. However, in the normally cycling endometrium, the progesterone exposure is not always sufficient to completely shut down PTEN expression. This potentially allows mutant clones to persist and become malignant [10]. In contrast, progestin exposure has the ability to quell expression of PTEN, and at therapeutic doses, it is actually capable of causing the involution of PTEN-negative latent precancers [3]. Further, progestin can act as an estrogen antagonist via the downregulation of the estrogen receptor [32].

Such ablation of latent precancers is thought to be one of the major mechanisms behind the decline in endometrial cancer prevalence [14] amongst women using either oral contraceptives [34, 35] or hormonal intrauterine devices [36]. When women are sampled cycle after cycle, three potential patterns of latent precursor expression occur. The first is "emergence" in which PTEN-null glands appear in a follow-up sample. The second is "persistence" in which PTEN-null glands remain in repeat samples. The final pattern is "regression" in which previously present PTEN-null glands are no longer present in follow-up samples [14]. Persistence and emergence are common patterns in normally cycling endometrium, with 53% of repeat samples demonstrating persistence and 37% of repeat samples demonstrating emergence [10]. In contrast, the dominant pattern is regression in women using progestins. Specifically, oral contraceptives have a regression rate of 75% [3] and intrauterine devices have a regression rate of 93% [32]. Interestingly, a similar regression rate is seen with the use of non-medicated (hormone-free) IUD implantation, likely secondary to inflammation [14].

Additional Obesity-Related Nongenetic Risk Modifiers

The link between obesity and both EIN and cancer likely also involves insulin homeostasis [2]. In both diabetes and insulin-resistant states, such as obesity, circulating levels of insulin and insulin-like growth factor (IGF) rise. Endometrial cancer is known to express receptors for both insulin and IGF, raising the possibility that these factors are involved to the development of EIN and carcinoma [37]. Furthermore, insulin plays a role in the induction of androgen synthesis by the adrenals and ovaries, thereby providing additional substrate for aromatase [38].

References

1. Mahabir S, et al. Usefulness of body mass index as a sufficient adiposity measurement for sex hormone concentration associations in postmenopausal women. Cancer Epidemiol Biomark Prev. 2006;15:2502–7.
2. O'Rourke RW. Endometrial hyperplasia, endometrial cancer, and obesity: convergent mechanisms regulating energy homeostasis and cellular proliferation. Surg Obes Relat Dis. 2014;10:926–8.
3. Zheng W, Baker HE, Mutter GL. Involution of PTEN-null endometrial glands with progestin therapy. Gynecol Oncol. 2004;92:1008–13.
4. Mutter GL. Pten, a protean tumor suppressor. Am J Pathol. 2001;158:1895–8.
5. Mutter GL, et al. Altered PTEN expression as a diagnostic marker for the earliest endometrial precancers. J Natl Cancer Inst. 2000;92:924–30.
6. Stambolic V, et al. High incidence of breast and endometrial neoplasia resembling human Cowden syndrome in pten+/− mice. Cancer Res. 2000;60:3605–11.
7. Liaw D, et al. Germline mutations of the PTEN gene in Cowden disease, an inherited breast and thyroid cancer syndrome. Nat Genet. 1997;16:64–7.
8. Marsh DJ, et al. Mutation spectrum and genotype-phenotype analyses in Cowden disease and Bannayan-Zonana syndrome, two hamartoma syndromes with germline PTEN mutation. Hum Mol Genet. 1998;7:507–15.
9. Eng C. Cowden Syndrome. J Genet Couns. 1997;6:181–92.
10. Mutter GL, et al. Molecular identification of latent precancers in histologically normal endometrium. Cancer Res. 2001;61:4311–4.
11. Mutter GL, Monte NM, Neuberg D, Ferenczy A, Eng C. Emergence, involution, and progression to carcinoma of mutant clones in normal endometrial tissues. Cancer Res. 2014;74:2796–802.
12. Ries LAG, Melbert D, Krapcho M, Stinchcomb DG, Howlader N, Horner MJ, et al. [Internet] SEER Cancer Statistics Review, 1975–2005 [updated 2008 March 17]. National Cancer Institute; Bethesda, M. [1 screen] A. from: http://seercancer gov/csr/1975_2005/. Accessed 18 Mar 2014.
13. Jemal A, Siegel R, Xu J, Ward E. Cancer statistics. CA Cancer J Clin. 2010;60:277–300.
14. Lin M, Burkholder KA, Viswanathan AN, Neuberg D, Mutter GL. Involution of latent endometrial precancers by hormonal and nonhormonal mechanisms. Cancer. 2009;115:2111–8.
15. Jarboe EA, Mutter GL. Endometrial intraepithelial neoplasia. Semin Diagn Pathol. 2010;27:215–25.
16. Kendall BS, et al. Reproducibility of the diagnosis of endometrial hyperplasia, atypical hyperplasia, and well-differentiated carcinoma. Am J Surg Pathol. 1998;22:1012–9.
17. Bergeron C, et al. A multicentric European study testing the reproducibility of the WHO classification of endometrial hyperplasia with a proposal of a simplified working classification for biopsy and curettage specimens. Am J Surg Pathol. 1999;23:1102–8.
18. Zaino RJ. Endometrial hyperplasia: is it time for a quantum leap to a new classification? Int J Gynecol Pathol. 2000;19:314–21.
19. Mutter GL, Zaino RJ, Baak JPA, Bentley RC, Robboy SJ. Benign endometrial hyperplasia sequence and endometrial intraepithelial Neoplasia. Int J Gynecol Pathol. 2007;26:103–14.
20. Baak JP, et al. The molecular genetics and morphometry-based endometrial intraepithelial neoplasia classification system predicts disease progression in endometrial hyperplasia more accurately than the 1994 World Health Organization classification system. Cancer. 2005;103:2304–12.
21. Mutter GL, Kauderer J, Baak JPA, Alberts D, Gynecologic Oncology Group. Biopsy histomorphometry predicts uterine myoinvasion by endometrial carcinoma: a gynecologic oncology group study. Hum Pathol. 2008;39:866–74.
22. Kurman RJ. Kaminski, P. F. & Norris, H. J. The behavior of endometrial hyperplasia. A long-term study of 'untreated' hyperplasia in 170 patients. Cancer. 1985;56:403–12.

23. Faquin WC, et al. Sporadic microsatellite instability is specific to neoplastic and preneoplastic endometrial tissues. Am J Clin Pathol. 2000;113:576–82.
24. Matias-Guiu X, Prat J. Molecular pathology of endometrial carcinoma. Histopathology. 2013;62:111–23.
25. Monte NM, Webster KA, Neuberg D, Dressler GR, Mutter GL. Joint loss of PAX2 and PTEN expression in endometrial Precancers and cancer. Cancer Res. 2010;70:6225–32.
26. Mutter GL, et al. Endometrial precancer diagnosis by histopathology, clonal analysis, and computerized morphometry. J Pathol. 2000;190:462–9.
27. Torres M, Gómez-Pardo E, Dressler GR, Gruss P. Pax-2 controls multiple steps of urogenital development. Development. 1995;121:4057–65.
28. Tong G-X, Chiriboga L, Hamele-Bena D, Borczuk AC. Expression of PAX2 in papillary serous carcinoma of the ovary: immunohistochemical evidence of fallopian tube or secondary Müllerian system origin? Mod Pathol. 2007;20:856–63.
29. Rabban JT, McAlhany S, Lerwill MF, Grenert JP, Zaloudek CJ. PAX2 distinguishes benign mesonephric and mullerian glandular lesions of the cervix from endocervical adenocarcinoma, including minimal deviation adenocarcinoma. Am J Surg Pathol. 2010;34:137–46.
30. Strissel PL, et al. Early aberrant insulin-like growth factor signaling in the progression to endometrial carcinoma is augmented by tamoxifen. Int J Cancer. 2008;123:2871–9.
31. Mutter GL, Lin MC, Fitzgerald JT, Kum JB, Eng C. Changes in endometrial PTEN expression throughout the human menstrual cycle. J Clin Endocrinol Metab. 2000;85:2334–8.
32. Orbo A. Regression of latent endometrial Precancers by progestin infiltrated intrauterine device. Cancer Res. 2006;66:5613–7.
33. Antunes CM, et al. Endometrial cancer and estrogen use. Report of a large case-control study. N Engl J Med. 1979;300:9–13.
34. Grimes DA, Economy KE. Primary prevention of gynecologic cancers. Am J Obstet Gynecol. 1995;172:227–35.
35. Weiderpass E, et al. Use of oral contraceptives and endometrial cancer risk (Sweden). Cancer Causes Control. 1999;10:277–84.
36. Curtis KM, Marchbanks PA, Peterson HB. Neoplasia with use of intrauterine devices. Contraception. 2007;75:S60–9.
37. Zhang G, et al. The expression and role of hybrid insulin/insulin-like growth factor receptor type 1 in endometrial carcinoma cells. Cancer Genet Cytogenet. 2010;200:140–8.
38. Fader AN, Arriba LN, Frasure HE, von Gruenigen VE. Endometrial cancer and obesity: epidemiology, biomarkers, prevention and survivorship. Gynecol Oncol. 2009;114:121–7.

Chapter 6
Obesity, Adipokines, and Gynecologic Cancer

Elizabeth V. Connor, Ofer Reizes, and Caner Saygin

Abstract The evidence that obesity and excess fat in adipose tissue lead to poor prognosis for gynecological cancers is overwhelming. Indeed, obese women are at two to fourfold greater risk of developing endometriod cancer than normal weight women. Further, obese women with a BMI greater than 40 have a sixfold increased relative risk of death from uterine cancer compared to women with BMI of 25 or less. Adipose tissue is now well recognized as an endocrine organ capable of secreting factors called adipokines that act locally and on other organ systems, tissues, and tumors. This chapter will review the existing evidence that adipose-derived factors promote both the initiation and progression of gynecological cancers. Where available, we will discuss the evidence for interaction with specific gynecological organs sites and define future directions for approaches to disrupt the obesity-cancer link.

Keywords Adipose tissue • Adipokines • Leptin • Adiponectin • Gynecological cancer • Uterine • Endometrial • Cervical • Ovarian

Introduction

Adipokines and the Adipose Organ

While the association between obesity and malignancy is well established, we seldom consider adipose tissue, the fat-storing organ, as a participant in the development of malignancy. Adipose tissue is composed of lipid-filled adipocytes, preadipocytes, loose connective tissue, surrounding collagen fibers, vasculature,

E.V. Connor, M.D.
Department of Obstetrics/Gynecology and Women's Health Institute,
Cleveland Clinic Foundation, 9500 Euclid Avenue, Cleveland, OH 44195, USA
e-mail: connore2@ccf.org

O. Reizes, Ph.D. (✉) • C. Saygin, M.D.
Department of Cellular and Molecular Medicine, Lerner Research Institute, Cleveland Clinic,
9500 Euclid Avenue, NC10, Cleveland, OH 44195, USA
e-mail: reizeso@ccf.org; sayginc@ccf.org

© Springer International Publishing AG 2018
N.A. Berger et al. (eds.), *Focus on Gynecologic Malignancies*, Energy Balance
and Cancer 13, DOI 10.1007/978-3-319-63483-8_6

fibroblasts, and immune cells. There are two types of adipose tissue: white adipose tissue (WAT) and brown adipose tissue (BAT). WAT primarily stores energy in the form of fatty acids and dominates the subcutaneous and visceral fat pads in the body. BAT is capable of generating heat by uncoupling of the respiratory chain in mitochondria, and though traditionally only found in neonates and infants, BAT has more recently been identified in visceral fat in adult humans [1]. In general, 85% of adipose tissue in humans is subcutaneous, approximately 10% is located in the omentum, and the remaining 5% is dispersed as visceral fat surrounding organs such as the heart, kidneys, and lymph nodes [2] (Fig. 6.1).

The discovery of the first adipokine two decades ago has led to a better understanding of the larger role that adipose tissue plays at both the cellular and systemic level. Adipokines (also known as adipocytokines) are proteins secreted by adipocytes that can act locally (through autocrine or paracrine function) or systemically (through endocrine function) to exert effects on steroidogenesis, immune response, and metabolism. Adipose tissue is known to secrete at least twenty of these effector proteins, making it a complex organ with key endocrine, metabolic, and immunomodulatory roles. Only recent investigation has linked adipokines to the development and course of malignancy.

Of the gynecologic cancers, ovarian and endometrial cancers are associated with obesity. For each 5 kg/m² increase in body mass index (BMI), risk of developing ovarian cancer increases by a factor of 1.03 compared to 1.52 for endometrial cancer [3]. These two gynecologic malignancies represent ideal models for the study of adipokines

Fig. 6.1 Adipose tissue distribution. Adipose tissue is primarily located in the subcutaneous fat, but is also present in the omentum and viscera

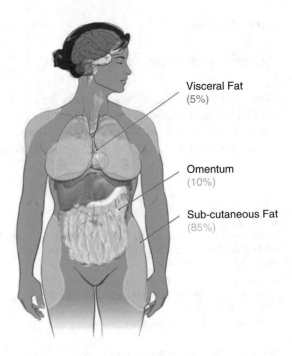

Visceral Fat
(5%)

Omentum
(10%)

Sub-cutaneous Fat
(85%)

as they relate to obesity, metabolic dysregulation, and cancer. This chapter will present the most well-studied adipokines, their mechanisms of action, and current evidence for involvement in the development of ovarian and endometrial cancers.

The Ovary

The ovary is the female gonadal organ and an active endocrine organ. The ovary is composed of an inner medulla, an outer cortex, and a hilum containing the ovarian vessels and lymphatics. The ovary is surrounded by an epithelial cell lining. The cortex houses the germinal epithelium and ovarian follicles. The medulla consists of connective tissue, contractile cells, and interstitial cells. The interstitial cells immediately surrounding a developing follicle undergo differentiation to become theca cells (Fig. 6.2).

Theca cells and granulosa cells are the hormone-producing machinery of the ovary. The theca cells express LH receptors and in response to LH convert cholesterol to progesterone and androstenedione, a weak androgen. Androstenedione diffuses across the basement membrane of the theca cell into the granulosa cell. In the granulosa cell, FSH activates aromatase conversion of the androstenedione to estrone and estradiol for systemic release (Fig. 6.3).

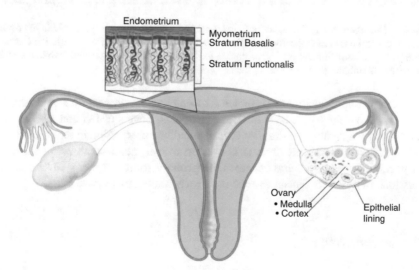

Fig. 6.2 Gynecologic osrgans. The structure of the ovary supports hormone production and hormone effects such as follicular development and ovulation. The layers of the endometrium respond to hormone fluctuations by proliferating and shedding

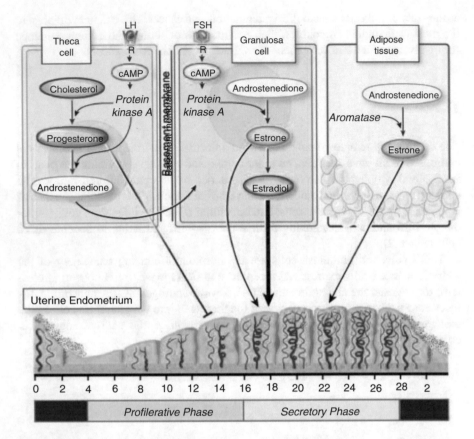

Fig. 6.3 Hormone production and effects. Progesterone and estradiol are produced in the ovarian theca and granulosa cells respectively. In the adipose tissue, androgens are converted to estrone, a weak estrogen. Estradiol and estrone promote proliferation of the endometrium, while progesterone promotes stability of the endometrium

In postmenopausal women, follicles are depleted and progesterone and estradiol production sharply declines as the ovary atrophies. Levels of LH and FSH are elevated, but are only able to stimulate androstenedione production in the ovarian stromal cells. This androstenedione is converted to estrone, a weak estrogen, in the peripheral adipose tissue and becomes the primary source of estrogen. Production of estrone in postmenopausal women is directly related to adipose mass.

The Endometrium

While the endometrium is not an endocrine organ, it is a dynamic hormone-responsive organ. The endometrium lines the cavity of the uterus and is composed of two layers: the basalis layer and the functionalis layer. As their names imply, the basalis layer forms a base along the uterine myometrium and provides stability through the menstrual cycle while the functionalis layer faces the uterine cavity and proliferates (proliferative phase) then sheds (secretory or luteal phase) with each cycle. Estradiol and progesterone drive the proliferative and luteal phases of the menstrual cycle respectively, and receptor expression is highly regulated over the course of the cycle.

At menopause, cyclic hormone production in the ovary ceases, and the decrease in estrogen causes the endometrium to atrophy. Instead of the potent estradiol released by the premenopausal ovary, estrone produced by peripheral conversion of androstenedione in the adipose tissue becomes the primary circulating estrogen. In the presence of endogenous or exogenous estrogen excess, the endometrium retains the ability to proliferate in response. Uncontrolled proliferation can lead to post-menopausal bleeding or may be visualized as a thickened endometrial stripe on transvaginal ultrasound.

Leptin

Douglas Coleman and Jeffrey Friedman are credited with the discovery of a novel hormone produced by adipocytes and capable of suppressing food intake and body weight in mice. The hormone was named "leptin" from the Greek word *leptos* meaning thin. Leptin is a 16 kDa (167 amino acid) peptide hormone encoded by the *obese* (*OB* or *LEP*) gene and secreted by adipocytes that acts in the hypothalamus to regulate satiety and control energy metabolism [4, 5]. Leptin circulates in the plasma either as a free hormone or bound to a soluble protein receptor.

The leptin receptor (Ob-R or LEPR) is a transmembrane receptor with six known isoforms (Ob-R$_a$-Ob-R$_f$) and a member of the class I cytokine receptor family. LEPR has been identified in multiple tissue sites including the hypothalamus, lung, kidney, and ovary [6]. The extracellular domain of LEPR is similar among isoforms, while the intracellular domain demonstrates variability as a result of alternative RNA splicing at the C-terminus. Isoforms are classified based on the length of the intracellular domain: long, short, or soluble. In the membrane-bound isoforms, structure of the intracellular domain affects downstream pathway activation. Activation of LEPR may result in JAK-STAT, MAPK, and PI3K pathway activation and is associated with transcription regulation, cell proliferation and survival.

Normally, circulating levels of leptin are proportional to fat mass and increase with increasing body weight. The ratio of free to bound leptin is variable and highest in obese individuals, in which free leptin is believed to act as a signal of satiety. In the case of either leptin deficiency or receptor deficiency, satiety is not conveyed and an obese phenotype results. When leptin reaches very high levels in obesity, intracellular signaling may be disrupted leading to leptin resistance. This results in reduced appetite suppression and paradoxically increasing adiposity.

Leptin and the Ovary

Leptin was first discovered as a secreted product of adipocytes; however, other tissues are now known to secrete leptin, including the placenta, ovaries, skeletal muscle, and stomach [7]. Leptin protein has been identified in ovarian granulosa, theca, stromal, and luteal cells as well as in follicular fluid [6, 8]. However, leptin mRNA has only been identified in granulosa and theca cells, suggesting that leptin is produced in these cells and transported to other sites in the ovary [6]. LEPR is expressed in human, rat, cattle, and porcine granulosa and theca cells [9]. LEPR mRNA has been identified in ovarian tissue, confirming production of the receptor in the ovary [6].

Leptin has been shown to affect steroidogenesis, and not surprisingly, has shown effects on ovulation in vitro and in vivo [10–13]. Interestingly, LEPR expression fluctuates in concert with the menstrual cycle, suggesting ties to the hormonal regulation of ovarian function [14]. Leptin increases serum luteinizing hormone (LH) and reduces estradiol [8, 14], which supports a more specific role in regulating ovulation. Leptin is additionally capable of facilitating oocyte maturation by activation of the MAPK pathway [9], and has been shown to increase meiotic resumption in pre-ovulatory oocytes [6].

Leptin Tumorigenic Effects and Pathways in Ovarian Cancer

In various malignancies, leptin has been shown to mediate tumorigenic effects through JAK/STAT, ERK, and PI3K pathways to promote cell proliferation, migration, invasion, angiogenesis and survival [15]. The PI3K pathway is the most extensively studied in ovarian cancer, and leptin-induced PI3K pathway activation is associated with proliferation in ovarian cancer cells [16–20]. Several investigators have demonstrated inhibition of leptin's tumorigenic effects through direct PI3K inhibition [17, 18, 20]. Additionally, gene silencing of the leptin receptor is associated with downregulation of phosphorylated Akt and the PI3K axis [20]. Leptin activation of the JAK/STAT pathway has also been demonstrated in ovarian cancer, as well as reversal of this effect with a STAT3 inhibitor [19, 21]. There is also support for leptin activation of MEK-ERK1/2 [16, 21] as well as p38 MAPK [21]. Leptin also has anti-apoptotic effects that promote cell survival. Leptin has been shown to suppress pro-apoptotic proteins Bad, tumor necrosis factor receptor (TNFR1), and caspase-6 [22]. Additionally, increased expression of the leptin receptor is associated with increased expression of pro-apoptotic proteins Bcl-XL and XIAP [20].

Given the close relationship between leptin and hormonal regulation of normal ovarian tissue, there has been some investigation into the hormone-dependent effects of leptin on ovarian cancer cells. Choi et al. reported increased leptin-induced proliferative effects on ovarian cancer cell lines OVCAR-3 and A2780 after transfection with estrogen receptor-α [17]. Kasiappan et al. demonstrated that leptin was capable of increasing cell proliferation through estrogen receptor-α activation, and this was suppressed by administration of vitamin D3 [23]. More investigation is needed to better establish the hormone-dependent and -independent mechanisms of leptin action in the ovary.

Leptin as a Biomarker in Ovarian Cancer

Despite the established tumorigenic potential of leptin, the majority of current research has demonstrated lower levels of leptin in ovarian cancer patients compared to controls [24–28]. This is opposite the trend seen in other cancers such as breast and endometrial cancer, and may reflect the poor nutritional status or cachexia that is characteristic of advanced stage disease. Given the difference in leptin levels in women with ovarian cancer, investigators have proposed that decreased leptin may be an independent predictor of ovarian malignancy in women with adnexal masses. However, two studies have failed to identify leptin as an independent predictor of ovarian malignancy [29, 30]. The predictive value of leptin has shown to be more promising when considered in combination with other analytes. Mor et al. reported that a panel of four analytes (leptin, prolactin, osteoponin and insulin-like growth factor II) was able to discriminate between malignant and benign controls with sensitivity and specificity of 95%, yielding a positive predictive value of 95% [26]. Visintin et al. later proposed a panel of six analytes (the four tested by Mor et al., as well as macrophage inhibitory factor and CA-125), and reported accuracy of 98.7% in distinguishing ovarian cancer patients from healthy controls [28]. In both studies, leptin was lower in women with ovarian cancer compared to controls.

More recently, leptin has been evaluated as a biomarker for the prediction of clinical outcomes in ovarian cancer. Most studies report that with disease progression, leptin levels further decrease while leptin receptors are over-expressed [19, 20, 25]. Grabowski et al. reported leptin levels in ovarian cancers at diagnosis, after cytoreductive surgery, and after adjuvant chemotherapy and remission. They found that leptin levels increased postoperatively and with remission, which suggests that leptin levels may be an effective marker of residual disease burden after cytoreductive surgery or a marker of response to chemotherapy. Leptin receptor expression has also been studied with regard to clinical outcomes. LEPR overexpression correlates with poorer progression-free survival [19, 20]. Additionally, one study found that leptin receptors are more highly expressed in metastases and ascites than in primary tumor tissue, further supporting that receptor overexpression correlates with progressive disease [19]. Taken together, these findings suggest that leptin and LEPR may be useful biomarkers for identifying risk of malignancy or guiding surveillance and treatment in women with ovarian cancer.

Leptin and the Endometrium

Both leptin and LEPR are expressed in the human endometrium [31]. Leptin modulates chemokine expression among endometrial stromal and epithelial cells and specifically increases secretion of IL-6, IL-8, GRO-α, MCP-1, and MIP-3α [32]. In endometrial epithelial cells, leptin stimulates proliferation in a dose-dependent fashion, but also enhances growth inhibition and DNA fragmentation, suggesting that it acts in a regulatory role to control growth of the endometrial lining [33].

There has been much investigation in the role of leptin as it relates to both fertility and endometriosis. Leptin expression is lower and LEPR expression is higher in women with infertility secondary to implantation failure, and leptin is believed to have a role in preparing the endometrial lining for successful implantation of the blastocyst [34]. Conversely, women with endometriosis exhibit higher levels of leptin in the serum and peritoneal fluid, even when controlling for BMI [35]. Leptin expression is also increased in endometriomas and endometriotic foci [36]. Leptin has demonstrated a stimulatory effect on proliferation, migration, and invasion in endometriotic epithelial cells and exerts this effect through JAK/STAT and ERK pathway activation [37, 38]. The higher levels of leptin in endometriosis and leptin's known pro-inflammatory and proliferative effects suggest that leptin may contribute to the initiation or progression of endometriosis in women.

Leptin as a Biomarker in Endometrial Cancer

Leptin level and leptin-to-adiponectin ratio are elevated in women with endometrial cancer, even after accounting for BMI [39–41]. Leptin level is associated with increasing depth of invasion and lymph node metastasis as well as poorer overall survival [42]. LEPR is more highly expressed in women with endometrial cancer [43], but there is inconsistent evidence supporting whether increased expression of LEPR correlates with higher grade and stage [42, 44, 45].

Leptin Pathway Activation in Endometrial Cancer

Several studies have demonstrated that leptin has a stimulatory effect on endometrial cancer cell proliferation and invasion via activation of JAK/STAT, MAPK and ERK1/2, and PI3K/Akt [46–48]. Leptin also decreases apoptosis of endometrial adenocarcinoma cells via NFκB pathway activation [45]. Further evidence has shown that leptin regulates VEGF and increases expression of VEGF and VEGF-R in endometrial cells, and that this effect is greater in malignant cell lines [49]. This pro-angiogenic effect is dependent on leptin activation of JAK2 and subsequent activation of the PI3K and MAPK pathways [49]. Thus, leptin has been shown to increase proliferation and invasion, increase release of pro-angiogenic factor VEGF, and decrease apoptosis, which may contribute to the development and progression of endometrial cancer.

Given that leptin is increased in women with endometrial cancer and given its well-established tumorigenic effects, leptin may represent a therapeutic target. In a recent prospective study, brief pre-operative treatment of women with endometrial cancer with metformin resulted in decreased serum level of leptin, demonstrating that leptin level is modifiable [50]. More investigation is needed to evaluate whether treatment with metformin has effects of tumorigenesis or clinical outcomes.

Adiponectin

Scherer et al. identified adiponectin in 1995 as the most highly expressed mRNA transcript in adipocytes [51]. Adiponectin is a 30 kDa protein (244 amino acids) that is encoded by the *AdipoQ* gene and secreted by adipocytes. Adiponectin is the only adipokine that is inversely proportional to fat mass. There are four described isoforms of adiponectin: a homotrimer (90 kDa), a hexamer composed of two homotrimers, a low molecular weight (LMW) form (180 kDa), and a high molecular weight (HMW) form (360–400 kDa) [52].

Adiponectin binds to adiponectin receptor 1 (AdipoR1) and adiponectin receptor 2 (AdipoR2), which are transmembrane receptors, as well as T-cadherin. Binding of adiponectin to AdipoR1 results in stimulation of the adenosine monophosphate-activated protein kinase (AMPK) pathway, which regulates lipid and glucose metabolism as well as cell proliferation, migration, and angiogenesis [53]. Binding to AdipoR2 activates peroxisome proliferator-activated receptor alpha (PPARα), which regulates glucose metabolism and insulin sensitivity [53]. PPARα further inhibits NFκB, thereby decreasing proliferation, survival, cell migration, as well as a cascade of inflammatory cytokines. Both AdipoR1 and AdipoR2 stimulate ceramidase, decreasing ceramide while increasing sphingosine 1-phosphate levels and protecting against apoptosis [54].

Normally, adiponectin increases glucose uptake and utilization in muscle tissue while suppressing glucose production in the liver and decreasing triglyceride concentrations through upregulation of AMPK [55]. Obesity is associated with lower adiponectin levels as well as decreased expression of its receptors [56, 57]. Conversely, weight loss has been shown to increase adiponectin levels [58].

Adiponectin and the Ovary

Adiponectin and its receptors AdipoR1 and AdipoR2 are produced in ovarian tissue and expressed differentially in ovarian tissue [59, 60]. Adiponectin mRNA and protein have been isolated in the theca, corpus luteum, oocyte, and follicular fluid.

AdipoR1 mRNA and protein have been isolated in granulosa cells, theca cells, the corpus luteum, and the oocyte whereas AdipoR2 has only been isolated in the granulosa cells, the corpus luteum, and the oocyte. As discussed previously, AMPK and PPARα are key effectors of adiponectin upon binding to its receptor. PPAR isoforms and AMPK have been demonstrated in multiple ovarian models [61–66]. Importantly, AMPK is known to have a regulatory role on steroidogenesis in the ovary by decreasing progesterone production in the granulosa cells [66, 67].

Given the downstream metabolic and hormonal regulation in the ovary, adiponectin has been extensively investigated in the context of Polycystic Ovary Syndrome (PCOS). Low adiponectin is predictive of PCOS in women independent of body mass, and is independently associated with insulin resistance and the metabolic syndrome [68–72]. Expression of adipokine receptors AdipoR1 and AdipoR2 is also lower in polycystic ovaries compared to normal ovaries [73]. Normally adiponectin suppresses steroidogenesis in the ovary, and low levels of adiponectin correlate with higher levels of estradiol, progesterone, and hyperandrogenism [73]. Conditions of androgen excess have been shown to inhibit adiponectin secretion by adipocytes in obese women with PCOS, further lowering adiponectin levels in these women [74]. Lower adiponectin in women with PCOS additionally correlates with increased folliculogenesis and polycystic appearing ovaries [75]. Metformin, a biguanide classically used to decrease insulin resistance in type II diabetes, activates AMPK pathway to decrease excess steroidogenesis and is now commonly used to increase ovulation in women with PCOS and infertility [76].

Adiponectin and Ovarian Cancer

Serum adiponectin levels are lower in patients with ovarian cancer compared to controls [24, 77]; however, adiponectin levels have not been shown to correlate with progression of disease [24]. One study found no difference in serum adiponectin in women with ovarian malignancy when compared to women with borderline or benign ovarian masses [78]. Two studies have reported on adiponectin receptor expression in ovarian cancer in chicken models. Ocón-Grove et al. demonstrated decreased adipoR1 mRNA expression in cancerous ovaries compared to normal ovarian tissue [79]. Tiwari et al. reported decreased mRNA levels of adiponectin, adipoR1, and adipoR2 in cancerous ovaries and ovarian cancer cell lines as compared to normal ovaries and cells [80]. However, in these studies protein expression was inconsistent with respect to malignancy. AdipoR1 protein expression was not different in malignancy versus controls, and adipoR2 protein was increased in cancerous ovarian tissue but decreased in the ovarian cancer cell line as compared to their respective controls. Notably, serum adiponectin did not vary between the groups, so results may not be reflective of a human population.

Currently there is only one study associating adiponectin level with clinical outcomes in women with ovarian cancer. Diaz et al. evaluated leptin and adiponectin levels in women with ovarian cancer and found that lower leptin-to-adiponectin ratios were associated with improved progression-free survival (57 months in lowest tertile, 49 months in median tertile, and 37 months in high tertile) [81].

Adiponectin and Targeted Pathways in Ovarian Cancer

Adiponectin's activation of AMPK and PPARα leads to respective inhibition of mTOR/PI3K-Akt and NFκB, cumulatively resulting in regulation of cell survival, proliferation, and migration. The direct tumor suppressor effects of adiponectin have been studied in a range of malignancies including breast, endometrial, and colorectal carcinomas. Particularly in breast cancer, adiponectin has been shown to decrease proliferation [82], invasion, migration [83], and increases apoptosis [84–86].

While studies investigating the direct effects of adiponectin in ovarian cancer are lacking, there is building evidence for the use of metformin to activate AMPK and PPARα pathways in an effort to suppress tumorigenic effects. Metformin has been shown to decrease tumor growth, tumor cell proliferation, angiogenesis, and metastasis in mouse models [87–89]. Metformin in combination with standard chemotherapy has also demonstrated ability to reduce tumor volume beyond the effect of cisplatin or paclitaxel alone in mice [87, 89]. Retrospective studies have shown that long-term metformin use is associated with a reduced risk of ovarian cancer and improved progression-free survival [90, 91]. Currently, metformin is being evaluated in combination with standard chemotherapy for safety and efficacy in the treatment of advanced ovarian, fallopian tube, and primary peritoneal carcinomas (NCT02312661, NCT02437812, NCT02122185).

Adiponectin and the Endometrium

The epithelial and stromal cells of the endometrium express adiponectin and its receptors, and expression of adipoR1 and adipoR2 increases in the midluteal phase of the menstrual cycle coincident with embryo implantation [92]. In the normal human endometrium, adiponectin receptor activation results in increased phosphorylation of AMPK and increased secretion of IL-6, IL-8, and monocyte chemoattractant protein 1 from the endometrial stromal cells [92]. For these reasons, adiponectin is believed to play a regulatory role in energy homeostasis and control of inflammation in the endometrial lining. High levels of adiponectin may represent stability of the endometrium and ideal conditions for regulated menstrual cycles and successful implantation of a developing embryo.

Adiponectin levels have been closely studied in the context of endometriosis, infertility, and PCOS, all of which involve dysregulation of the endometrium. Takemura et al. reported that adiponectin is significantly lower in women with endometriosis compared to controls, suggesting a link between adiponectin and the increased inflammation and endometrial dysfunction seen in endometriosis [93]. Given the suspected role of adiponectin in endometrial stability, Dos Santos et al. investigated expression of adiponectin and its receptors in the endometrial lining of women diagnosed with implantation failure as a cause of infertility. They found that while endometrial adiponectin was similar in these women compared to controls, women with implantation failure had significantly lower expression of adipoR1 and adipoR2 [34]. Adiponectin and adiponectin receptor expression are lower in women with PCOS, even when accounting for BMI [94, 95]. In vitro studies have shown that increased levels of testosterone and insulin lower adiponectin and its receptors in endometrial stromal cells, which suggests that the hyperandrogenism and hyperinsulinemia in PCOS cause endometrial dysfunction through reduction of adiponectin and subsequent inflammation [95].

Adiponectin as a Biomarker in Endometrial Cancer

Multiple large meta-analyses of almost 2000 women with endometrial cancer have demonstrated lower serum adiponectin levels in women with endometrial cancer [40, 96, 97]. This finding is further supported by a prospective study of 99 postmenopausal women with either vaginal bleeding or thickened endometrial stripe on imaging who underwent dilation and curettage followed by hysterectomy [98]. Both adiponectin and adiponectin/leptin index were predictive of endometrial cancer in this population, and adiponectin/leptin index demonstrated higher discrimination than adiponectin alone [98]. While adiponectin level has not been shown to correlate with clinical stage, adiponectin is lower in high grade cancers [99]. Given these relationships, adiponectin demonstrates potential utility in identifying women at risk of developing endometrial cancer and predicting more aggressive variants of this cancer.

There is less consistency on the relationship between adipoR1 and adipoR2 expression in endometrial cancers. Moon et al. in 2011 reported that overall adipoR expression was not significantly different in endometrial cancer compared to normal endometrial tissue [100]. Alternatively, Yamauchi et al. reported that both adipoR1 and adipoR2 were significantly decreased in endometrial cancers compared to controls, and that lower levels of adipoR1 and adipoR2 expression correlated with higher grade, increased myometrial invasion, and lymph node metastasis [101]. More investigation is needed to better understand patterns of receptor expression in endometrial cancers.

Adiponectin and Targeted Pathways in Endometrial Cancer

Adiponectin has a suppressive effect on proliferation and increases apoptosis in endometrial cancer cell lines [100, 102, 103]. Similar to its actions in other cells, adiponectin activates AMPK in endometrial cancer cells, thereby inhibiting the Akt/

mTOR pathway to suppress proliferation [100, 102]. Addition of an AMPK inhibitor counteracts this effect and leads to cell proliferation [103].

As previously discussed with regard to ovarian cancer, metformin has emerged as a therapeutic agent in endometrial cancer for its ability to exert anti-tumorigenic effects similar to adiponectin. Retrospective evidence demonstrates improved overall survival and recurrence-free survival for women with endometrial cancer taking metformin [104]. One prospective study demonstrated that even short-term metformin treatment for 4–6 weeks prior to surgery for endometrial cancer resulted in decreased endometrial growth as determined by immunohistochemical evaluation of the tumor specimen with Ki-67 and topoisomerase IIα [105]. There are multiple ongoing clinical trials assessing metformin as an adjunct to treatment for endometrial cancer in both operative and non-operative patients.

Emerging Adipokines and Relevance to Gynecologic Cancers

Visfatin (Table 6.1)

Rongvaux et al. discovered in 2002 that two molecules currently under investigation, Pre-B-cell colony enhancing factor (PBEF) and nampt, were actually the same molecule [106]. PBEF was identified as a cytokine secreted by leukocytes that increased expression of several inflammatory mediators: TNF-α, IL-1B, and IL-6 [107, 108]. Nampt was identified as an enzyme with multiple roles, including immune signaling and biosynthesis of NAD [108]. This 52 kDa molecule was later termed visfatin, and was noted to be secreted by adipocytes [109].

Visfatin directly correlates with obesity and is also associated with insulin resistance, adiposity, metabolic syndrome, type II diabetes, and cardiovascular disease [110]. Transcription of visfatin is regulated by TNF, IL-6, and glucocorticoids [111]. Neutrophils, monocytes, and macrophages are all capable of visfatin secretion. Visfatin induces IL-6 and CD36 expression via the JNK and NFκB pathways leading to differentiation of monocytes and macrophages [112]. Thus, visfatin represents a direct link between obesity and inflammation (Fig. 6.4).

Visfatin and Ovarian Cancer

Visfatin is expressed in ovarian granulosa cells, human cumulus cells, and oocytes [113]. Visfatin is known to increase IGF-1-induced steroidogenesis as well as cell proliferation [113]. Not surprisingly, PCOS is associated with elevated serum levels of visfatin, and visfatin correlates with higher total cholesterol, LDL cholesterol, triglycerides, lipoprotein a, and homocysteine [114, 115].

Visfatin is more highly expressed in ovarian cancers as compared to benign tissue controls [116]. Additionally, an elevated level of visfatin in the ascites of women

Table 6.1 Mechanism and actions of adipokines in gynecologic cancers

	Mechanism of action	Physiological effects	Pathophysiological effects	Ovary	Endometrium
Leptin	JAK-STAT, MEK/ERK, MAPK, PI3K pathways	Inhibits hunger, stimulates satiety	Increased cell proliferation, growth, survival, angiogenesis, invasion/migration, inflammation and dysregulated cytokine signaling	Decreased in ovarian cancer, increases LH, decreases E2	Increased in Endometrial Cancer Decreased In Infertility, Increased In Endometriosis
Adiponectin	AMPK and PPARα/NFκB pathways, Increased ceramidase activity	Glucose and lipid homeostasis, Insulin sensitivity	Hypoadiponectinemia causes insulin resistance and loss of inhibitory effect on cell proliferation, survival, migration and inflammation	Decreased in ovarian cancer, decreased in PCOS	Decreased in endometrial cancer, decreased in endometriosis
Visfatin	ERK, MAPK, PI3K and cytokine pathways	B cell and vascular smooth muscle maturation, NAD biosynthesis	Increased cell survival, cytokine production, migration, increased antioxidative enzymes	Increased in ovarian cancer, increased in PCOS	Increased in endometrial cancer
Resistin	MAPK, PI3K, and NFκB pathways	Energy homeostasis, inflammatory response	Increased inflammation, cell survival, adhesion, migration and metastasis, insulin resistance (?)	(?)Increased in PCOS	Increased in endometrial cancer
Chemerin	G protein-coupled receptor, MAPK/ERK pathways	Adipocyte differentiation, chemoattractant	Increased inflammation and invasion, recruitment of immune cells	Increased in PCOS	Increased in endometriosis
Omentin	Akt and AMPK pathways	Modulation of insulin action, increased cell differentiation and suppression of inflammation	Promotes apoptosis, glucose intolerance (?)	Decreased in PCOS	Unknown
Apelin	G protein-coupled receptor, PI3K/Akt and MEK/ERK pathways	Blood pressure control and angiogenesis, histamine and insulin release, fluid homeostasis	Increased cell proliferation, migration, survival, lymphangiogenesis and angiogenesis	Unknown	Increased in endometrial cancer

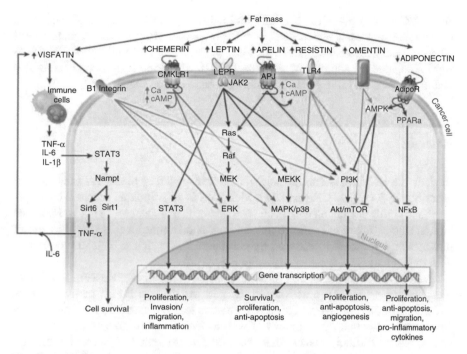

Fig. 6.4 Adipokine effects. The adipokines mediate their various effects through multiple pathways affecting cell growth and survival

with ovarian cancer is associated with more extensive intraperitoneal dissemination [117]. In vitro, ascites-derived visfatin increases migration in ovarian cancer cell line CAOV-3 and this effect is reversed with Rho/ROCK inhibition [117]. More recently, a visfatin inhibitor (FK866) demonstrated effective reduction of tumor cell proliferation in vivo alone and in combination with a CD73 inhibitor [118]. More investigation is needed to better evaluate visfatin as a potential therapeutic target in ovarian cancer.

Visfatin and Endometrial Cancer

There are currently no studies documenting the effect of visfatin on the normal endometrium. However, the human endometrium does express visfatin and both serum level and endometrial tissue expression of visfatin are higher in women with endometrial cancer [119–121]. Higher endometrial tissue expression of visfatin correlates with advanced stage, increased depth of myometrial invasion, and poorer overall survival [121]. Higher serum visfatin level correlates with increased myometrial invasion and increased lymph node metastasis [119]. Thus, visfatin may be a useful predictive or prognostic biomarker.

Recent in vitro studies have demonstrated that visfatin exposure increases proliferation and decreases apoptosis in endometrial cancer cell lines [122]. Visfatin increases expression of the insulin receptor and activates the PI3K/Akt and MAPK and ERK1/2 pathways [122]. These findings were subsequently confirmed in an in vivo mouse model, which demonstrated increased proliferation of cancer cells when treated with visfatin [122]. In vitro proliferative and anti-apoptotic effects were abrogated by addition of PI3K and MEK inhibitors, further suggesting that visfatin may be useful in guiding therapy for endometrial cancer [122].

Resistin

Resistin is a 12.5 kDa (92 amino acid) molecule encoded by the *RETN* gene and first described in 2001 [123]. Resistin was identified as an adipokine secreted by adipocytes and highly correlated with insulin resistance in a mouse model [123]. However, human studies failed to replicate this finding, and further investigation has shown that resistin is primarily produced by peripheral mononuclear cells and correlates with inflammatory state rather than adiposity [124].

Resistin drives inflammation through multiple mechanisms. Resistin binds Toll-like receptor 4 (TLR4) to activate PI3K, p38 MAPK and NFκB pathways [125, 126]. Activation of PI3K and MAPK pathways leads to a subsequent release of a cascade of inflammatory mediators as well as factors to promote cell proliferation and survival. Further, resistin has been shown to enhance secretion of pro-inflammatory cytokines TNF-α and IL-12 in macrophages via the NFκB pathway [125]. Resistin also promotes epithelial cell activation by promoting endothelin-1 (ET-1) release, upregulating adhesion molecules, and downregulating TRAF-3, an inhibitor of CD40 signaling [127].

Resistin and Ovarian Cancer

Resistin expression has been demonstrated in both human and animal ovarian models [14]. Porcine studies did not show any effect of resistin on granulosa cell proliferation, but did show inhibition of caspase activity and DNA fragmentation suggesting an effect on cell survival [128]. While there is conflicting evidence of whether serum resistin is elevated in women with PCOS, resistin does independently correlate with insulin resistance, increasing BMI, and elevated testosterone in these women [129–131].

There are minimal studies investigating the role of resistin in ovarian malignancy. A single study showed that resistin increased expression of VEGF mRNA and protein in an ovarian cancer cell line via a PI3K/Akt dependent pathway [132]. More investigation is needed to better assess the possible pro-angiogenic effects of resistin in ovarian cancer.

Resistin and Endometrial Cancer

There are even fewer investigations into the relationship between resistin and endometrial cancer. Two small studies demonstrated higher serum resistin in women with endometrial cancer compared to matched controls [119, 133]. Additionally, higher resistin levels in one study correlated with increased lymph node metastasis [119]. Especially given the established ability of resistin to promote an inflammatory microenvironment, more investigation is warranted to explore the impact of visfatin on the development and progression of endometrial cancer.

Chemerin

Chemerin is a 16 kDa protein that was discovered as a chemoattractant for immune cells including natural killer cells, macrophages, and dendritic cells [134]. Chemerin binds to a G protein-coupled receptor (CMKLR1) expressed on the surface of adipocytes and immune cells to induce Ca2+ influx, increase in intracellular cAMP, and activation of MAPK and ERK 1/2 [15]. This cascade promotes adipocyte differentiation and chemotaxis of additional CMKLR-1-expressing cells [135]. Chemerin is also highly associated with increasing BMI and metabolic syndrome [136]. Thus, chemerin represents a link between metabolic dysregulation and the chronic inflammatory state.

Chemerin and the Ovary

Chemerin and its receptor CMKLR1 are expressed in human ovarian granulosa cells [137]. Serum chemerin is increased in obese women and is particularly elevated in women with PCOS [138–142]. Chemerin levels also correlate independently with BMI, abdominal fat content, insulin resistance, androgen levels, ovarian volume, triglyceride level, total cholesterol, LDL cholesterol, in women with PCOS [138, 140, 142–144]. This is at least in part due to direct effect of chemerin on steroidogenesis in the ovary. Chemerin reduces progesterone and estradiol production in ovarian granulosa cells via a MAPK-dependent pathway [145]. Chemerin also suppresses aromatase expression in granulosa cells and inhibits progesterone and estradiol secretion in ovarian follicles [146]. Taken as a whole, this supports that dysfunctional secretion of chemerin has direct impact on hormonal production and effect in the ovary. Additionally, chemerin levels are higher in the peritoneal fluid of women with endometriosis and are associated with higher levels of inflammatory cytokines TNF-α and IL-6 in these women [147]. So, in addition to demonstrating steroidogenic effects on the ovary, chemerin is also associated with pro-inflammatory conditions in the ovary and peritoneum. Despite this, there are currently no data to support a relationship between chemerin and ovarian cancer.

Chemerin and the Endometrium

Chemerin also has yet to be linked to endometrial cancer. However, chemerin has been shown to have higher expression in endometrial stromal cells in early pregnancy and is known to support natural killer cell migration to the endometrium and decidualization of the endometrial tissue to prepare for pregnancy [148]. This seems to suggest that chemerin is capable of both regulating immune response in the endometrium and inducing vascular remodeling in the endometrial tissue, both of which may affect malignant development and progression.

Chemerin and Malignancy

The majority of current research linking chemerin to malignancy is in the context of gastric and esophageal cancers. Elevated chemerin levels are associated with increased risk of developing colorectal cancer [149]. In patients with gastric cancer, increased chemerin level is associated with advanced stage and poorer prognosis [144, 150]. At the cellular level, this is believed to be due to chemerin's ability to stimulate invasion in both gastric cancer and esophageal squamous cancers [151, 152].

Omentin

Discovered in 2006, omentin-1 is a 31 kDa protein secreted from adipocytes that enhances insulin sensitivity and regulates glucose metabolism via Akt signaling [153]. Omentin also mediates the inflammatory response through activation of AMPK and suppression of JNK pathway [154]. Omentin levels are lower in conditions of obesity and insulin resistance [155].

Omentin and the Ovary

While ovarian tissue studies of omentin have not been reported, there has been investigation into the relationship between omentin and PCOS. Several studies have reported decreased omentin levels in women with PCOS independent of BMI [156–158]. Omentin is inversely correlated with androgen levels in women with PCOS, supporting a possible link between omentin, steroidogenesis, and hyperandrogenism [156]. Interestingly, treatment of these women with metformin resulted in increased serum omentin [159]. Despite these findings, there are no published studies investigating the effects of omentin in the ovary at the cellular or tissue level.

Omentin and the Endometrium

There are currently no studies reporting omentin expression in the endometrium, or omentin levels as they relate to endometrial cancer. One recent prospective trial did demonstrate that pre-operative treatment of endometrial cancer patients with metformin lowered omentin levels [50]; however, the clinical relevance of this is yet to be determined.

Omentin and Malignancy

While there are no data relating omentin to gynecologic cancers, there are published data in hepatocellular carcinoma, colorectal, and prostate cancers. Omentin has been shown to inhibit cellular proliferation and induce apoptosis through Sirt1 deacetylase and JNK signaling in hepatocellular carcinoma cell lines [160]. Despite these demonstrated tumor suppressive effects, omentin levels are known to be higher in patients with colorectal cancer and prostate cancer [161–163]. Evidently, more investigation is needed to better elucidate the role of omentin in human malignancy.

Apelin

Apelin was first discovered by Tatemoto et al. in 1998 after they successfully isolated apelin peptide from bovine stomach and demonstrated binding to the APJ G protein-coupled receptor [164]. Apelin circulates as one of three active forms, ranging from 13 to 36 amino acids in size [165]. When bound to the APJ receptor, apelin is believed to activate ERK and Akt pathways, promoting cellular proliferation [165]. There is also evidence that activation of the APJ receptor may lead to intracellular cAMP accumulation [165].

Since its discovery, apelin has been identified as an important regulator of the cardiovascular system. Apelin promotes proliferation and migration of endothelial cells and is a potent angiogenic factor in tissues [14, 165]. At the systemic level, apelin is believed to play a role in cardiovascular remodeling and fluid homeostasis. In the peripheral adipose tissue, apelin increases glucose uptake and decreases insulin resistance and adiposity. However, levels of apelin are paradoxically higher in obese individuals and those with type II diabetes [166].

Apelin and the Ovary

Apelin and its receptor APJ are expressed in the theca cells of bovine ovaries, and the APJ receptor is expressed in granulosa cells [167]. In the theca cells, LH induces increased expression of apelin and APJ, suggesting that conditions of elevated LH such as ovulation and PCOS may increase apelin [167]. Apelin may play a regulatory role in follicular selection, as expression of apelin and APJ are both increased in mature follicles [168].

Apelin and the Endometrium

Apelin is expressed by the glandular cells of the endometrium and exhibits higher level of expression during the secretory phase of the menstrual cycle [169]. A comparison of apelin expression in women with and without endometriosis did not demonstrate any differences [169]. There is a single study evaluating associating apelin level with endometrial cancer. Altinkaya et al. found that women with endometrial cancer demonstrated higher serum levels of apelin even when controlling for BMI [170].

Apelin and Malignancy

Apelin has demonstrated higher expression in colon adenomas and adenocarcinomas [171]. Apelin has been more extensively studied in the context of lymphangiogenesis. Apelin has been shown to bind APJ in lymphatic endothelial cells with subsequent increased migration, survival, and formation of microvessels in vitro via ERK and PI3K pathway activation [172]. In vivo, apelin overexpression is associated with accelerated tumor growth, lymphangiogenesis, and lymph node metastasis [172]. Thus, apelin may play a role in progression of disease and may be useful as a biomarker or therapeutic target particular in malignancies such as ovarian cancer that progress quickly and often present in an advanced stage.

Conclusion

The discovery of adipokines has expanded our current understanding of the relationship between obesity, metabolism, immune and endocrine function. With that knowledge, adipokines are now being explored for their role in the development of human malignancy. While obesity has long been associated with the development of ovarian and endometrial cancers, investigation into the roles that adipokines play in the diagnosis, course, and treatment of these cancers will hopefully bring us to a better understanding of their nature and will help us to develop more effective management strategies for the women affected by these cancers.

Acknowledgements We would like to thank VeloSano Bike to Cure and the Laura J. Fogarty Endowment for Uterine Cancer Research at the Cleveland Clinic for their support of our research endeavors in gynecologic malignancy. We would also like to acknowledge Amanda Mendelsohn of the Cleveland Clinic Center for Medical Art and Photography for the figures presented in this chapter.

References

1. Nedergaard J, Bengtsson T, Cannon B. Unexpected evidence for active brown adipose tissue in adult humans. Am J Physiol Endocrinol Metab. 2007;293(2):E444–52.
2. Exley MA, Hand L, O'Shea D, Lynch L. Interplay between the immune system and adipose tissue in obesity. J Endocrinol. 2014;223(2):41–8.
3. Renehan AG, Tyson M, Egger M, Heller RF, Zwahlen M. Body-mass index and incidence of cancer: a systematic review and meta-analysis of prospective observational studies. Lancet. 2008;371(9612):569–78.
4. Hamilton BS, Paglia D, Kwan AY, Deitel M. Increased obese mRNA expression in omental fat cells from massively obese humans. Nat Med. 1995;1(9):953–6.
5. Lonnqvist F, Arner P, Nordfors L, Schalling M. Overexpression of the obese (ob) gene in adipose tissue of human obese subjects. Nat Med. 1995;1(9):950–3.
6. Ryan NK, Woodhouse CM, Van der Hoek KH, Gilchrist RB, Armstrong DT, Norman RJ. Expression of leptin and its receptor in the murine ovary: possible role in the regulation of oocyte maturation. Biol Reprod. 2002;66(5):1548–54.
7. Margetic S, Gazzola C, Pegg GG, Hill RA. Leptin: a review of its peripheral actions and interactions. Int J Obes Relat Metab Disord. 2002;26(11):1407–33.
8. Agarwal SK, Vogel K, Weitsman SR, Magoffin DA. Leptin antagonizes the insulin-like growth factor-I augmentation of steroidogenesis in granulosa and theca cells of the human ovary. J Clin Endocrinol Metab. 1999;84:1072–6.
9. Craig J, Zhu H, Dyce PW, Petrik J, Li J. Leptin enhances oocyte nuclear and cytoplasmic maturation via the mitogen-activated protein kinase pathway. Endocrinology. 2004;145:5355–63.
10. Duggal PS, Van Der Hoek KH, Milner CR, Ryan NK, Armstrong DT, Magoffin DA, Norman RJ. The in vivo and in vitro effects of exog enous leptin on ovulation in the rat. Endocrinology. 2000;141:1971–6.
11. Spicer LJ, Francisco CC. The adipose obese gene product, leptin: evidence of a direct inhibitory role in ovarian function. Endocrinology. 1997;138:3374–9.
12. Spicer LJ, Francisco CC. Adipose obese gene product, leptin, inhibits bovine ovarian thecal cell steroidogenesis. Biol Reprod. 1998;58:207–12.
13. Zachow RJ, Magoffin DA. Direct intraovarian effects of leptin: impairment of the synergistic action of insulin-like growth factor-I on follicle-stimulating hormone-dependent estradiol-17 beta production by rat ovarian granulosa cells. Endocrinology. 1997;138:847–50.
14. Dupont J, Reverchon M, Cloix L, Froment P, Rame C. Involvement of adipokines, AMPK, PI3K and the PPAR signaling pathways in ovarian follicle development and cancer. Int J Dev Biol. 2012;56:959–67.
15. Booth A, Magnuson A, Fouts J, Foster M. Adipose tissue, obesity and adipokines: role in cancer promotion. Horm Mol Biol Clin Investig. 2015;21(1):57–74.
16. Chen C, Chang YC, Lan MS, Breslin M. Leptin stimulates ovarian cancer cell growth and inhibits apoptosis by increasing cyclin D1 and Mcl-1 expression via the activation of the MEK/ERK1/2 and PI3K/Akt signaling pathways. Int J Oncol. 2013;42(3):1113–9.
17. Choi JH, Lee KT, Leung PC. Estrogen receptor alpha pathway is involved in leptin-induced ovarian cancer cell growth. Carcinogenesis. 2011;32(4):589–96.
18. Hoffmann M, Fiedor E, Ptak A. 17β-Estradiol reverses leptin-inducing ovarian cancer cell migration by the PI3K/Akt signaling pathway. Reprod Sci. 2016;23(11):1600–8.
19. Kato S, Abarzua-Catalan L, Trigo C, Delpiano A, Sanhueza C, García K, Ibañez C, Hormazábal K, Diaz D, Brañes J, Castellón E, Bravo E, Owen G, Cuello MA. Leptin stimulates migration and invasion and maintains cancer stem-like properties in ovarian cancer cells: an explanation for poor outcomes in obese women. Oncotarget. 2015;6(25):21100–19.
20. Uddin S, Bu R, Ahmed M, Abubaker J, Al-Dayel F, Bavi P, Al-Kuraya KS. Overexpression of leptin receptor predicts an unfavorable outcome in Middle Eastern ovarian cancer. Mol Cancer. 2009;18(8):74.

21. Choi JH, Park SH, Leung PC, Choi KC. Expression of leptin receptors and potential effects of leptin on the cell growth and activation of mitogen-activated protein kinases in ovarian cancer cells. J Clin Endocrinol Metab. 2005;90(1):207–10.
22. Ptak A, Rak-Mardyła A, Gregoraszczuk EL. Cooperation of bisphenol A and leptin in inhibition of caspase-3 expression and activity in OVCAR-3 ovarian cancer cells. Toxicol In Vitro. 2013;27(6):1937–43.
23. Kasiappan R, Sun Y, Lungchukiet P, Quarni W, Zhang X, Bai W. Vitamin D suppresses leptin stimulation of cancer growth through microRNA. Cancer Res. 2014;74(21):6194–204.
24. Jin JH, Kim HJ, Kim CY, Kim YH, Ju W, Kim SC. Association of plasma adiponectin and leptin levels with the development and progression of ovarian cancer. Obstet Gynecol Sci. 2016;59(4):279–85.
25. Macciò A, Madeddu C, Massa D, Mudu MC, Lusso MR, Gramignano G, Serpe R, Melis GB, Mantovani G. Hemoglobin levels correlate with interleukin-6 levels in patients with advanced untreated epithelial ovarian cancer: role of inflammation in cancer-related anemia. Blood. 2005;106(1):362–7.
26. Mor G, Visintin I, Lai Y, Zhao H, Schwartz P, Rutherford T, Yue L, Bray-Ward P, Ward DC. Serum protein markers for early detection of ovarian cancer. Proc Natl Acad Sci U S A. 2005;102(21):7677–82.
27. Nick AM, Sood AK. The ROC 'n' role of the multiplex assay for early detection of ovarian cancer. Nat Clin Pract Oncol. 2008;5(10):568–9.
28. Visintin I, Feng Z, Longton G, Ward DC, Alvero AB, Lai Y, Tenthorey J, Leiser A, Flores-Saaib R, Yu H, Azori M, Rutherford T, Schwartz PE, Mor G. Diagnostic markers for early detection of ovarian cancer. Clin Cancer Res. 2008;14(4):1065–72.
29. Sen S, Kuru O, Akbayır O, Oğuz H, Yasasever V, Berkman S. Determination of serum CRP, VEGF, Leptin, CK-MB, CA-15-3 and IL-6 levels for malignancy prediction in adnexal masses. J Turk Ger Gynecol Assoc. 2011;12(4):214–9.
30. Serin IS, Tanriverdi F, Yilmaz MO, Ozcelik B, Unluhizarci K. Serum insulin-like growth factor (IGF)-I, IGF binding protein (IGFBP)-3, leptin concentrations and insulin resistance in benign and malignant epithelial ovarian tumors in postmenopausal women. Gynecol Endocrinol. 2008;24(3):117–21.
31. González RR, Caballero-Campo P, Jasper M, Mercader A, Devoto L, Pellicer A, Simon C. Leptin and leptin receptor are expressed in the human endometrium and endometrial leptin secretion is regulated by the human blastocyst. J Clin Endocrinol Metab. 2000;85(12):4883–8.
32. Fukuda J, Nasu K, Sun B, Shang S, Kawano Y, Miyakawa I. Effects of leptin on the production of cytokines by cultured human endometrial stromal and epithelial cells. Fertil Steril. 2003;80(S2):783–7.
33. Tanaka T, Umesaki N. Leptin regulates the proliferation and apoptosis of human endometrial epithelial cells. Int J Mol Med. 2008;22(5):683–9.
34. Dos Santos E, Serazin V, Morvan C, Torre A, Wainer R, de Mazancourt P, Dieudonné MN. Adiponectin and leptin systems in human endometrium during window of implantation. Fertil Steril. 2012;97(3):771–8.
35. Matarese G, Alviggi C, Sanna V, Howard JK, Lord GM, Carravetta C, Fontana S, Lechler RI, Bloom SR, De Placido G. Increased leptin levels in serum and peritoneal fluid of patients with pelvic endometriosis. J Clin Endocrinol Metab. 2000;85(7):2483–7.
36. Choi YS, Oh HK, Choi JH. Expression of adiponectin, leptin, and their receptors in ovarian endometrioma. Fertil Steril. 2013;100:135–41.
37. Ahn JH, Choi YS, Choi JH. Leptin promotes human endometriotic cell migration and invasion by up-regulating MMP-2 through the JAK2/STAT3 signaling pathway. Mol Hum Reprod. 2015;21(10):792–802.
38. Oh HK, Choi YS, Yang YI, Kim JH, Leung PC, Choi JH. Leptin receptor is induced in endometriosis and leptin stimulates the growth of endometriotic epithelial cells through the JAK2/STAT3 and ERK pathways. Mol Hum Reprod. 2013;19(3):160–8.

39. Ashizawa N, Yahata T, Quan J, Adachi S, Yoshihara K, Tanaka K. Serum leptin-adiponectin ratio and endometrial cancer risk in postmenopausal female subjects. Gynecol Oncol. 2010;119(1):65–9.
40. Gong TT, Wu QJ, Wang YL, Ma XX. Circulating adiponectin, leptin and adiponectin-leptin ratio and endometrial cancer risk: evidence from a meta-analysis of epidemiologic studies. Int J Cancer. 2015;137(8):1967–78.
41. Wang PP, He XY, Wang R, Wang Z, Wang YG. High leptin level is an independent risk factor of endometrial cancer: a meta-analysis. Cell Physiol Biochem. 2014;34(5):1477–84.
42. Zhang Y, Lil U, Li C, Ai H. Correlation analysis between the expressions of leptin and its receptor (ObR) and clinicopathology in endometrial cancer. Cancer Biomark. 2014;14(5):353–9.
43. Mantzos F, Vanakara P, Samara S, Wozniak G, Kollia P, Messinis I, Hatzitheofilou C. Leptin receptor expression in neoplastic and normal ovarian and endometrial tissue. Eur J Gynaecol Oncol. 2011;32(1):84–6.
44. Yuan SS, Tsai KB, Chung YF, Chan TF, Yeh YT, Tsai LY, Su JH. Aberrant expression and possible involvement of the leptin receptor in endometrial cancer. Gynecol Oncol. 2004;92(3):769–75.
45. Zhou X, Li H, Chai Y, Liu Z. Leptin Inhibits the apoptosis of endometrial carcinoma cells through activation of the nuclear factor κB-inducing kinase/IκB kinase pathway. Int J Gynecol Cancer. 2015;25(5):770–8.
46. Gao J, Tian J, Lv Y, Shi F, Kong F, Shi H, Zhao L. Leptin induces functional activation of cyclooxygenase-2 through JAK2/STAT3, MAPK/ERK, and PI3K/AKT pathways in human endometrial cancer cells. Cancer Sci. 2009;100(3):389–95.
47. Sharma D, Saxena NK, Vertino PM, Anania FA. Leptin promotes the proliferative response and invasiveness in human endometrial cancer cells by activating multiple signal-transduction pathways. Endocr Relat Cancer. 2006;13(2):629–40.
48. Wu X, Yan Q, Zhang Z, Du G, Wan X. Acrp30 inhibits leptin-induced metastasis by down-regulating the JAK/STAT3 pathway via AMPK activation in aggressive SPEC-2 endometrial cancer cells. Oncol Rep. 2012;27(5).1488–96.
49. Carino C, Olawaiye AB, Cherfils S, Serikawa T, Lynch MP, Rueda BR, Gonzalez RR. Leptin regulation of proangiogenic molecules in benign and cancerous endometrial cells. Int J Cancer. 2008;123(12):2782–90.
50. Soliman PT, Zhang Q, Broaddus RR, Westin SN, Iglesias D, Munsell MF, Schmandt R, Yates M, Ramondetta L, Lu KH. Prospective evaluation of the molecular effects of metformin on the endometrium in women with newly diagnosed endometrial cancer: a window of opportunity study. Gynecol Oncol. 2016;143(3):466–71.
51. Scherer PE, Williams S, Fogliano M, Baldini G, Lodish HF. A novel serum protein similar to C1q, produced exclusively in adipocytes. J Biol Chem. 1995;270(45):26746–9.
52. Hada Y, Yamauchi T, Waki H, Tsuchida A, Hara K, Yago H, et al. Selective purification and characterizaton of adponectin multimer species from human plasma. Biochem Biophys Res Commun. 2007;356:487–93.
53. Yamauchi T, Kamon J, Ito Y, Tsuchida A, Yokomizo T, Kita S, Sugiyama T, Miyagishi M, Hara K, Tsunoda M, Murakami K, Ohteki T, Uchida S, Takekawa S, Waki H, Tsuno NH, Shibata Y, Terauchi Y, Froguel P, Tobe K, Koyasu S, Taira K, Kitamura T, Shimizu T, Nagai R, Kadowaki T. Cloning of adiponectin receptors that mediate antidiabetic metabolic effects. Nature. 2003;423:762–9.
54. Holland WL, Miller RA, Wang ZV, Sun K, Barth BM, Bui HH, Davis KE, Bikman BT, Halberg N, Rutkowski JM, Wade MR, Tenorio VM, Kuo MS, Brozinick JT, Zhang BB, Birnbaum MJ, Summers SA, Scherer PE. Receptor-mediated activation of cer- amidase activity initiates the pleiotropic actions of adiponectin. Nat Med. 2003;17:55–63.
55. Yamauchi T, Kamon J, Waki H, Terauchi Y, Kubota N, Hara K, Mori Y, Ide T, Murakami K, Tsuboyama-Kasaoka N, Ezaki O, Akanuma Y, Gavrilova O, Vinson C, Reitman ML, Kagechika H, Shudo K, Yoda M, Nakano Y, Tobe K, Nagai R, Kimura S, Tomita M, Froguel

P, Kadowaki T. The fat-derived hormone adiponectin reverses insulin resistance associated with both lipoatrophy and obesity. Nat Med. 2001;7:941–6.

56. Arita Y, Kihara S, Ouchi N, Takahashi M, Maeda K, Miyagawa J, Hotta K, Shimomura I, Nakamura T, Miyaoka K, Kuriyama H, Nishida M, Yamashita S, Okubo K, Matsubara K, Muraguchi M, Ohmoto Y, Funahashi T, Matsuzawa Y. Paradoxical decrease of an adipose-specific protein, adiponectin, in obesity. Biochem Biophys Res Commun. 1999;257:79–83.

57. Kadowaki T, Yamauchi T. Adiponectin and adiponectin receptors. Endocr Rev. 2005;26:439–51.

58. Chandran M, Phillips SA, Ciaraldi T, Henry RR. Adiponectin: more than just another fat cell hormone. Diabet Care. 2003;26:2442–50.

59. Chabrolle C, Tosca L, Dupont J. Regulation of adiponectin and its receptors in rat ovary by human chorionic gonadotrophin treatment and potential involvement of adiponectin in granulosa cell steroidogenesis. Reproduction. 2007;133(4):719–31.

60. Ledoux S, Campos DB, Lopes FL, Dobias-Goff M, Palin MF, Muphy BD. Adiponectin induces periovulatory changes in ovarian follicular cells. Endocrinology. 2006;147(11):5178–86.

61. Downs SM, Hudson ER, Hardie DG. A potential role for AMP-activated protein kinase in meiotic induction in mouse oocytes. Dev Biol. 2002;245(1):200–12.

62. Komar CM, Braissant O, Wahli W, Curry TE. Expression and localization of PPARs in the rat ovary during follicular development and the periovulatory period. Endocrinology. 2001;142(11):4831–8.

63. Mayes MA, Laforest MF, Guillemette C, Gilchrist RB, Richard FJ. Adenosine 5'-monophosphate kinase-activated protein kinase (PRKA) activators delay meiotic resumption in porcine oocytes. Biol Reprod. 2007;76(4):589–97.

64. Tosca L, Crochet S, Ferre P, Foufelle F, Tesseraud S, Dupont J. AMP-activated protein kinase activation modulates progesterone secretion in granulosa cells from hen preovulatory follicles. J Endocrinol. 2006;190(1):85–97.

65. Tosca L, Crochet S, Uzbekova S, Dupont J. Effects of metformin on bovine granulosa cells steroidogenesis: possible involvement of adenosine 5'monophosphate-activated protein kinade (AMPK). Biol Reprod. 2007;76(3):368–78.

66. Tosca L, Froment P, Solnais P, Ferre P, Foufelle F, Dupont J. Adenosine 5'-monophosphate-activated protein kinase regulates progesterone secretion in rat granulosa cells. Endocrinology. 2005;146(10):4500–13.

67. Dupont J, Chabrolle C, Ramé C, Tosca L, Coyral-Castel S. Role of the peroxisome proliferator-activated receptors, adenosine monophosphate-activated kinase, and adiponectin in the ovary. PPAR Res. 2008, 2008:162275.

68. Cankaya S, Demir B, Aksakal SE, Dilbaz B, Demirtas C, Goktolga U. Insulin resistance and its relationship with high molecular weight adiponectin in adolescents with polycystic ovary syndrome and a maternal history of polycystic ovary syndrome. Fertil Steril. 2014;102(3):826–30.

69. Chen CI, Hsu MI, Lin SH, Chang YC, Hsu CS, Tzeng CR. Adiponectin and leptin in overweight/obese and lean women with polycystic ovary syndrome. Gynecol Endocrinol. 2015;31(4):264–8.

70. Ko JK, Li HW, Lam KS, Tam S, Lee VC, Yeung TW, Ho PC, Ng EH. Serum adiponectin is independently associated with the metabolic syndrome in Hong Kong, Chinese women with polycystic ovary syndrome. Gynecol Endocrinol. 2016;32(5):390–4.

71. Sarray S, Madan S, Saleh LR, Mahmoud N, Almawi WY. Validity of adiponectin-to-leptin and adiponectin-to-resistin ratios as predictors of polycystic ovary syndrome. Fertil Steril. 2015;104(2):460–6.

72. Trolle B, Lauszus FF, Frystyk J, Flyvbjerg A. Adiponectin levels in women with polycystic ovary syndrome: impact of metformin treatment in a randomized controlled study. Fertil Steril. 2010;94(6):2234–8.

73. Comim FV, Hardy K, Franks S. Adiponectin and its receptors in the ovary: further evidence for a link between obesity and hyperandrogenism in polycystic ovary syndrome. PLoS One. 2013;8(11):e80416.
74. Luque-Ramírez M, Alvarez-Blasco F, Escobar-Morreale HF. Antiandrogenic contraceptives increase serum adiponectin in obese polycystic ovary syndrome patients. Obesity. 2009;17(1):3–9.
75. Tao T, Xu B, Liu W. Ovarian HMW adiponectin is associated with folliculogenesis in women with polycystic ovary syndrome. Reprod Biol Endocrinol. 2013;11:99.
76. Nestler JE, Jakubowicz DJ, Evans WS, Pasquali R. Effects of metformin on spontaneous and clomiphene-induced ovulation in the polycystic ovary syndrome. NEJM. 1998;338(26):1876–80.
77. Otokozawa S, Tanaka R, Akasaka H, Ito E, Asakura S, Ohnishi H, Saito S, Miura T, Saito T, Mori M. Associations of serum isoflavone, adiponectin and insulin levels with risk for epithelial ovarian cancer: results of a case-control study. Asian Pac J Cancer Prev. 2015;16(12):4987–91.
78. Aune G, Stunes AK, Lian AM, Reseland J, Tingulstad S, Torp SH, et al. Circulating interleukin-8 and plasminogen activator inhibitor-1 are increased in women with ovarian carcinoma. Results Immunol. 2012;2:190–5.
79. Ocon-Grove OM, Krzysik-Walker SM, Giles J, Johnson P, Hendricks GL, Ramachandran R. Expression of adiponectin and its receptors, AdipoR1, AdipoR2 and T-cadherin, in chicken ovarian tumors. Biol Reprod. 2008;78(S1):139–40.
80. Tiwari A, Ocon-Grove OM, Hadley JA, Giles JR, Johnson PA, Ramachandran R. Expression of adiponectin and its receptors is altered in epithelial ovarian tumors and ascites-derived ovarian cancer cell lines. Int J Gynecol Cancer. 2015;25(3):399–406.
81. Diaz ES, Karlan BY, Li AJ. Obesity-associated adipokines correlate with survival in epithelial ovarian cancer. Gynecol Oncol. 2013;129(2):353–7.
82. Grossmann ME, Nkhata KJ, Mizuno NK, Ray A, Cleary MP. Effects of adiponectin on breast cancer cell growth and signaling. Br J Cancer. 2008;98:370–9.
83. Surmacz E. Leptin and adiponectin: emerging therapeutic targets in breast cancer. J Mammary Gland Biol Neoplasia. 2013;18:321–32.
84. Dieudonne MN, Bussiere M, Dos Santos E, Leneveu MC, Giudicelli Y, Pecquery R. Adiponectin mediates antiproliferative and apoptotic responses in human MCF7 breast cancer cells. Biochem Biophys Res Commun. 2006;345:271–9.
85. Dos Santos E, Benaitreau D, Dieudonne MN, Leneveu MC, Serazin V, Giudicelli Y, Pecquery R. Adiponectin mediates an antiproliferative response in human MDA-MB 231 breast cancer cells. Oncol Rep. 2008;20:971–7.
86. Nakayama S, Miyoshi Y, Ishihara H, Noguchi S. Growth-inhibitory effect of adiponectin via adiponectin receptor 1 on human breast cancer cells through inhibition of S-phase entry without inducing apoptosis. Breast Cancer Res Treat. 2008;112:405–41.
87. Lengyel E, Litchfield LM, Mitra AK, Nieman KM, Mukherjee A, Zhang Y, Johnson A, Bradaric M, Lee W, Romero IL. Metformin inhibits ovarian cancer growth and increases sensitivity to paclitaxel in mouse models. Am J Obstet Gynecol. 2015;212(4):479.e1–10.
88. Rattan R, Graham RP, Maguire JL, Giri S, Shridhar V. Metformin suppresses ovarian cancer growth and metastasis with enhancement of cisplatin cytotoxicity in vivo. Neoplasia. 2011;13(5):483–91.
89. Shank JJ, Yang K, Ghannam J, Cabrera L, Johnston CJ, Reynolds RK, Buckanovich RJ. Metformin targets ovarian cancer stem cells in vitro and in vivo. Gynecol Oncol. 2012;127(2):390–7.
90. Bodmer M, Becker C, Meier C, Jick SS, Meier CR. Use of metformin and the risk of ovarian cancer: a case-control analysis. Gynecol Oncol. 2011;123(2):200–4.
91. Kumar S, Meuter A, Thapa P, Langstraat C, Giri S, Chien J, Rattan R, Cliby W, Shridhar V. Metformin intake is associated with better survival in ovarian cancer: a case-control study. Cancer. 2013;119(3):555–62.

92. Takemura Y, Osuga Y, Yamauchi T, Kobayashi M, Harada M, Hirata T, Morimoto C, Hirota Y, Yoshino O, Koga K, Yano T, Kadowaki T, Taketani Y. Expression of adiponectin receptors and its possible implication in the human endometrium. Endocrinology. 2006;147(7):3203–10.
93. Takemura Y, Osuga Y, Harada M, Hirata T, Koga K, Morimoto C, Hirota Y, Yoshino O, Yano T, Taketani Y. Serum adiponectin concentrations are decreased in women with endometriosis. Hum Reprod. 2005;20(12):3510–3.
94. Artimani T, Saidijam M, Aflatoonian R, Ashrafi M, Amiri I, Yavangi M, SoleimaniAsl S, Shabab N, Karimi J, Mehdizadeh M. Downregulation of adiponectin system in granulosa cells and low levels of HMW adiponectin in PCOS. J Assist Reprod Genet. 2016;33(1):101–10.
95. García V, Oróstica L, Poblete C, Rosas C, Astorga I, Romero C, Vega M. Endometria from obese PCOS women with hyperinsulinemia exhibit altered adiponectin signaling. Horm Metab Res. 2015;47(12):901–9.
96. Lin T, Zhao X, Kong WM. Association between adiponectin levels and endometrial carcinoma risk: evidence from a dose-response meta-analysis. BMJ Open. 2015;5(9):e008541.
97. Zeng F, Shi J, Long Y, Tian H, Li X, Zhao AZ, Li RF, Chen T. Adiponectin and endometrial cancer: a systematic review and meta-analysis. Cell Physiol Biochem. 2015;36(4):1670–8.
98. Nowosielski K, Pozowski J, Ulman-Włodarz I, Romanik M, Poręba R, Sioma-Markowska U. Adiponectin to leptin index as a marker of endometrial cancer in postmenopausal women with abnormal vaginal bleeding: an observational study. Neuro Endocrinol Lett. 2012;33(2):217–23.
99. Rzepka-Górska I, Bedner R, Cymbaluk-Płoska A, Chudecka-Głaz A. Serum adiponectin in relation to endometrial cancer and endometrial hyperplasia with atypia in obese women. Eur J Gynaecol Oncol. 2008;29(6):594–7.
100. Moon HS, Chamberland JP, Aronis K, Tseleni-Balafouta S, Mantzoros CS. Direct role of adiponectin and adiponectin receptors in endometrial cancer: in vitro and ex vivo studies in humans. Mol Cancer Ther. 2011;10(12):2234–43.
101. Yamauchi N, Takazawa Y, Maeda D, Hibiya T, Tanaka M, Iwabu M, Okada-Iwabu M, Yamauchi T, Kadowaki T, Fukayama M. Expression levels of adiponectin receptors are decreased in human endometrial adenocarcinoma tissues. Int J Gynecol Path. 2012;31(4):352–7.
102. Cong L, Gasser J, Zhao J, Yang B, Li F, Zhao AZ. Human adiponectin inhibits cell growth and induces apoptosis in human endometrial carcinoma cells, HEC-1-A and RL95 2. Endocr Relat Cancer. 2007;14(3):713–20.
103. Zhang L, Wen K, Han X, Liu R, Qu Q. Adiponectin mediates antiproliferative and apoptotic responses in endometrial carcinoma by the AdipoRs/AMPK pathway. Gynecol Oncol. 2015;137(2):311–20.
104. Ko EM, Walter P, Jackson A, Clark L, Franasiak J, Bolac C, Havrilesky LJ, Secord AA, Moore DT, Gehrig PA, Bae-Jump V. Metformin is associated with improved survival in endometrial cancer. Gynecol Oncol. 2014;132(2):438–42.
105. Mitsuhashi A, Kiyokawa T, Sato Y, Shozu M. Effects of metformin on endometrial cancer cell growth in vivo: a preoperative prospective trial. Cancer. 2014;120(19):2986–95.
106. Rongvaux A, Shea RJ, Mulks MH, Gigot D, Urbain J, Leo O, Andris F. Pre-B-cell colony-enhancing factor, whose expression is up-regulated in activated lymphocytes, is a nicotinamide phosphoribosyltransferase, a cytosolic enzyme involved in NAD biosynthesis. Eur J Immunol. 2002;32(11):3225–34.
107. Samal B, Sun Y, Stearns G, Xie C, Suggs S, McNiece I. Cloning and characterization of the cDNA encoding a novel human pre-B-cell colony-enhancing factor. Mol Cell Biol. 1994;14(2):1431–7.
108. Luk T, Malam Z, Marshall JC. Pre-B cell colony-enhancing factor (PBEF)/visfatin: a novel mediator of innate immunity. J Leukoc Biol. 2008;83(4):804–16.
109. Chen MP, Chung FM, Chang DM, Tsai JC, Huang HF, Shin SJ, Lee YJ. Elevated plasma level of visfatin/pre-B cell colony-enhancing factor in patients with type 2 diabetes mellitus. J Clin Endocrinol Metab. 2006;91(1):295–9.

110. Chang YC, Chang TJ, Lee WJ, Chuang LM. The relationship of visfatin/pre-B-cell colony-enhancing factor/nicotinamide phosphoribosyltransferase in adipose tissue with inflammation, insulin resistance, and plasma lipids. Meta. 2010;59(1):93–9.

111. Andrade-Oliveira V, NOS C, Moraes-Vieira PM. Adipokines as drug targets in diabetes and underlying disturbances. J Diabet Res. 2015;2015:681612.

112. Yun MR, JM SEO, Park HY. Visfatin contributes to the differentiation of monocytes into macrophages through the differential regulation of inflammatory cytokines in THP-1 cells. Cell Signal. 2014;26(4):705–15.

113. Reverchon M, Cornuau M, Cloix L, Ramé C, Guerif F, Royère D, Dupont J. Visfatin is expressed in human granulosa cells: regulation by metformin through AMPK/SIRT1 pathways and its role in steroidogenesis. Mol Hum Reprod. 2013;19(5):313–26.

114. Plati E, Kouskouni E, Malamitsi-Puchner A, Boutsikou M, Kaparos G, Baka S. Visfatin and leptin levels in women with polycystic ovaries undergoing ovarian stimulation. Fertil Steril. 2010;94(4):1451–6.

115. Tsouma I, Kouskouni E, Demeridou S, Boutsikou M, Hassiakos D, Chasiakou A, Hassiakou S, Baka S. Correlation of visfatin levels and lipoprotein lipid profiles in women with polycystic ovary syndrome undergoing ovarian stimulation. Gynecol Endocrinol. 2014;30(7):516–9.

116. Shackelford RE, Bui MM, Coppola D, Hakam A. Over-expression of nicotinamide phosphoribosyltransferase in ovarian cancers. Int J Clin Exp Pathol. 2010;3(5):522–7.

117. Li Y, Li X, Liu KR, Zhang JN, Liu Y, Zhu Y. Visfatin derived from ascites promotes ovarian cancer cell migration through Rho/ROCK signaling-mediated actin polymerization. Eur J Cancer Prev. 2015;24(3):231–9.

118. Sociali G, Raffaghello L, Magnone M, Zamporlini F, Emionite L, Sturla L, Bianchi G, Vigliarolo T, Nahimana A, Nencioni A, Raffaelli N, Bruzzone S. Antitumor effect of combined NAMPT and CD73 inhibition in an ovarian cancer model. Oncotarget. 2016;7(3):2968–84.

119. Ilhan TT, Kebapcilar A, Yilmaz SA, Ilhan T, Kerimoglu OS, Pekin AT, Akyurek F, Unlu A, Celik C. Relations of serum visfatin and resistin levels with endometrial cancer and factors associated with its prognosis. Asian Pac J Cancer Prev. 2015;16(11):4503–8.

120. Nergiz Avcioglu S, Altinkaya SO, Küçük M, Yüksel H, Ömürlü IK, Yanik S. Visfatin concentrations in patients with endometrial cancer. Gynecol Endocrinol. 2015;31(3):202–7.

121. Tian W, Zhu Y, Wang Y, Teng F, Zhang H, Liu G, Ma X, Sun D, Rohan T, Xue F. Visfatin, a potential biomarker and prognostic factor for endometrial cancer. Gynecol Oncol. 2013;129(3):505–12.

122. Wang Y, Gao C, Zhang Y, Gao J, Teng F, Tian W, Yang W, Yan Y, Xue F. Visfatin stimulates endometrial cancer cell proliferation via activation of PI3K/Akt and MAPK/ERK1/2 signalling pathways. Gynecol Oncol. 2016;143(1):168–78.

123. Steppan CM, Bailey S, Bhat S, Brown EJ, Banerjee RR, Wright CM, Patel HR, Ahima RS, Lazar MA. The hormone resistin links obesity to diabetes. Nature. 2001;409(6818):307–12.

124. Lehrke M, Reilly M, Millington SC, Iqbal N, Rader DJ, Lazar MA. An inflammatory cascade leading to hyperresistinemia in humans. PLoS Med. 2004;1(2):e45.

125. Silswal N, Singh AK, Aruna B, Mukhopadhyay S, Ghosh S, Ehtesham NZ. Human resistin stimulates the pro-inflammatory cytokines TNF-alpha and IL-12 in macrophages by NF-kappaB-dependent pathway. Biochem Biophys Res Commun. 2005;334(4):1092–101.

126. Hsieh YY, Shen CH, Huang WS, Chin CC, Kuo YH, Hsieh MC, Yu HR, Chang TS, Lin TH, Chiu YW, Chen CN, Kuo HC, Tung SY. Resistin-induced stromal cell-derived factor-1 expression through Toll-like receptor 4 and activation of p38 MAPK/NFκB signaling pathway in gastric cancer cells. J Biomed Sci. 2014;21:59.

127. Verma S, Li SH, Wang CH, Fedak PW, Li RK, Weisel RD, Mickle DA. Resistin promotes endothelial cell activation: further evidence of adipokine-endothelial interaction. Circulation. 2003;108(6):736–40.

128. A R, Drwal E, Wróbel A, Gregoraszczuk E. Resistin is a survival factor for porcine ovarian follicular cells. Reproduction. 2015;150(4):343–55.

129. Munir I, Yen H, Baruth T, Tarkowski R, Azziz R, Magoffin DA, Jakimiuk AJ. Resistin stimulation of 17alpha-hydroxylase activity in ovarian theca cells in vitro: relevance to polycystic ovary syndrome. J Clin Endocrinol Metab. 2005;90(8):4852–7.
130. Seow KM, Juan CC, Hsu YP, Ho LT, Wang YY, Hwang JL. Serum and follicular resistin levels in women with polycystic ovarian syndrome during IVF-stimulated cycles. Hum Reprod. 2005;20(1):117–21.
131. Yilmaz M, Bukan N, Demirci H, Oztürk C, Kan E, Ayvaz G, Arslan M. Serum resistin and adiponectin levels in women with polycystic ovary syndrome. Gynecol Endocrinol. 2009;25(4):246–52.
132. Pang L, Zhang Y, Yu Y, Zhang S. Resistin promotes the expression of vascular endothelial growth factor in ovary carcinoma cells. Int J Mol Sci. 2013;14(5):9751–66.
133. Hlavna M, Kohut L, Lipkova J, Bienertova-Vasku J, Dostalova Z, Chovanec J, Vasku A. Relationship of resistin levels with endometrial cancer risk. Neoplasma. 2011;58(2):124–8.
134. Wittamer V, Franssen JD, Vulcano M, Mirjolet JF, Le Poul E, Migeotte I, Brézillon S, Tyldesley R, Blanpain C, Detheux M, Mantovani A, Sozzani S, Vassart G, Parmentier M, Communi D. Specific recruitment of antigen-presenting cells by chemerin, a novel processed ligand from human inflammatory fluids. J Exp Med. 2003;198(7):977–85.
135. Goralski KB, TC MC, Hanniman EA, Zabel BA, Butcher EC, Parlee SD, Muruganandan S, Sinal CJ. Chemerin, a novel adipokine that regulates adipogenesis and adipocyte metabolism. J Biol Chem. 2007;282(38):28175–88.
136. Bozaoglu K, Bolton K, McMillan J, Zimmet P, Jowett J, Collier G, Walder K, Segal D. Chemerin is a novel adipokine associated with obesity and metabolic syndrome. Endocrinology. 2007;148(10):4687–94.
137. Reverchon M, Cornuau M, Ramé C, Guerif F, Royère D, Dupont J. Chemerin inhibits IGF-1-induced progesterone and estradiol secretion in human granulosa cells. Hum Reprod. 2012;27(6):1790–800.
138. Guvenc Y, Var A, Goker A, Kuscu NK. Assessment of serum chemerin, vaspin and omentin-1 levels in patients with polycystic ovary syndrome. J Int Med Res. 2016;44(4):796–805.
139. Guzel EC, Celik C, Abali R, Kucukyalcin V, Celik E, Guzel M, Yilmaz M. Omentin and chemerin and their association with obesity in women with polycystic ovary syndrome. Gynecol Endocrinol. 2014;30(6):419–22.
140. Huang R, Yue J, Sun Y, Zheng J, Tao T, Li S, Liu W. Increased serum chemerin concentrations in patients with polycystic ovary syndrome: Relationship between insulin resistance and ovarian volume. Clin Chim Acta. 2015;450:366–9.
141. Tan BK, Chen J, Farhatullah S, Adya R, Kaur J, Heutling D, Lewandowski KC, O'Hare JP, Lehnert H, Randeva HS. Insulin and metformin regulate circulating and adipose tissue chemerin. Diabetes. 2009;58(9):1971–7.
142. Yang S, Wang Q, Huang W, Song Y, Feng G, Zhou L, Tan J. Are serum chemerin levels different between obese and non-obese polycystic ovary syndrome women? Gynecol Endocrinol. 2016;32(1):38–41.
143. Kort DH, Kostolias A, Sullivan C, Lobo RA. Chemerin as a marker of body fat and insulin resistance in women with polycystic ovary syndrome. Gynecol Endocrinol. 2015;31(2):152–5.
144. Wang L, Zhong Y, Ding Y, Shi X, Huang J, Zhu F. Elevated serum chemerin in Chinese women with hyperandrogenic PCOS. Gynecol Endocrinol. 2014;30(10):746–50.
145. Reverchon MBM, Ramé C, Froment P, Dupont J. Chemerin (RARRES2) decreases in vitro granulosa cell steroidogenesis and blocks oocyte meiotic progression in bovine species. Biol Reprod. 2014;90(5):102.
146. Wang Q, Bertoldo MJ, Xue K, Liu JY, Leader A, Tsang BK. Chemerin, a novel regulator of follicular steroidogenesis and its potential involvement in polycystic ovarian syndrome. Endcrinology. 2012;153(11):5600–11.
147. Jin CH, Yi KW, Ha YR, Shin JH, Park HT, Kim T, Hur JY. Chemerin expression in the peritoneal fluid, serum, and ovarian endometrioma of women with endometriosis. Am J Reprod Immunol. 2015;74(4):379–86.

148. Carlino C, Trotta E, Stabile H, Morrone S, Bulla R, Soriani A, Iannitto ML, Agostinis C, Mocci C, Minozzi M, Aragona C, Perniola G, Tedesco F, Sozzani S, Santoni A, Gismondi A. Chemerin regulates NK cell accumulation and endothelial cell morphogenesis in the decidua during early pregnancy. J Clin Endocrinol Metab. 2012;97(10):3603–12.
149. Erdogan S, Yilmaz FM, Yazici O, Yozgat A, Sezer S, Ozdemir N, Uysal S, Purnak T, Sendur MA, Ozaslan E. Inflammation and chemerin in colorectal cancer. Tumour Biol. 2016;37(5):6337–42.
150. Zhang J, Jin HC, Zhu AK, Ying RC, Wei W, Zhang FJ. Prognostic significance of plasma chemerin levels in patients with gastric cancer. Peptides. 2014;61:7–11.
151. Kumar JD, Kandola S, Tiszlavicz L, Reisz Z, Dockray GJ, Varro A. The role of chemerin and ChemR23 in stimulating the invasion of squamous oesophageal cancer cells. Br J Cancer. 2016;114(10):1152–9.
152. Wang C, Wu WK, Liu X, To KF, Chen GG, Yu J, Ng EK. Increased serum chemerin level promotes cellular invasiveness in gastric cancer: a clinical and experimental study. Peptides. 2014;51:131–8.
153. Yang RZ, Li MJ, Hu H, Pray J, Wu HB, Hansen BC, Shuldiner AR, Fried SK, McLenithan JC, Gong DW. Identification of omentin as a novel depot-specific adipokine in human adipose tissue: possible role in modulating insulin action. Am J Physiol Endocrinol Metab. 2006;290:E1253–61.
154. Ohashi K, Shibata R, Murohara T, Ouchi N. Role of anti-inflammatory adipokines in obesity-related diseases. Trends Endocrinol Metab. 2014;25:348–55.
155. Shibata R, Ouchi N, Takahashi R, Terakura Y, Ohashi K, Ikeda N, Higuchi A, Terasaki H, Kihara S, Murohara T. Omentin as a novel biomarker of metabolic risk factors. Diabet Metab Synd. 2012;4:37.
156. Choi JH, Rhee E, Kim KH, Woo HY, Lee WY, Sung KC. Plasma omentin-1 levels are reduced in non-obese women with normal glucose tolerance and polycystic ovary syndrome. Eur J Endocrinol. 2011;165(5):789–96.
157. Güneş M, Bunkan K. Examination of angiopoietin-like protein 4, neuropeptide Y, omentin-1 levels of obese and non-obese patients with polycystic ovary syndrome. Gynecol Endocrinol. 2015;31(11):903–6.
158. Tan BK, Adya R, Farhatullah S, Lewandowski KC, O'Hare P, Lehnert H, Randeva HS. Omentin-1, a novel adipokine, is decreased in overweight insulin-resistant women with polycystic ovary syndrome: ex vivo and in vivo regulation of omentin-1 by insulin and glucose. Diabetes. 2008;57(4):801–8.
159. Tan BK, Adya R, Farhatullah S, Chen J, Lehnert H, Randeva HS. Metformin treatment may increase omentin-1 levels in women with polycystic ovary syndrome. Diabetes. 2010;59(12):3023–31.
160. Zhang YY, Zhou LM. Omentin-1, a new adipokine, promotes apoptosis through regulating Sirt1-dependent p53 deacetylation inhepatocellular carcinoma cells. Eur J Pharm. 2013;698:137–44.
161. Aleksandrova K, di Giuseppe R, Isermann B, Biemann R, Schulze M, Wittenbecher C, Fritsche A, Lehmann R, Menzel J, Weikert C, Pischon T, Boeing H. Circulating omentin as a novel biomarker for colorectal cancer risk: data from the EPIC-Potsdam cohort study. Cancer Res. 2016;76(13):3862–71.
162. Fazeli MS, Dashti H, Akbarzadeh S, Assadi M, Aminian A, Keramati MR, Nabipour I. Circulating levels of novel adipocytokines in patients with colorectal cancer. Cytokine. 2013;62(1):81–5.
163. Uyeturk U, Uyeturk U, Kın Tekce B, Eroglu M, Kemahlı E, Uyeturk U, Gucuk A. Serum omentin level in patients with prostate cancer. Med Oncol. 2014;31(4):923.
164. Tatemoto K, Hosoya M, Habata Y, Fujii R, Kakegawa T, Zou MX, Kawamata Y, Fukusumi S, Hinuma S, Kitada C, Kurokawa T, Onda H, Fujino M. ISolation and characterization of a novel endogenous peptide ligand for the human APJ receptor. Biochem Biophys Res Commun. 1998;251(2):471–6.

165. Carpéné CDC, Attané C, Valet P, Portillo MP, Churruca I, Milagro FI, Castan-Laurell I. Expanding role for the apelin/APJ system in physiopathology. J Physiol Biochem. 2007;63(4):359–73.
166. Castan-Laurell I, Dray C, Attane C, Duparc T, Knauf C, Valet P. Apelin, diabetes, and obesity. Endocrine. 2011;40:1–9.
167. Shimizu T, Kosaka N, Murayama C, Tetsuka M, Miyamoto A. Apelin and APJ receptor expression in granulosa and theca cells during different stages of follicular development in the bovine ovary: involvement of apoptosis and hormonal regulation. Anim Reprod Sci. 2009;116(1):28–37.
168. Schilffarth S, Antoni B, Schams D, Meyer HH, Berisha B. The expression of apelin and its receptor APJ during different physiological stages in the bovine ovary. Int J Biol Sci. 2009;5(4):344–50.
169. Ozkan ZS, Ciljin H, Simsek M, Cobanoglu B, Ilhan N. Investigation of apelin expression in endometriosis. J Reprod Infertil. 2013;14(2):50–5.
170. Altinkaya SO, Nergiz S, Kucuk M, Yuksel H. Apelin levels are higher in obese patients with endometrial cancer. J Obstet Gynaecol Res. 2015;41:294–300.
171. Picault FX, Chaves-Almagro C, Projetti F, Prats H, Masri B, Audigier Y. Tumour co-expression of apelin and its receptor is the basis of an autocrine loop involved in the growth of colon adenocarcinomas. Eur J Cancer. 2014;50(3):663–74.
172. Berta J, Hoda MA, Laszlo V, Rozsas A, Garay T, Torok S, Grusch M, Berger W, Paku S, Renyi-Vamos F, Masri B, Tovari J, Groger M, Klepetko W, Hegedus B, Dome B. Apelin promotes lymphangiogenesis and lymph node metastasis. Oncotarget. 2014;5:4426–37.

Chapter 7
Adipose Derived Stromal Cells in Gynecologic Cancers

Aparna Mitra and Ann H. Klopp

Abstract Adipose stem cells or adipose derived stromal cells (ASC) are a unique population of multipotent mesenchymal cells within adipose tissue which can be readily isolated, expanded and differentiated in culture. When injected systemically or regionally, ASC migrate into sites of injury, forming supportive mesenchymal tissues, which contribute to wound healing. The capacity for expansion and homing has made ASC a focus of investigation in regenerative medicine to repair injury to organs, including the heart, joints or nervous tissues. ASC tropism for sites of injury is driven by chemotactic cytokines, such as CXCL1 and SDF-1, which are also secreted by tumors, which can similarly drive ASC into tumor stroma. Once engrafted in tumors, ASC contribute to the formation of cancer stroma. ASC may be particularly relevant in gynecologic cancers, which are surrounded by adipose tissues, providing ample source of ASC to form tumor stroma.

Keywords Adipose stem cells—immune response • Adipose stem cells—obesity • Pericytes • Adipose stem cells—ovarian cancer • Adipose stem cells—endometrial cancer

Defining Adipose Derived Stromal Cells

In 2001, adipose tissue was reported to be a plentiful source of mesenchymal stem cells, which morphologically and functionally resemble bone marrow derived mesenchymal stem cells. These cells were named adipose derived stromal cells (ADSC) or adipose stem cells (ASC) [1]. The International Federation for Adipose Therapeutics

A. Mitra
Department of Experimental Radiation Oncology, M.D. Anderson Cancer Center,
1515 Holcombe Blvd, Houston, TX 77030, USA
e-mail: AMitra1@mdanderson.org

A.H. Klopp, M.D., Ph.D. (✉)
Department of Radiation Oncology, MD Anderson Cancer Center,
1515 Holcombe Blvd, Houston, TX 77030, USA
e-mail: AKlopp@mdanderson.org

© Springer International Publishing AG 2018
N.A. Berger et al. (eds.), *Focus on Gynecologic Malignancies*, Energy Balance and Cancer 13, DOI 10.1007/978-3-319-63483-8_7

and Science (IFATS) defines ASC as plastic-adherent, multipotent cell population that have characteristic cell surface marker expression (CD45⁻CD235a⁻CD31 ⁻CD34⁺). ASC can be easily propagated in culture [2, 3]. In vivo, they can home to tumors [4] where they contribute to cancer stroma [5]. ASC have similar morphology and differentiation potential as bone marrow derived MSC with a similar cell surface marker expression. [6]. ASC are isolated by enzymatically digesting adipose tissue, centrifugation to remove mature adipocytes and culturing the remaining cells, known as the stromal vascular fraction. These plastic adherent cells have characteristic cell surface marker expression including expression of the hematopoietic lineage marker, CD34, with absence of CD45 [7, 8]. ASC can be stimulated to differentiate into mesenchymal lineage cells, including adipocytes, chondrocytes, cardiac and skeletal myocytes through culture with specific growth factors. Reports of differentiation into insulin producing β cells, hepatocytes and neuronal cells are less reproducible.

ASC in Regenerative Medicine

BM-MSC and ASC have been shown to function in repair of normal tissue damage through growth factor secretion and differentiation into mesenchymal lineage cells. ASCs are an appealing source of stem cells in regenerative medicine due to ease of isolation, genomic stability, high expansion potential and low immunogenicity. The high concentration of ASC results in fewer passages to generate sufficiently high numbers of ASC for therapeutics and subsequently less risk of developing chromosomal abnormalities [9–11]. ASC promote neovascularization through secretion of growth factors including vascular endothelial growth factor (VEGF), granulocyte/macrophage colony-stimulating factor (GM-CSF), cell-derived stromal factor 1-alpha (SDF-1α, hepatocyte growth factor (HGF), transforming growth factor β (TGF β), and fibroblast growth factor 2 (FGF2).

The capacity of ASC to speed repair of normal tissue injury has led to investigation into ASC to treat cardiac, orthopedic and neurologic injury. Clinical trials are testing the capacity of ASC to treat disease as diverse as diabetes, liver cirrhosis, fistulas, cardiovascular disease, Crohn's disease, atherosclerosis and bone [12]. Delivery of ASCs to infarcted heart of nude rats reduced infarct volume after 28 days by increasing local angiogenesis along with cardiac nerve sprouting [13]. Intraglandular transplant of ASCs into submandibular glans of SD rats showed alleviation of xerostomia caused by radiation [14].

ASC may find applications in repair normal tissue injury to gynecologic organs after cancer treatment. In rodent models of stress incontinence, periurethral injection of ASC increased sphincter muscle volume and increased in maximum bladder volume [15]. ASC may also have potential to regenerate the function of the ovary or endometrium to restore fertility. ASC injected into chemotherapy damaged ovaries, engrafted into the thecal layers, resulting in an increased number of corpus lutea and ovarian follicles [16]. Treatment of thin endometrium in a rat model with ASC did not have significant effects on endometrial gland density of volume, likely due to low rates of engraftment in this model [17].

Obesity and Adipose Derived Stromal Cells

Obesity increases ASC mobilization and impairs ASC differentiation potential. Obesity is defined by expansion in adipose volume with adipocyte hypertrophy, with accompanying metabolic, immune and cardiovascular abnormalities [18]. When the lipid storing capacity of the subcutaneous adipose tissue reaches saturation, then fat is deposited in the visceral adipose that surrounds the abdominal organs. Increase in visceral adipose volume is accompanied by concomitant increase in secretion of adipokines from visceral fat cells [19]. As visceral and subcutaneous adipose tissue expands, the population of pre-adipocytes within the adipose tissue increases [20, 21] but the number of ASC within adipose tissue decreases [11]. This hypertrophy induced decline in the number of ASCs within tissue may be due to need to support remodeling of the extracellular matrix in response to obesity as well as to accommodate the demand for adipocyte filling and hyperplastic expansion [22].

High-fat diet-induced obesity increases adipose expansion in obesity through MMP3 signaling ([23]). MMP3 has been reported to regulate stem cells function in mammary tissue through inactivation of wnt5b, suggesting that MMP3 effects on ECM remodeling in adipose tissue may be due to changes in stem cell function [24].

Increase in adipose volume is also accompanied by an increase in the number of circulating ASC. [25] The number of circulating ASC, detected with flow cytometry as C34+ leukocytes, was significantly higher in obese patients as compared to lean patients colorectal cancer [26].

Interestingly, addition of ASC improves dyslipidemia via activation of AMPK and white fat tissue browning [27]. ASCs or umbilical cord derived stem cells were administered via physiological saline into mice once a week for a total of three weeks. ASC treated mice showed improved dyslipidemia and lower body weight.

Obesity can impair the stem cell characteristics of ASC, including differentiation potential. Obese and visceral derived ASC have impaired capacity to differentiate into cartilage, bone and adipocytes [27]. Obesity and depot source also impacts the presence of stem cell markers in ASCs. Subcutaneous derived ASC from obese individuals demonstrated marked reduction in stem cell markers, Oct4, Sal, Sox15, Klf4 and BMI1 [28].

ASC and the Immune Response

ASC, like MSC, have immunosuppressive effects. MSC and ASC lack expression of HLA-DR which renders them non-immunogenic [29]. The immunosuppressive effect of MSC and ASC has been exploited to treat auto-immune disease, including graft vs host disease, inflammatory bowel disease and systemic lupus erythematosus. The same pathways that ASC utilize to suppress auto-immunity may suppress the anti-tumor immune response and play a role in the tumor promoting effects of

ASC observed in some models. Jagged 2, a ligand for Notch, appears to regulate the immunomodulatory effects of ASC [30].

ASCs from obese individuals polarize T cell towards the pro-inflammatory TH17 lineage, thus creating a more inflammatory milieu [31]. Additionally, ASC from obese individuals reduce insulin response in adipocytes through regulation of Th1/Th17 balance and monocyte activation [32]. The impact of this immune modulation in cancer progression has not been well studied.

ASCs directly inhibit cytotoxic T-lymphocyte proliferation and increase proliferation of the suppressive regulatory T-cell population (Tregs). One important mechanism by which this occurs is through expression of indole amine 2, 3-dioxygenase (IDO) [33]. IDO converts tryptophan into kynurenine which inhibits T cell activation and induces the proliferation of immunosuppressive Tregs. Prostaglandin E2 may also mediate the immunosuppressive effects of ASC [34]. ASCs inhibited proliferation of lymphocytes in ASC/T lymphocyte co-cultures. Inhibition of PGE2 allowed for T lymphocyte proliferation by decreasing IL10 secretion [33]. ASC have also been shown to suppress B-cells. Co-culture with ASC reduces the formation of antibody producing plasma cells, suggesting that ASC may have therapeutic potential in treatment of proliferative disease of B cell disorders and preventing B-cell mediated rejection of organ transplants [35].

Impact of Adipose Depot on ASC Source

Visceral fat is intra-abdominal adipose tissue deposited around major abdominal organs, including liver, pancreas and kidney. The major secretory product of visceral fat is NEFA (Non esterified fatty acid) which promotes the liver to increase production of triglycerides. Deposition of visceral adipose at abnormally high levels can trigger many disease, including cardiovascular disease, metabolic syndromes and hypertension. Assessing fasting triglycerides along with waist circumference is important in evaluating the risk of developing these diseases.

Visceral adiposity may be particularly relevant in gynecologic cancers. Visceral adipose surrounds gynecologic cancers and is a frequent site of metastasis for ovarian and endometrial cancers. Visceral adipose is heavily infiltrated with immune cells, as well as lymphatic and nervous tissue. The immunosuppressive regulatory T-cells (Tregs) are more common in visceral adipose tissues. Tregs are a subset of CD4+ cells positive for CD25 and expressing FoxP3, CTLA4 and GITR (glucocorticoid induced tumor necrosis factor receptor), which have immunosuppressive effects [36]. Adipose-derived Tregs are involved in lymphocyte migration, extravasation and lipid metabolism and have a more anti-inflammatory role than lymph node derived Tregs owing to the abundant expression of IL10.

These unique features of visceral adipose are likely to alter ASC populations, resulting in unique phenotype of ASC derived from visceral adipose. ASC may retain some phenotypic changes after weight loss. In previously obese mice, elevated levels of mTOR persisted in adipose tissue [37].

ASC and Cancers

ASC effects on tumor growth vary as a function of the model used and the technique to introduce ASC [38]. This is likely due to the complex interplay between growth factors, vascularization and hypoxia and the immune response. ASC universally home to the tumor microenvironment and contribute to the stroma and vascularization of tumors. In breast cancer models, ASCs home to the tumor microenvironment and promote breast cancer growth [39]. ASCs have also been found to home to gliomas, suggesting that ASC have the potential to be used as vehicles for delivering anti-tumor agents [40].

Several mechanisms of ASC support for tumor growth have been identified. ASC form pericytes which support tumor growth by supporting vascularization [41]. Hypoxia, present in the tumor microenvironment, augments secretion of the angiogenic cytokine, VEGF [42].

ASC are more likely to contribute directly to the formation of tumor vasculature than bone marrow derived MSC. Bone marrow derived MSC preferentially contribute to the formation of fibroblast specific protein (FSP) positive and fibroblast activation protein (FAP) positive tumor associated fibroblasts. The vascular and fibrovascular stroma (pericytes, alpha-SMA(+) myofibroblasts, and endothelial cells) originates from stromal cells derived from neighboring adipose tissue [43].

ASC and Ovarian Cancers

Omental derived ASC promote the proliferation, migration, chemotherapy, and radiation response of ovarian cancer cells [44]. ASCs increase growth and invasive properties of ovarian cancer by activation of matrix-metalloproteinase which may facilitate development of omental metastasis. Bidirectional communication between ovarian cancer and its microenvironment is critical for tumor growth and may have potential as a therapeutic strategy to re-educate elements of the tumor microenvironment [45].

ASC and Endometrial Cancers

ASC derived paracrine factors have been shown to increase endometrial cancer cell growth rate and enhance tumor angiogenesis [41]. Nitric oxide signaling can mediate ASC effects on proliferation of ovarian and endometrial cancer. Visceral derived ASC secrete arginine which is taken up by cancer cells, leading to increase intracellular NO synthesis and subsequent citrulline generation. The secreted citrulline causes increased adipogenesis of the ASCs thus leading to a metabolic coupling between ASCs and cancer cells [46].

ASC and Cervical, Vaginal and Vulvar Cancers

The role of adipose derived stromal cells in HPV associated cancers has been less well studied. Human uterine cervical stromal cells or hUCESCs have been reported to abrogate tumor growth in mouse xenograft model. Conditioned media collected from cervical stromal cells could reduce cell proliferation, invasion and induced apoptosis of breast cancer cells. They also showed inhibitory effects on cancer associated fibroblast proliferation and could revert differentiation of macrophages [47].

ASC as a Target for Anti-cancer Treatment

Targeting ASC may be a therapeutic strategy to treat cancer. One strategy to accomplish this depleted ASCs in mice stroma using a bimodal proteolytic resistant peptide comprising of cyclic WAT7 and a pro-apoptotic domain [48]. This suggests ASC targeting drugs could be used to complement available cancer treatments for better outcomes.

ASC as a Delivery Vehicle for Anti-cancer Agents

Many features of ASC make them uniquely suited to serve as a delivery vehicle for anti-cancer agents. ASC are tumor tropic so they can be delivered intravenously or intraperitoneally and will home to sites of tumor. Once engrafted, they will persist and will not be eliminated by the immune system. This approach has been tested in mouse models with many agents, include TRAIL and IFNβ. ASCs engineered to express TRAIL using nanoparticles have been tested to treat glioblastomas [49]. Similar approaches have been used to target human cervical, pancreatic, colon and breast cancers [50]. ASCs engineered to deliver cytosine deaminase::uracil phosphoribosyl transferase (CD::UPRT) to treat prostate cancer cells has been shown to significantly inhibit growth further [51]. This approach using autologous MSC is being tested in trials for women with platinum resistant ovarian cancer.

Conclusions

ASC are a unique population of stem cells, which can migrate into gynecologic cancers, supporting tumor growth by forming stroma, providing metabolic support and suppressing anti-tumor immunity. The impact of obesity in ASC is complex but appears to increase the availability of ASC to form tumor stroma. ASC may become increasingly clinically relevant as a target for therapeutic strategies, or perhaps as a vehicle to deliver anti-cancer agents directly into gynecologic cancers.

References

1. Zuk PA, Zhu M, Mizuno H, Huang J, Futrell JW, Katz AJ, et al. Multilineage cells from human adipose tissue: implications for cell-based therapies. Tissue Eng. 2001;7(2):211–28. doi:10.1089/107632701300062859.
2. Dykstra JA, Facile T, Patrick RJ, Francis KR, Milanovich S, Weimer JM, Kota DJ. Concise review: fat and furious: harnessing the full potential of adipose-derived stromal vascular fraction. Stem Cells Transl Med. 2017;6(4):1096–108. doi:10.1002/sctm.16-0337.
3. Linkov F, Kokai L, Edwards R, Sheikh MA, Freese KE, Marra KG, Rubin JP. The role of adipose-derived stem cells in endometrial cancer proliferation. Scand J Clin Lab Invest Suppl. 2014;244:54–58.; discussion 57–8. doi:10.3109/00365513.2014.936682.
4. Chabot V, Dromard C, Rico A, Langonne A, Gaillard J, Guilloton F, et al. Urokinase-type plasminogen activator receptor interaction with beta1 integrin is required for platelet-derived growth factor-AB-induced human mesenchymal stem/stromal cell migration. Stem Cell Res Ther. 2015;6:188. doi:10.1186/s13287-015-0163-5.
5. Kidd S, Spaeth E, Dembinski JL, Dietrich M, Watson K, Klopp A, et al. Direct evidence of mesenchymal stem cell tropism for tumor and wounding microenvironments using in vivo bioluminescent imaging. Stem Cells. 2009;27(10):2614–23. doi:10.1002/stem.187.
6. Bunnell BA, Estes BT, Guilak F, Gimble JM. Differentiation of adipose stem cells. Methods Mol Biol. 2008;456:155 71. doi:10.1007/978-1-59745-245-8_12.
7. Scherberich A, Di Maggio ND, McNagny KM. A familiar stranger: CD34 expression and putative functions in SVF cells of adipose tissue. World J Stem Cells. 2013;5(1):1–8. doi:10.4252/wjsc.v5.i1.1.
8. Varma MJ, Breuls RG, Schouten TE, Jurgens WJ, Bontkes HJ, Schuurhuis GJ, et al. Phenotypical and functional characterization of freshly isolated adipose tissue-derived stem cells. Stem Cells Dev. 2007;16(1):91–104. doi:10.1089/scd.2006.0026.
9. De Jong OG, Van Balkom BW, Schiffelers RM, Bouten CV, Verhaar MC. Extracellular vesicles: potential roles in regenerative medicine. Front Immunol. 2014;5:608. doi:10.3389/fimmu.2014.00608.
10. Nakagami T, Yamazaki Y, Hayamizu F. Prognostic factors for progression of visual field damage in patients with normal-tension glaucoma. Jpn J Ophthalmol. 2006;50(1):38–43. doi:10.1007/s10384-005-0273-1.
11. Uzbas F, May ID, Parisi AM, Thompson SK, Kaya A, Perkins AD, Memili E. Molecular physiognomies and applications of adipose-derived stem cells. Stem Cell Rev. 2015;11(2):298–308. doi:10.1007/s12015-014-9578-0.
12. Bajek A, Gurtowska N, Olkowska J, Kazmierski L, Maj M, Drewa T. Adipose-derived stem cells as a tool in cell-based therapies. Arch Immunol Ther Exp. 2016;64(6):443–54. doi:10.1007/s00005-016-0394-x.
13. Cai L, Johnstone BH, Cook TG, Tan J, Fishbein MC, Chen PS, March KL. IFATS collection: human adipose tissue-derived stem cells induce angiogenesis and nerve sprouting following myocardial infarction, in conjunction with potent preservation of cardiac function. Stem Cells. 2009;27(1):230–7. doi:10.1634/stemcells.2008-0273.
14. Xiong X, Shi X, Chen F. Human adipose tissuederived stem cells alleviate radiationinduced xerostomia. Int J Mol Med. 2014;34(3):749–55. doi:10.3892/ijmm.2014.1837.
15. Wu G, Song Y, Zheng X, Jiang Z. Adipose-derived stromal cell transplantation for treatment of stress urinary incontinence. Tissue Cell. 2011;43(4):246–53. doi:10.1016/j.tice.2011.04.003.

16. Takehara Y, Yabuuchi A, Ezoe K, Kuroda T, Yamadera R, Sano C, et al. The restorative effects of adipose-derived mesenchymal stem cells on damaged ovarian function. Lab Investig. 2013;93(2):181–93. doi:10.1038/labinvest.2012.167.

17. Hunter RK 2nd, Nevitt CD, Gaskins JT, Keller BB, Bohler HC Jr, LeBlanc AJ. Adipose-derived stromal vascular fraction cell effects on a rodent model of thin endometrium. PLoS One. 2015;10(12):e0144823. doi:10.1371/journal.pone.0144823.

18. Hamdy O, Porramatikul S, Al-Ozairi E. Metabolic obesity: the paradox between visceral and subcutaneous fat. Curr Diabetes Rev. 2006;2(4):367–73.

19. Tchoukalova Y, Koutsari C, Jensen M. Committed subcutaneous preadipocytes are reduced in human obesity. Diabetologia. 2007;50(1):151–7. doi:10.1007/s00125-006-0496-9.

20. De Girolamo L, Stanco D, Salvatori L, Coroniti G, Arrigoni E, Silecchia G, et al. Stemness and osteogenic and adipogenic potential are differently impaired in subcutaneous and visceral adipose derived stem cells (ASCs) isolated from obese donors. Int J Immunopathol Pharmacol. 2013;26(1 Suppl):11–21. doi:10.1177/03946320130260S103.

21. Isakson P, Hammarstedt A, Gustafson B, Smith U. Impaired preadipocyte differentiation in human abdominal obesity: role of Wnt, tumor necrosis factor-alpha, and inflammation. Diabetes. 2009;58(7):1550–7. doi:10.2337/db08-1770.

22. Pincu Y, Huntsman HD, Zou K, De Lisio M, Mahmassani ZS, Munroe MR, et al. Diet-induced obesity regulates adipose-resident stromal cell quantity and extracellular matrix gene expression. Stem Cell Res. 2016;17(1):181–90. doi:10.1016/j.scr.2016.07.002.

23. Wu Y, Lee MJ, Ido Y, Fried SK. High-fat diet-induced obesity regulates MMP3 to modulate depot- and sex-dependent adipose expansion in C57BL/6J mice. Am J Physiol Endocrinol Metab. 2017;312(1):E58–71. doi:10.1152/ajpendo.00128.2016.

24. Kessenbrock K, Dijkgraaf GJ, Lawson DA, Littlepage LE, Shahi P, Pieper U, Werb Z. A role for matrix metalloproteinases in regulating mammary stem cell function via the Wnt signaling pathway. Cell Stem Cell. 2013;13(3):300–13. doi:10.1016/j.stem.2013.06.005.

25. Zhang Y, Daquinag A, Traktuev DO, Amaya-Manzanares F, Simmons PJ, March KL, et al. White adipose tissue cells are recruited by experimental tumors and promote cancer progression in mouse models. Cancer Res. 2009;69(12):5259–66. doi:10.1158/0008-5472.CAN-08-3444.

26. Bellows CF, Zhang Y, Chen J, Frazier ML, Kolonin MG. Circulation of progenitor cells in obese and lean colorectal cancer patients. Cancer Epidemiol Biomark Prev. 2011;20(11):2461–8. doi:10.1158/1055-9965.EPI-11-0556.

27. Liu GY, Liu J, Wang YL, Liu Y, Shao Y, Han Y, et al. Adipose-derived mesenchymal stem cells ameliorate lipid metabolic disturbance in mice. Stem Cells Transl Med. 2016;5(9):1162–70. doi:10.5966/sctm.2015-0239.

28. Patel RS, Carter G, El Bassit G, Patel AA, Cooper DR, Murr M, Patel NA. Adipose-derived stem cells from lean and obese humans show depot specific differences in their stem cell markers, exosome contents and senescence: role of protein kinase C delta (PKCdelta) in adipose stem cell niche. Stem Cell Investig. 2016;3:2. doi:10.3978/j.issn.2306-9759.2016.01.02.

29. Leto Barone AA, Khalifian S, Lee WP, Brandacher G. Immunomodulatory effects of adipose-derived stem cells: fact or fiction? Biomed Res Int. 2013;2013:383685. doi:10.1155/2013/383685.

30. Xishan Z, Bin Z, Haiyue Z, Xiaowei D, Jingwen B, Guojun Z. Jagged-2 enhances immunomodulatory activity in adipose derived mesenchymal stem cells. Sci Rep. 2015;5:14284. doi:10.1038/srep14284.

31. Chchimi M, Robert M, Bechwaty ME, Vial G, Rieusset J, Vidal H, et al. Adipocytes, like their progenitors, contribute to inflammation of adipose tissues through promotion of Th-17 cells and activation of monocytes, in obese subjects. Adipocytes. 2016;5(3):275–82. doi:10.1080/21623945.2015.1134402.

32. Eljaafari A, Robert M, Chehimi M, Chanon S, Durand C, Vial G, et al. Adipose tissue-derived stem cells from obese subjects contribute to inflammation and reduced insulin response in adipocytes through differential regulation of the Th1/Th17 balance and monocyte activation. Diabetes. 2015;64(7):2477–88. doi:10.2337/db15-0162.

33. Yanez R, Oviedo A, Aldea M, Bueren JA, Lamana ML. Prostaglandin E2 plays a key role in the immunosuppressive properties of adipose and bone marrow tissue-derived mesenchymal stromal cells. Exp Cell Res. 2010;316(19):3109–23. doi:10.1016/j.yexcr.2010.08.008.
34. Spaggiari GM, Abdelrazik H, Becchetti F, Moretta L. MSCs inhibit monocyte-derived DC maturation and function by selectively interfering with the generation of immature DCs: central role of MSC-derived prostaglandin E2. Blood. 2009;113(26):6576–83. doi:10.1182/blood-2009-02-203943.
35. Franquesa M, Mensah FK, Huizinga R, Strini T, Boon L, Lombardo E, et al. Human adipose tissue-derived mesenchymal stem cells abrogate plasmablast formation and induce regulatory B cells independently of T helper cells. Stem Cells. 2015;33(3):880–91. doi:10.1002/stem.1881.
36. Feuerer M, Herrero L, Cipolletta D, Naaz A, Wong J, Nayer A, et al. Lean, but not obese, fat is enriched for a unique population of regulatory T cells that affect metabolic parameters. Nat Med. 2009;15(8):930–9. doi:10.1038/nm.2002.
37. De Angel RE, Conti CJ, Wheatley KE, Brenner AJ, Otto G, Degraffenried LA, Hursting SD. The enhancing effects of obesity on mammary tumor growth and Akt/mTOR pathway activation persist after weight loss and are reversed by RAD001. Mol Carcinog. 2013;52(6):446–58. doi:10.1002/mc.21878.
38. Klopp AH, Gupta A, Spaeth E, Andreeff M, Marini F III. Concise review: dissecting a discrepancy in the literature: do mesenchymal stem cells support or suppress tumor growth? Stem Cells. 2011;29(1):11–9. doi:10.1002/stem.559.
39. Razmkhah M, Jaberipour M, Erfani N, Habibagahi M, Talei AR, Ghaderi A. Adipose derived stem cells (ASCs) isolated from breast cancer tissue express IL-4, IL-10 and TGF-beta1 and upregulate expression of regulatory molecules on T cells: do they protect breast cancer cells from the immune response? Cell Immunol. 2011;266(2):116–22. doi:10.1016/j.cellimm.2010.09.005.
40. Lamfers M, Idema S, van Milligen F, Schouten T, van der Valk P, Vandertop P, et al. Homing properties of adipose-derived stem cells to intracerebral glioma and the effects of adenovirus infection. Cancer Lett. 2009;274(1):78–87. doi:10.1016/j.canlet.2008.08.035.
41. Klopp AH, Zhang Y, Solley T, Amaya-Manzanares F, Marini F, Andreeff M, et al. Omental adipose tissue-derived stromal cells promote vascularization and growth of endometrial tumors. Clin Cancer Res. 2012;18(3):771–82. doi:10.1158/1078-0432.CCR-11-1916.
42. Rasmussen JG, Frobert O, Pilgaard L, Kastrup J, Simonsen U, Zachar V, Fink T. Prolonged hypoxic culture and trypsinization increase the pro-angiogenic potential of human adipose tissue-derived stem cells. Cytotherapy. 2011;13(3):318–28. doi:10.3109/14653249.2010.506505.
43. Kidd S, Spaeth E, Watson K, Burks J, Lu H, Klopp A, et al. Origins of the tumor microenvironment: quantitative assessment of adipose-derived and bone marrow-derived stroma. PLoS One. 2012;7(2):e30563. doi:10.1371/journal.pone.0030563.
44. Nowicka A, Marini FC, Solley TN, Elizondo PB, Zhang Y, Sharp HJ, et al. Human omental-derived adipose stem cells increase ovarian cancer proliferation, migration, and chemoresistance. PLoS One. 2013;8(12):e81859. doi:10.1371/journal.pone.0081859.
45. Quail DF, Joyce JA. Microenvironmental regulation of tumor progression and metastasis. Nat Med. 2013;19(11):1423–37. doi:10.1038/nm.3394.
46. Salimian Rizi B, Caneba C, Nowicka A, Nabiyar AW, Liu X, Chen K, et al. Nitric oxide mediates metabolic coupling of omentum-derived adipose stroma to ovarian and endometrial cancer cells. Cancer Res. 2015;75(2):456–71. doi:10.1158/0008-5472.CAN-14-1337.
47. Eiro N, Vizoso FJ. Inflammation and cancer. World J Gastrointest Surg. 2012;4(3):62–72. doi:10.4240/wjgs.v4.i3.62.
48. Daquinag AC, Zhang Y, Kolonin MG. Vascular targeting of adipose tissue as an anti-obesity approach. Trends Pharmacol Sci. 2011;32(5):300–7. doi:10.1016/j.tips.2011.01.004.

49. Jiang X, Fitch S, Wang C, Wilson C, Li J, Grant GA, Yang F. Nanoparticle engineered TRAIL-overexpressing adipose-derived stem cells target and eradicate glioblastoma via intracranial delivery. Proc Natl Acad Sci U S A. 2016;113(48):13857–62. doi:10.1073/pnas.1615396113.
50. Grisendi G, Bussolari R, Cafarelli L, Petak I, Rasini V, Veronesi E, et al. Adipose-derived mesenchymal stem cells as stable source of tumor necrosis factor-related apoptosis-inducing ligand delivery for cancer therapy. Cancer Res. 2010;70(9):3718–29. doi:10.1158/0008-5472.CAN-09-1865.
51. Cavarretta IT, Altanerova V, Matuskova M, Kucerova L, Culig Z, Altaner C. Adipose tissue-derived mesenchymal stem cells expressing prodrug-converting enzyme inhibit human prostate tumor growth. Mol Ther. 2010;18(1):223–31. doi:10.1038/mt.2009.237.

Chapter 8
Obesity and Endometrial Cancer: Mouse Models for Preclinical Prevention Studies

Rosemarie E. Schmandt and Katherine A. Naff

Abstract Endometrial cancer risk is more strongly associated with obesity than any other cancer type and it is estimated that well over half of endometrial cancer cases in the US are attributable to being overweight and obese. The evaluation of new therapeutic regimens for the prevention and treatment of human endometrial cancer patients is dependent on the development of relevant preclinical models. This chapter will examine the animal models available for endometrial cancer studies in the lab, with a focus on mouse models. Mice and other rodents represent the front line for early preclinical studies in cancer research. We will discuss specific mouse models of endometrial cancer and will further present techniques that can be used to study the role of diet, obesity, and exercise on the normal endometrium and on the pathogenesis of endometrial cancer in the lab.

Keywords Immune compromised mouse models • Immune competent mouse models • Diet induced obesity • Energy balance protocols in mice • Voluntary versus forced exercise

Choice of Mouse Model

Most preclinical evaluations of behavioral and pharmaceutical interventions in endometrial cancer research are initially performed in mice and rats [1, 2]. While the effects of obesity and/or exercise on the biology of the endometrium can theoretically be assessed in any animal model, it is important to recognize that not all rodent strains are susceptible to diet induced obesity [3–6], nor are they all

R.E. Schmandt, Ph.D. (✉)
Department of Gynecologic Oncology and Reproductive Medicine, UT MD
Anderson Cancer Center, Unit 1362, P.O. Box 301439, Houston, TX 77230-1439, USA
e-mail: rschmand@mdanderson.org

K.A. Naff, D.V.M
Unit 63, Department of Veterinary Medicine and Surgery, UT MD Anderson Cancer Center,
1515 Holcombe Blvd, Houston, TX 77030, USA
e-mail: kanaff@mdanderson.org

enthusiastic exercisers [7–10]. Furthermore, care must be taken when assessing bio-markers and their relationship to obesity and cancer as sexually dimorphic responses have been observed. Indeed, male mice have been used preferentially for many of the published studies evaluating the physiologic and biochemical mechanisms underlying the beneficial effects of diet, obesity and exercise [11, 12].

Mouse Strains

Immunodeficient Mouse Models for Xenografts

Nude, SCID and NSG Mice

Current pre-clinical models of endometrial cancer typically involve intrauterine or intra-peritoneal injection of human tumor cells, or subcutaneous and intrauterine implantation of patient derived xenografts (PDX) into athymic nude, SCID (severe combined immu-nodeficient) or NSG (NOD scid gamma) mice [13–17]. Because these mice are not fully immune-competent, they will not "reject" tumor cells or tumor explants derived from humans. These models have been used successfully for the preclinical testing of a variety of targeted therapies and chemotherapeutic agents for endometrial cancer [18–20].

While immune-compromised mice are useful for the evaluation of some chemo-therapeutic agents, the role of the immune microenvironment in disease response and progression cannot be fully studied in this context. Furthermore, and significant to the study of endometrial cancer prevention, nude, SCID, and NSG mice are resis-tant to diet induced obesity and cannot be practically used for obesity studies. Because obesity and exercise are both associated with inflammatory responses, immune-deficient mice also have limited utility in the study of lifestyle changes on endometrial cancer risk and progression. Genetically engineered NSG mice with "humanized" immune systems are now available from several commercial sources, including Jackson Labs, however they are costly at the present time [21].

Immune compromised mice have, however, found use in deciphering the role of adipose tissue on the tumor microenvironment and tumor progression [22]. Studies performed in vitro demonstrated that adipose-derived stem cell (ASC) conditioned media is a rich source of growth factors that promote endometrial cancer cell growth [23]. By injecting human omental ASCs into mice, Klopp et al. [24] were able to demonstrate in vivo the recruitment of omental ASCs to human endometrial xeno-graft (HEC1A) tumors in these animals, accompanied by increased tumor vascula-ture and growth. Interestingly, the effects on tumor growth and vascularization were greater with omental ASCs than those observed with subcutaneous ASCs. These findings emphasize the importance of fat distribution and the specific role of vis-ceral adipose tissue on endometrial cancer progression.

Immune-compromised mice have been used to demonstrate the therapeutic effects of exercise on tumor growth for a variety of tumor allografts and xenografts including breast cancer [25, 26], lung cancer [27, 28], pancreatic cancer [29], and prostate cancer [29], suggesting the involvement of additional exercised-induced factors in cancer prevention.

C57BL/6 Nude Mice

This less common, immune deficient strain of mice is derived from a spontaneous athymic mutant of the standard inbred C57BL/6 mouse. Unlike the parental strain, described in greater detail below, these animals will not reject human tumor cell lines, and can be used to passage xenografts of normal and malignant human tissue. When housed under thermoneutral conditions (33 °C), these mice, like the C57BL/6 parental strain, are susceptible to diet induced obesity, increased hepatic triglyceride accumulation, adipose tissue inflammation and glucose intolerance [30]. While costly, this model system would permit the study of patient derived endometrial cancer xenografts and cell lines in the context of obesity and a pre-diabetic setting.

Immune-Competent Mice

C57BL/6 Mice

As shown on Fig. 8.1, C57BL/6 mice are a commonly used and comparatively inexpensive inbred laboratory mouse strain. They are immune-competent, good breeders, and are the most commonly used background strain for the creation of genetically modified mouse models. Indeed, because of its wide-spread use, the C57BL/6J mouse genome was fully sequenced [31]. Unlike many mouse strains, which are resistant to diet induced obesity (DIO), the C57BL/6 and particularly the C57BL/6J sub-strain of mice have been widely used in the study of obesity, exercise and metabolism [32]. They are susceptible to high fat diet (HFD) induced obesity, and like humans, they develop hyperinsulinemia, hyperglycemia, "fatty liver", and a resistance to leptin sensitivity with increasing weight gain [3, 33–36]. Similarly, C57BL/6 mice fed a fructose-enriched diet develop increased adiposity, elevated hepatic triglyceride (TAG) accumulation and glucose intolerance [37]. Furthermore, C57BL/6 mice have also been used extensively for exercise and metabolism studies and their behaviors are well characterized.

The genes governing obesity and insulin sensitivity in the C57BL/6 mice have been mapped to chromosome 14, and have been shown to be "dominant acting" [3]. When C57BL/6 mice are crossed with the 129S6/SvEvTac (129) mouse strain, which is less susceptible to DIO, C57BL/6 × 129 offspring inherit the predisposition to increased body weight and glucose intolerance of the C57BL/6 mice. Therefore, transgenic mice, which are resistant to DIO, can be made more sensitive by back-crossing to the C57BL/6 strain. This breeding strategy can be utilized by investigators to the study the influence of obesity on the penetrance of cancer susceptibility genes in transgenic mouse models of endometrial cancer.

Unfortunately, because human xenografts are not possible in this animal model, it is important that well-characterized C57BL/6 endometrial cancer cell lines be established for pre-clinical drug testing, by either genetically modifying normal C57BL/6 endometrial epithelial cells, or by culturing cells isolated from primary tumors isolated from C57BL/6 mice. These cell lines are under development and are being characterized in several academic labs and are expected available to the scientific community in the near future.

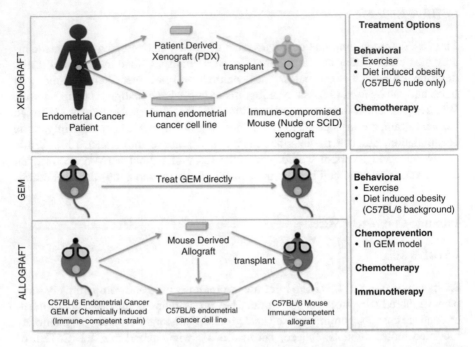

Fig. 8.1 Selecting mouse models for endometrial cancer prevention studies. While the effect of exercise, such as voluntary wheel running, can be studied in all xenograft, allograft and genetically modified mouse models of endometrial cancer, certain strains of mice are not equally susceptible to diet-induced obesity. C57BL/6 is one of the most commonly used laboratory mouse strains and, like humans, these mice are susceptible to diet-induced obesity and insulin resistance. Xenograft tumors from primary human tumors and cell lines can be grown in nude C57BL/6 mice, but this immune-deficient strain limits the study of tumor growth and progression in the context of obesity. Mouse endometrial cancer cell lines that grow in immune-competent animals are under development in several laboratories, and will be useful for the study of obesity and exercise on endometrial cancer recurrence and progression. Genetically modified mouse (GEM) models of endometrial cancer bred to a C57BL/6 background can be used to study the role of exercise and obesity on the penetrance and progression of familial cancers

Other Strains Susceptible to Diet Induced Obesity

Wild Type Inbred Strains

The body composition of a variety of mouse strains has been extensively studied [6], and susceptibility to diet induced obesity is noted in several strains. While less commonly used than C57BL/6 for cancer research, the AKR/J and DBA/2J mouse strains are susceptible to obesity and have been utilized for studies involving behaviors affecting metabolism and weight gain [38, 39]. Both strains are immune competent with AKR mice demonstrating a high incidence of leukemia, while DBA mice are used as a model of rheumatoid arthritis. These strains may be useful for the study of the effects of diet and obesity on endometrial proliferation and molecular changes influencing cancer risk, however they are not commonly used for genetic engineering or for tissue explants in the study of endometrial cancer.

Therefore strain-specific cell lines that can be used to establish preclinical models of recurrent endometrial cancer will need to be established by the investigator.

Wild Type Outbred Strains

ICR and CD-1 mice are outbred strains of laboratory mice that are susceptible to diet induced obesity and metabolic syndrome [40, 41]. While no syngeneic endometrial cancer cell lines exist from these strains, both have been used to study the effects of chemical carcinogens on the endometrium [42–44].

Chemically-Induced Mouse Model of Endometrial Cancer

Several models of chemically-induced endometrial hyperplasia and endometrial cancer have been developed. Neonatal exposure to diethylstilbestrol (DES) and other chemicals with estrogenic activity including tamoxifen and bisphenol A (BPA), have been shown to produce ovarian and oviductal abnormalities and endometrial hyperplasia in CD-1 mice with age [42, 45–47]. Endometrial cancers develop within 30 weeks following early treatment with N-methyl-N-nitrosourea (NMU) or estradiol in the outbred ICR mouse strain. Disease onset in this model can be accelerated further if animals are treated concurrently with both agents [43, 44].

Whether diet, obesity or exercise influence chemically induced endometrial cancer has not yet been reported, however studies using these models may be relevant to the evaluation of whether healthy lifestyle changes are protective against environmental carcinogen-induced endometrial cancer in humans.

Transgenic Mouse Models of Endometrial Cancer

A comprehensive review of genetically modified mouse models of endometrial cancer and their phenotypes has previously been published by Friel et al. [1]. With the exception of the PTEN knock out mice, the role of obesity and exercise on the pathogenesis of endometrial cancer has not been extensively reported in transgenic and knock-out mouse models of the disease. Current evidence suggests that certain driver mutations produce tumors that are less responsive to behavioral changes. These tumors may ultimately only respond to targeted chemotherapies. There is evidence, however, supporting improved response to chemotherapy with exercise in several cancer types [48, 49].

The effects of voluntary exercise on the biology of the endometrium can be studied on any genetically modified mouse model, despite some variation in activity between strains, however all mice are not equally susceptible to diet induced obesity. This can be remedied by back-crossing resistant mouse strains to C57BL/6 mice. First generation offspring should be susceptible to high fat diet-induced obesity [3].

Endometrial Hyperplasia

Endometrial hyperplasia describes a heterogeneous group of lesions that begin as regions of mild proliferation of glandular tissues, and progresses over time with increased crowding of glands and nuclear atypia to precancerous cells [50–53]. Because, in its earliest stages, endometrial hyperplasia can be often be reversed, this represents a period in which behavioral interventions may significantly reduce endometrial cancer risk. The modulation of localized estrogen and systemic insulin levels that occur as a consequence of weight loss and exercise would be expected to change the endometrial milieu and reduce endometrial proliferation.

In addition to the previously described chemically-induced mouse models of endometrial hyperplasia, several genetically modified models of endometrial hyperplasia have been developed. With the exception of the PTEN knock out mice, the effects of diet, obesity, and exercise on the progression of endometrial hyperplasia to cancer are not well-studied.

Loss of the PTEN tumor suppressor gene is one of the most common mutations observed in human endometrial cancer, and it is believed to be an early event in the pathogenesis of the disease. Systemic PTEN knock out mice die of variety of cancers in other organs, limiting the usefulness of this system for the extended timelines required for the development of endometrial hyperplasia. Tissue-specific knock out mice have been created to overcome this obstacle. Mice heterozygous for floxed PTEN in which cre-recombinase is driven by the progesterone promoter (C57BL6/129SV PR cre/+ PTEN f/f) demonstrate tissue specific loss of PTEN in the pituitary, ovary, endometrium, and mammary gland. [54]. Female mice with homozygous PTEN loss (Pten −/−) develop endometrial hyperplasia by 3 weeks of age and progress to in situ carcinoma by 3 months [54]. Female mice with heterozygous loss of the PTEN gene (Pten +/−) develop endometrial hyperplasia by 28 weeks and 20% progress to well-differentiated endometrial cancer by 10 months [55, 56].

In females with a systemic Pten +/− genotype, obesity has been reported to increase focal glandular hyperplasia with atypia to 78% as compared to 58% observed in lean mice at 28 weeks [57]. This effect was not observed in the tissue-specific knock-out mouse model [58]. The limited effects of obesity on this model system, suggests that once tumors have acquired mutations in the PTEN gene, the progression of hyperplasia cannot be reversed with weight regulation alone. The impact of exercise on disease progression in this model has not yet been studied.

In addition to the mouse models of chemically-induced endometrial hyperplasia described above, several other genetically modified mouse models of endometrial hyperplasia have been described [1]. These models mimic genetic mutations observed in human endometrial cancer. Female mice lacking the progesterone receptor develop endometrial hyperplasia in addition to other reproductive and behavioral abnormalities [59]. Accelerated endometrial hyperplasia might be expected in obese PR knock out mice as a consequence of increased estrogen synthesis and unopposed ER signaling associated with obesity. Conditionally dominant stabilized and conditional ablation of β-catenin demonstrate altered endometrial differentiation and proliferation [60]. Specific BRCA mutations are associated with endometrial hyperplasia [61], while targeted deletion of Mig6, a negative regulator of epidermal growth factor signaling, produced endometrial hyperplasia by 9 months of age [62]. Recently, overexpression of Sox9 in the uterine epithelium has been shown to result in simple and complex cystic glandular structures resembling human endometrial hyperplasia [63]. The ability of weight and exercise to reverse disease progression in these models remains unstudied.

Endometrial Cancer

Many of the genetically modified mouse models of hyperplasia will progress to endometrial cancer over time. There are other genetic modifications that lead to more aggressive phenotypes.

Over 10% of women with Peutz Jeghers Syndrome, characterized by a loss of the serine-threonine kinase, LKB1 (STK11), develop gynecologic cancers, including endometrial cancer [64, 65] Lkb1 acts as a tumor suppressor gene, and phosphorylates AMPK, a key regulator in cellular metabolism, that suppresses growth and proliferation under circumstances of nutrient depletion. In mice, while systemic homozygous deletion of Lkb1 (Lkb−/−) is embryonic lethal, Contreras et al. have described that greater than 50% of Lkb−/+ mice develop endometrial cancer [64]. Tissue specific deletion of LKB1 (Lkb−/−) in the endometrium results in well-differentiated, but invasive endometrial cancer by 9 months of age in 65% of mice [64].

Models of accelerated endometrial cancer have been developed by cross-breeding animals with mutations associated with endometrial hyperplasia. For example, conditional ablation of both Mig6 and PTEN [66] in progesterone receptor positive cells (using PR-cre) results in a phenotype of endometrial cancer at two weeks and adenocarcinoma at four weeks. While these models demonstrate the role of specific genes in the pathogenesis of endometrial cancer, with such a rapid onset of disease, it is unlikely these animals would be useful for behavioral prevention studies involving diet and exercise.

Important Considerations: Mouse Versus Human Menopause

The majority of endometrial cancers occur in post-menopausal women, although the incidence in premenopausal women is increasing. In premenopausal women, it is thought that estrogen is protective against visceral adiposity and prevents obesity-associated hyperinsulinemia and type 2-diabetes, both of which increase the risk of endometrial cancer. Loss of ovarian hormone production during menopause is associated with overall weight gain and with a redistribution of fat to the abdomen, similar to that observed in men. This sexual dimorphism of obesity is observed in both humans and mice [12, 67, 68], and should be considered when planning to study the effects of obesity, diet and exercise on the endometrium in a preclinical model.

Mice do not undergo menopause in the same manner humans do [69]. Although their fertility decreases over time, mice do not achieve the very low levels of estrogen observed in humans. In order to eliminate the effects of estrogen, and to mimic post-menopausal conditions, mice used in endometrial cancer studies are often ovariectomized [70]. Estrogen levels typically fall to low levels within 1–2 weeks in ovariectomized mice.

For those interested in characterizing molecular changes in the endometrium during the transition through menopause, and the response of the endometrium to diet and exercise, rodent models that mimic the progression through peri-menopause to menopause have been developed [70–72]. Chemically induced ovarian failure can be achieved following a 15-day course of treatment with the ovotoxic chemical, 4-vinylcyclohexene diepoxide (VCD). At low doses, mature follicles are depleted, the ovaries begin to fail and VCD selectively causes apoptosis for primordial follicles with no detectable effect on other peripheral tissues [72, 73]. This technique can successfully induce "menopause" in normal wild-type or genetically modified mice and rats.

Finally, genetically modified "menopausal" mice are under development. These include heterozygous knockouts of the Follicle Stimulating Hormone Receptor, which demonstrate time dependent loss of reproductive functions similar to that observed during menopause [71]. The Aryl-hydrocarbon receptor KO mouse demonstrates low fertility and develops uterine tumors at 6–13 months. Follotropin Receptor Knock Out Mice (FORKO) are anovulatory and have atrophic ovaries which do not secrete estrogen, similar to what is observed in aging women [74]. Studies evaluating the effects of obesity and exercise on the endometrium in these models are not yet described in the literature. The effects of these single gene modifications on overall endometrial physiology have also not been described.

Diet Induced Obesity

The first model of diet-induced obesity (DIO) was described in 1949, when a palatable liquid diet was used to induce obesity in rats [75]. While offering a palatable diet often results in increased body fat due to hyperphagia, a growing body of evidence from human and animal research showed that diets with a higher proportion of calories from fat induce obesity more efficiently, independently of the quantity consumed. Manipulation of macronutrient densities within the diet is now the standard method for induction of obesity in experimental rodents.

The Western Diet

DIO is reliably produced in susceptible mouse and rat stocks and strains by feeding commercially available, Western-type diets. The term "Western" in this context refers to the similarities between these diets and the calorically dense, high fat and high carbohydrate diets available to much of the Western world [33]. In theory, any existing diet may be "Westernized" simply by adding fats and sugars; however, this will alter the density of other dietary components, creating nutrient imbalances between experimental and control groups. It is also difficult to interpret the relative contributions of fat and carbohydrates to the development of obesity in a typical Western diet, since each component may independently influence palatability, satiety, and metabolic outcomes [76].

An alternative to this approach is to increase the fat and/or carbohydrate components of open-source, purified diets. In purified diets, protein, fat, and carbohydrate components are supplied by separate, purified ingredients; for example, protein may be supplied by casein, fat by palm oil, and carbohydrates by fructose. The formulas of open source diets are non-proprietary and are published and available to the public. This permits the investigator to increase the caloric density of a diet by altering the proportions of macronutrients, without otherwise changing the caloric content or diluting the availability of nutrients.

A second critical consideration when working with DIO models is the choice of control diet. Purified diets are more expensive to produce than standard rodent chows, and using a chow for control groups may appear to be an economical choice. Nevertheless, it is impossible to draw meaningful comparisons between groups fed a Westernized, purified diet and a chow [75]. Unlike purified diets that are created from specific and standardized ingredients, chows are created from complex ingredients, largely plant-based, that vary from batch to batch due to sourcing, time of harvest, soil conditions, farming methods, and other variables beyond the investigator's knowledge or control. The impact of these conditions on the nutrient and non-nutrient components of the chow are unpredictable and unmeasurable. In addition, most chows are proprietary formulas rather than open-source; therefore the exact proportions of each component are typically unknown to the investigator and are not publishable. By feeding Westernized and standard versions of the same open-source, purified diet to experimental and control groups respectively, dietary variables are reduced, and repeatability is enhanced.

Other Dietary Factors Affecting the Endometrium

Non-nutritive components must also be taken into account when choosing an appropriate diet for DIO models. The isoflavones present in plant-based chows are highly bioavailable and known to exert estrogenic effects on the genital tract of female mice and rats, including increased uterine weights, premature vaginal opening, and estrus induction, potentially confounding studies of gynecologic cancers [77, 78]. Soy isoflavones also exert non-reproductive effects that may impact both obesity models and cancer studies. In a study conducted by Mezei et al. [79], fatty Zucker rats fed a diet high in soy isoflavones demonstrated improved lipid metabolism in both sexes, and improved glucose tolerance in females, compared to control animals fed a diet low in isoflavones. Cell culture models in the same study demonstrated that soy isoflavones activate peroxisome proliferator-activated (PPAR) receptors. PPAR activation is known to modulate PTEN expression. While the role of this pathway in development of endometrial cancer is not fully understood, loss of PTEN is thought to be an early event in the pathogenesis of endometrial cancer, in both humans and mice. Furthermore, studies in transgenic mice and humans suggest that upregulation of PTEN via PPAR activation exerts anti-hyperplasia effects on the endometrium [80–82]. These findings illustrate the need for the investigator to look beyond the simple goal of obesity induction, by selecting diets with known ingredients and controlled proportions of nutritive and non-nutritive components, especially where studies of gynecologic cancers are concerned.

Custom Diets for Obesity Studies

The use of purified ingredient, open-source diets allows the investigator to customize a diet to meet specific study criteria. While C57Bl/6 mice fed a diet of 60% of calories from any fat source will show similar increases in total body fat and weight under controlled conditions, the source and type of fat significantly influences the expression of metabolic syndrome [83]. In one study comparing the effects of animal fat, saturated vegetable fat, and polyunsaturated vegetable fat in the C57Bl/6 DIO model, butterfat produced the highest levels of glucose and cholesterol, but lower levels of triglycerides compared to coconut oil and lard [84]. These distinctions are critical to developing the animal models necessary for gaining a full understanding of the risk factors for endometrial cancer. The variability in effects between different types of carbohydrate is less well studied, but it seems reasonable to control for this variable as well via selection of experimental and control diets with known and purified sources of carbohydrates as well as fat.

Standardization of Obesity Protocols in Mice

In order to practically compare the effects of diet-induced obesity and type 2-diabetes in mice, Heydemann proposed a standardized protocol for scientific studies [33]. Some of the suggested criteria seem equally applicable to the study of diet-induced obesity and its contribution to endometrial cancer risk and progression in mouse models. For the purposes of endometrial cancer research, a modified list would include (1) using C57BL/6J mice for xenograft studies, and transgenic mice backcrossed to this strain; (2) using mice from 4 to 20 weeks of age for xenograft studies, to avoid the effects of age; (3) Using a HFD plus high fructose to more accurate reflect the human diet.

Models of Exercise

Exercise is defined by the CDC as "A subcategory of physical activity that is planned, structured, repetitive, and purposive in the sense that the improvement or maintenance of one or more components of physical fitness is the objective". To date, the role of exercise on the pathogenesis of endometrial cancer has not been well studied in any animal species. The American Physiological Society has published an online resource book outlining the design of animal exercise protocols for a wide range of large and small research animals [85].

For the purposes of this chapter, we will focus on common exercise regimens used in mice and rats. A variety of equipment is currently available for rodents, which facilitates the study of aerobic and resistance training on obesity, type 2 diabetes, cardiovascular disease as well as cancer risk in the lab [86–88].

Running

Treadmill Running

Treadmills are rolling belts with an adjustable speed and slope, enabling forced/regulated exercise training for rodents. A variety of treadmills are commercially available, and many can be modified to accommodate multiple mice or rats (Touchscreen Treadmill, Harvard Apparatus, Holliston, MA; Rota-Rod Treadmill, Med Associates, Fairfax VT).

One advantage of treadmill running is that the investigator can design a fixed workout for all animals in the study. The investigator regulates running speed, duration and incline, such that all animals undergo identical exercise regimens and allowing for a direct comparison between treatment groups. Typically, animals are acclimatized to the apparatus using a "training program" where animals are exposed to the wheel and are trained to run faster and farther over a period of time, until the desired "workout" is achieved. Animals must be monitored for the duration of their time on the treadmill.

As an example, Jones et al. describe a treadmill protocol in which exercising animals began training at a speed of 10 m/min, 0% grade, for 10 min for 5 days per week on weeks 1 and 2, and progressively increased to the desired exercise "dose" of 18 m/min at 0% grade for 45 min, 5 days for 8 weeks. This training intensity was previously demonstrated to correspond to 70–75% of murine maximal oxygen uptake [89] and was shown to delay tumor growth in a xenograft model of breast cancer in nude mice [90]. Control mice are exposed to the exercise apparatus for the same amount of time daily, without treadmill running.

While moderate to high levels of exercise has demonstrated beneficial effects on the overall health of animals, intense and excessive exercising can produce inflammation, free radicals, and tissue damage, conditions thought to contribute to tumor progression. Furthermore, because stress and fatigue can counter the physiologic benefits of exercise in cancer prevention [91–94], investigators must be careful to optimize their exercise program for their model system, so that the dose can be easily maintained and reproduced between animals and is not stressful.

Treadmills are often equipped with electrical shock grids or "air-puff" accessories, which are intended to motivate activity and force exercise, but which may in fact, stress the animals. In the protocol described above, Jones et al. specifically avoid the use of "electrical stimulation to encourage the animals to run" [90].

Voluntary Wheel Running

In a comparison of endurance training of mice using forced treadmill versus voluntary wheel running, Knab et al. reported high intra-mouse variability between repeated endurance tests in mice run on enclosed treadmills with shock as a motivation. Voluntary wheel running, however, was shown to be stable and repeatable within individual mice [95]. This emphasizes the importance of carefully designed treadmill protocols for individual studies, which do not necessitate the use of shock, and which may be mouse-strain specific. Furthermore, treadmill running requires constant monitoring during exercise periods, to ensure mice are not injured, or do not escape. Voluntary wheel running is an attractive alternative form of exercise.

For voluntary running protocols, mice are housed individually with a wheel, or given individual access to a running wheel for a fixed amount of time daily. Animals run freely in a non-stressful environment, and the number of revolutions of the wheel are counted either mechanically or electronically and converted to distance.

Older versions of voluntary running wheels are incorporated as a module into the structure of the mouse and rat cages, count wheel rotations mechanically, and require specialized cage racks. Newer voluntary running wheels, commercially available through Med Associates (Fairfax VT), fit into the standard shoebox style mouse cages used by most animal facilities [96, 97]. The number rotations are wirelessly transmitted to a USB hub, so that not only the distance run by each mouse is measured, but also the frequency and duration of runs performed by each mouse are captured and recorded by a computer over time. This system also allows the investigator to monitor the training response of each mouse over time, so that tumors can be initiated once mice are acclimatized to the wheel. While individual mice may run different distances daily, decreasing distance run may indicate tumor progression, and tumor size can be ultimately be correlated to overall mouse activity. Finally, because the mouse does not need constant monitoring by the investigator during "wheel time", the investigator is free to do other work.

Female mice, in particular, prefer group housing conditions, and many animal care committees request justification for the individual housing of animals to avoid the effects of social isolation. Rather than housing individual mice with a wheel, animals can be removed from their cages and allowed to run for a fixed amount of time daily. Optimal wheel running times can be set by the investigator, after which animals are returned to social housing conditions. Control mice are housed individually with locked wheels for the same amount of time daily, therefore mimicking the same isolation period as exercising mice, and are returned to their home cage for social housing.

Several studies have been published demonstrating the effects of voluntary wheel running on cancer initiation and progression, and the mechanisms underlying the cancer preventive effects of voluntary exercise are being elucidated. Pedersen et al. have recently shown that four weeks of voluntary running decreases a subcutaneous model of melanoma in both athymic and C57BL/6 mice, with a greater response to exercise seen in the immune-competent animals, attributed to mobilization of IL-6 sensitive NK cells. Similarly, the Lewis Lung cancer model was inhibited by exercise. Voluntary wheel running also significantly reduced the number of lung metastases following tail vein injection of melanoma cells, and prevents the incidence and progression of diethylnitrosamine-induced liver cancer [28].

Specifically in female mice, voluntary exercise has been shown to decrease cancer progression in a syngeneic (4T1 cell) model of breast cancer in BALB/c mice [48, 98]. Pre-tumor exercise was shown to decrease 4T1 breast cancer cell tumor growth in elderly mice in a distance-dependent manner [25], and has been shown to inhibit tumor growth in the transgenic polyoma middle T oncoprotein (PyMT) mice which are a genetically modified mouse model of invasive breast cancer [99]. In both cases, in addition to metabolic changes, exercise-induced changes in the immune microenvironment are implicated in the attenuation of disease.

With the development of syngeneic xenografts and transgenic mouse models of endometrial cancer, we anticipate that the role of exercise on the prevention of both primary and recurrent endometrial cancer can conveniently be investigated using voluntary wheel running.

Swimming

Rodents are natural swimmers. Rats have been shown to swim continuously or stay afloat for more than 2 days, while mice have been shown to swim continuously for up to 3 h with little difficulty. Rodent swimming protocols used for laboratory studies include speed-swimming, maze-swimming and swimming to exhaustion [86].

High intensity interval training in the form of swimming has been shown to ameliorate the metabolic co-morbidities associated with diet-induced obesity [100], while aerobic swim training starting at 6 min five times weekly, increasing to 60 min, five times weekly over a 12 week period, is protective against fatty liver disease associated with a high fat diet [101]. With respect to cancer, Zhang et al. have shown that moderate swimming (8 min per day over 9 weeks), suppressed growth and metastasis of human liver cancer cells in nude mice, and murine liver cancer in C57BL/6 mice [102]. Animals forced to swim for longer periods, by creating a current, for 16 and 32 min, demonstrated the opposite effect, underscoring the deleterious effects of chronic stress on cancer progression.

Swimming, as a training method, is inexpensive and requires little specialized equipment, but the investigator's ability to quantitate effort or to standardize training is more limited, as compared to running protocols. Of course, like treadmill running, swimming animals must be constantly monitored, water should be maintained at a warm temperature (32–36 °C) and animals may be dried and given supplemental warmth after exercise training to avoid cold-induced stress. As illustrated by the previously described mouse experiments, lack of standardized protocols makes it difficult to compare data between investigators. Furthermore, it should be noted that swimming has been used as a stressor and as a measure of depression, as well as an exercise model in rats and mice [103–105]. Both swimming and treadmill running are forced activities and produce a stress response, as indicated by increases in corticosterone and ACTH in rats [106]. Protocols which incorporate an acclimatization period for regular moderate swim training are necessary to reduce stress levels, if swimming is to be used effectively as a form of exercise in cancer prevention studies.

Strength Training (Resistance Exercise)

Progressive resistance training protocols have been designed specifically to increase muscular strength and endurance in rodents in the study of muscular hypertrophy [88, 107, 108]. The techniques have been applied to study the effects of exercise on mental health and cognition (reviewed by Strickland and Smith [109]). Studies in mice have also demonstrated beneficial effects of resistance exercise training on insulin resistance and obesity [110], both of which are risk factors for endometrial cancer in humans. Although unreported to date, these methods may have utility in the study of endometrial cancer prevention in genetically modified and xenograft rodent models of endometrial cancer.

Resistance Wheel Training and Treadmill Running

Wireless exercise wheels can be fitted with a servo brake, which will respond to the rpm transmission of the wheel and can alter the intensity of the workout. Treatment groups can be set up such that one group can run unhindered, while a second group can have their activity restricted when running above a predefined velocity [111]. Similarly, for rats, mechanical wheel motion can be restricted using a weighted system (up to 200 g) to increase load [109, 112]. Because running is voluntary, animals may decrease their distance run as a consequence of weighted wheels.

Weights can also be added to tail of mice or rats undergoing treadmill training to increase the resistance while running. In weight pulling models, animals are typically incentivized to move with electric shock or a puff of air, although this is not strictly necessary. This technique therefore, has the same advantages and disadvantages as those described in regular treadmill running, and necessitates careful study design to accurately assess the beneficial effects of exercise on cancer prevention.

Ladder Climbing

Ladder climbing serves primarily to build hind-limb strength in rodents. Animals are placed at the base of a vertical ladder and encouraged to climb either via shock or with a food incentive. Weights can be added to the tail to increase resistance. [88, 109].

This model is not extensively used as model of exercise in cancer prevention models, however ladder climbing has been used to examine the effects resistance training as compared to aerobic motorized wheel running on skeletal muscle, and its effects on cancer cachexia in the colon-26 mouse model [113]. Resistance training was performed 3 days per week with a starting load of 50% of body weight followed by 10% increase every 2 weeks through 11 weeks.

While neither aerobic nor resistance training reduced tumor associated weight loss in these mice, tissue analysis revealed that resistance training actually induced the expression of genes associated with muscle damage and repair. This suggests the importance of experimental design, and determination of appropriate dose for maximal beneficial effect. Furthermore, as previously described, shock "encouragement" may produce a stress response in animals, and work in opposition to the desired effect, therefore for cancer prevention studies, positive reinforcement is suggested.

Considerations

For investigators wishing to study the effect of exercise on normal endometrial proliferation and gene transcription using a mouse model, it is worth noting different mouse strains demonstrate considerable variability in activity, including voluntary wheel running [7–10, 95]. Age also plays a role in running distance and intensity in mice [114] emphasizing the importance of age-matched controls and standardization of conditions between animal experiments, to allow for comparisons between studies utilizing the same strains.

Mice are nocturnal and are most active at night [96]. Because 12-h light cycles are regulated in most animal colonies (frequently lights on from 6 a.m. to 6 p.m.), it may be most convenient for investigators and their staff to request a room that is on a reverse light cycle. Studies that involve voluntary exercise can be conducted during regular work hours, which correspond to nighttime for the mice, allowing for maximal mouse activity. Most university or hospital rodent colonies are agreeable to setting up rooms on reverse light cycles for animals participating in behavioral studies.

Measuring Changes in Body Composition and Metabolism in the Mouse

In humans, abdominal or visceral fat gain is most closely associated with metabolic syndrome and type-2 diabetes, which are risk factors associated with endometrial cancer.

Magnetic Resonance Imaging (MRI), Computerized Tomography (CT) and Dual energy X-ray absorptiometry (DEXA) are all techniques used to identify and quantify fat deposits and distribution in humans [115, 116]. For investigators wishing to study these parameters in mice, and who desire to specifically and quantitatively correlate fat distribution with changes in the endometrium and endometrial cancer risk, these same non-invasive techniques can be used. Unlike direct measurement of visceral fat distribution by dissection, these technologies can be used to monitor changes in fat distribution and body composition longitudinally in response to diet and exercise.

Dual Energy X-Ray Absorptiometry (DEXA)

Dual energy X-ray absorptiometry (DEXA) is a methodology originally used in humans to evaluate bone mineral density. It has since been shown to effectively measure body composition and fat distribution both humans and rodents [117, 118]. In comparison to other techniques described in this section, including μCT and μMRI, DEXA densitometers for small animal studies are commercially available for individual laboratory use (GE Lunar PIXImus Densitometer). Analyses are completed in a short (5 min per scan) time frame with low radiation levels. This technique has been used to measure visceral versus non-visceral fat accumulation to define obese mouse phenotypes fed control and high fat diets. Using DEXA, visceral fat burden could be associated with glucose intolerance in C57BL/6 mice fed a high fat diet (Chen et al.). DEXA can therefore be used to estimate changes in obesity in live animals, before and after treatment. This is in contrast to direct measurement by dissection, which would necessitate the use of twice the number of animals and "before" and "after" treatment groups.

Micro-computed Tomography (μCT)

While more costly and less readily available to individual researchers, micro-computed tomography (μCT) is available as a component of some institutional metabolic core and imaging facilities. Compared to DEXA and μMRI, μCT is a moderate to high radiation technique. However it is a non-invasive, quantitative tool that can evaluate changes in total, visceral, and subcutaneous adiposity in longitudinal studies, and is considered as a gold standard method of body composition analysis.

Advocates of μCT argue that compared to current imaging techniques with similar capabilities, such as μMRI or the combination of DEXA with MRI (NMR), it may also be more cost-effective and offer higher spatial resolutions [119, 120].

Micro Magnetic Resonance Imaging (μMRI)

Micro Magnetic Resonance Imaging (μMRI) have previously been used, in combination with proton magnetic resonance spectroscopy (¹H-MRS) to characterize the morphological and biochemical aspects of adipose tissues and other visceral organs in the ob/ob mouse model [121]. ¹H-MRS has the capability to evaluate the polyunsaturation degree of the lipid chains and evaluate the presence of lipids in different organs in addition to fat deposits. Like μCT, these technologies are unlikely to be housed in individual labs, and located in a core imaging facility.

In summary, multiple imaging techniques are available to track diet and exercised induced changes in total fat stores, adipose distribution, and in the case of ¹H-MRS, even lipid composition in mouse models in response to diet and exercise. Because these changes may be relevant to endometrial cancer initiation, progression, and treatment response in humans, advanced imaging technologies should be applied to rodent models when possible.

Conclusion

In humans, obesity is the major risk factor for endometrial cancer, and is thought to contribute to more than half of the cases diagnosed. The development of new interventional strategies for the prevention and treatment of endometrial cancer patients are dependent on the availability of animal models that accurately reflect human disease. While careful consideration must be given to the predisposition of specific mouse strains to diet induced obesity, several novel mouse models of endometrial cancer are currently available that can be used to evaluate the role of diet and obesity in the pathogenesis of endometrial cancer. These pre-clinical models may yield important insights into the biological and molecular mechanisms by which behavioral interventions can be best applied to endometrial cancer prevention in women.

References

1. Friel AM, Growdon WB, McCann CK, Olawaiye AB, Munro EG, Schorge JO, Castrillon DH, Broaddus RR, Rueda BR. Mouse models of uterine corpus tumors: clinical significance and utility. Front Biosci (Elite Ed). 2010;2:882–905.
2. Vollmer G. Endometrial cancer: experimental models useful for studies on molecular aspects of endometrial cancer and carcinogenesis. Endocr Relat Cancer. 2003;10:23–42.
3. Almind K, Kahn CR. Genetic determinants of energy expenditure and insulin resistance in diet-induced obesity in mice. Diabetes. 2004;53:3274–85.
4. Brockmann GA, Bevova MR. Using mouse models to dissect the genetics of obesity. Trends Genet. 2002;18:367–76.

5. Fellmann L, Nascimento AR, Tibirica E, Bousquet P. Murine models for pharmacological studies of the metabolic syndrome. Pharmacol Ther. 2013;137:331–40.
6. Reed DR, Bachmanov AA, Tordoff MG. Forty mouse strain survey of body composition. Physiol Behav. 2007;91:593–600.
7. Jung AP, Curtis TS, Turner MJ, Lightfoot JT. Physical activity and food consumption in high- and low-active inbred mouse strains. Med Sci Sports Exerc. 2010;42:1826–33.
8. Kilikevicius A, Venckunas T, Zelniene R, Carroll AM, Lionikaite S, Ratkevicius A, Lionikas A. Divergent physiological characteristics and responses to endurance training among inbred mouse strains. Scand J Med Sci Sports. 2013;23:657–68.
9. Lerman I, Harrison BC, Freeman K, Hewett TE, Allen DL, Robbins J, Leinwand LA. Genetic variability in forced and voluntary endurance exercise performance in seven inbred mouse strains. J Appl Physiol (1985). 2002;92:2245–55.
10. Massett MP, Berk BC. Strain-dependent differences in responses to exercise training in inbred and hybrid mice. Am J Physiol Regul Integr Comp Physiol. 2005;288:R1006–13.
11. Dakin RS, Walker BR, Seckl JR, Hadoke PW, Drake AJ. Estrogens protect male mice from obesity complications and influence glucocorticoid metabolism. Int J Obes. 2015;39:1539–47.
12. Griffin C, Lanzetta N, Eter L, Singer K. Sexually dimorphic myeloid inflammatory and metabolic responses to diet-induced obesity. Am J Physiol Regul Integr Comp Physiol. 2016;311:R211–6.
13. Belizario JE. Immunodeficient mouse models: an overview. Open Immunol J. 2009;2:79–85.
14. Cabrera S, Llaurado M, Castellvi J, Fernandez Y, Alameda F, Colas E, Ruiz A, Doll A, Schwartz S Jr, Carreras R, et al. Generation and characterization of orthotopic murine models for endometrial cancer. Clin Exp Metastasis. 2012;29:217–27.
15. Haldorsen IS, Popa M, Fonnes T, Brekke N, Kopperud R, Visser NC, Rygh CB, Pavlin T, Salvesen HB, McCormack E, et al. Multimodal imaging of orthotopic mouse model of endometrial carcinoma. PLoS One. 2015;10:e0135220.
16. Ruggeri BA, Camp F, Miknyoczki S. Animal models of disease: pre-clinical animal models of cancer and their applications and utility in drug discovery. Biochem Pharmacol. 2014;87:150–61.
17. Tentler JJ, Tan AC, Weekes CD, Jimeno A, Leong S, Pitts TM, Arcaroli JJ, Messersmith WA, Eckhardt SG. Patient-derived tumour xenografts as models for oncology drug development. Nat Rev Clin Oncol. 2012;9:338–50.
18. Iwadate R, Inoue J, Tsuda H, Takano M, Furuya K, Hirasawa A, Aoki D, Inazawa J. High expression of p62 protein is associated with poor prognosis and aggressive phenotypes in endometrial cancer. Am J Pathol. 2015;185:2523–33.
19. Lee JW, Stone RL, Lee SJ, Nam EJ, Roh JW, Nick AM, Han HD, Shahzad MM, Kim HS, Mangala LS, et al. EphA2 targeted chemotherapy using an antibody drug conjugate in endometrial carcinoma. Clin Cancer Res. 2010;16:2562–70.
20. Theisen ER, Gajiwala S, Bearss J, Sorna V, Sharma S, Janat-Amsbury M. Reversible inhibition of lysine specific demethylase 1 is a novel anti-tumor strategy for poorly differentiated endometrial carcinoma. BMC Cancer. 2014;14:752.
21. Morton JJ, Bird G, Refaeli Y, Jimeno A. Humanized mouse xenograft models: narrowing the tumor-microenvironment gap. Cancer Res. 2016;76(21):6153–8.
22. Freese KE, Kokai L, Edwards RP, Philips BJ, Sheikh MA, Kelley J, Comerci J, Marra KG, Rubin JP, Linkov F. Adipose-derived stems cells and their role in human cancer development, growth, progression, and metastasis: a systematic review. Cancer Res. 2015;75:1161–8.
23. Linkov F, Kokai L, Edwards R, Sheikh MA, Freese KE, Marra KG, Rubin JP. The role of adipose-derived stem cells in endometrial cancer proliferation. Scand J Clin Lab Invest Suppl. 2014;244:54–8. discussion 57–8
24. Klopp AH, Zhang Y, Solley T, Amaya-Manzanares F, Marini F, Andreeff M, Debeb B, Woodward W, Schmandt R, Broaddus R, et al. Omental adipose tissue-derived stromal cells promote vascularization and growth of endometrial tumors. Clin Cancer Res. 2012;18:771–82.
25. Goh J, Endicott E, Ladiges WC. Pre-tumor exercise decreases breast cancer in old mice in a distance-dependent manner. Am J Cancer Res. 2014;4:378–84.

26. Welsch MA, Cohen LA, Welsch CW. Inhibition of growth of human breast carcinoma xeno-grafts by energy expenditure via voluntary exercise in athymic mice fed a high-fat diet. Nutr Cancer. 1995;23:309–18.
27. Higgins KA, Park D, Lee GY, Curran WJ, Deng X. Exercise-induced lung cancer regression: mechanistic findings from a mouse model. Cancer. 2014;120:3302–10.
28. Pedersen L, Idorn M, Olofsson GH, Lauenborg B, Nookaew I, Hansen RH, Johannesen HH, Becker JC, Pedersen KS, Dethlefsen C, et al. Voluntary running suppresses tumor growth through epinephrine- and IL-6-dependent NK cell mobilization and redistribution. Cell Metab. 2016;23:554–62.
29. Zheng X, Cui XX, Huang MT, Liu Y, Shih WJ, Lin Y, Lu YP, Wagner GC, Conney AH. Inhibitory effect of voluntary running wheel exercise on the growth of human pan-creatic Panc-1 and prostate PC-3 xenograft tumors in immunodeficient mice. Oncol Rep. 2008;19:1583–8.
30. Stemmer K, Kotzbeck P, Zani F, Bauer M, Neff C, Muller TD, Pfluger PT, Seeley RJ, Divanovic S. Thermoneutral housing is a critical factor for immune function and diet-induced obesity in C57BL/6 nude mice. Int J Obes. 2015;39:791–7.
31. Mouse Genome Sequencing C, Waterston RH, Lindblad-Toh K, Birney E, Rogers J, Abril JF, Agarwal P, Agarwala R, Ainscough R, Alexandersson M, et al. Initial sequencing and comparative analysis of the mouse genome. Nature. 2002;420:520–62.
32. Fontaine DA, Davis DB. Attention to background strain is essential for metabolic research: C57BL/6 and the international knockout mouse consortium. Diabetes. 2016;65:25–33.
33. Heydemann A. An overview of murine high fat diet as a model for type 2 diabetes mellitus. J Diabetes Res. 2016;2016:2902351.
34. Lin S, Thomas TC, Storlien LH, Huang XF. Development of high fat diet-induced obesity and leptin resistance in C57Bl/6J mice. Int J Obes Relat Metab Disord. 2000;24:639–46.
35. Montgomery MK, Hallahan NL, Brown SH, Liu M, Mitchell TW, Cooney GJ, Turner N. Mouse strain-dependent variation in obesity and glucose homeostasis in response to high-fat feeding. Diabetologia. 2013;56:1129–39.
36. Wu Y, Wu T, Wu J, Zhao L, Li Q, Varghese Z, Moorhead JF, Powis SH, Chen Y, Ruan XZ. Chronic inflammation exacerbates glucose metabolism disorders in C57BL/6J mice fed with high-fat diet. J Endocrinol. 2013;219:195–204.
37. Montgomery MK, Fiveash CE, Braude JP, Osborne B, Brown SH, Mitchell TW, Turner N. Disparate metabolic response to fructose feeding between different mouse strains. Sci Rep. 2015;5:18474.
38. Alexander J, Chang GQ, Dourmashkin JT, Leibowitz SF. Distinct phenotypes of obesity-prone AKR/J, DBA2J and C57BL/6J mice compared to control strains. Int J Obes. 2006;30:50–9.
39. Wang CY, Liao JK. A mouse model of diet-induced obesity and insulin resistance. Methods Mol Biol. 2012;821:421–33.
40. Gao M, Ma Y, Liu D. High-fat diet-induced adiposity, adipose inflammation, hepatic steatosis and hyperinsulinemia in outbred CD-1 mice. PLoS One. 2015;10:e0119784.
41. Li Z, Jin H, Oh SY, Ji GE. Anti-obese effects of two Lactobacilli and two Bifidobacteria on ICR mice fed on a high fat diet. Biochem Biophys Res Commun. 2016;480:222–7.
42. Newbold RR, Jefferson WN, Padilla-Banks E. Long-term adverse effects of neonatal expo-sure to bisphenol A on the murine female reproductive tract. Reprod Toxicol. 2007;24:253–8.
43. Niwa K, Murase T, Furui T, Morishita S, Mori H, Tanaka T, Mori H, Tamaya T. Enhancing effects of estrogens on endometrial carcinogenesis initiated by N-methyl-N-nitrosourea in ICR mice. Jpn J Cancer Res. 1993;84:951–5.
44. Niwa K, Tanaka T, Mori H, Yokoyama Y, Furui T, Mori H, Tamaya T. Rapid induction of endometrial carcinoma in ICR mice treated with N-methyl-N-nitrosourea and 17 beta-estradiol. Jpn J Cancer Res. 1991;82:1391–6.
45. Gray K, Bullock B, Dickson R, Raszmann K, Walmer D, McLachlan J, Merlino G. Potentiation of diethylstilbestrol-induced alterations in the female mouse reproductive tract by transform-ing growth factor-alpha transgene expression. Mol Carcinog. 1996;17:163–73.
46. Newbold RR, Jefferson WN, Padilla-Burgos E, Bullock BC. Uterine carcinoma in mice treated neonatally with tamoxifen. Carcinogenesis. 1997;18:2293–8.

47. Wordinger RJ, Morrill A. Histology of the adult mouse oviduct and endometrium following a single prenatal exposure to diethylstilbestrol. Virchows Arch B Cell Pathol Incl Mol Pathol. 1985;50:71–9.
48. Betof AS, Lascola CD, Weitzel D, Landon C, Scarbrough PM, Devi GR, Palmer G, Jones LW, Dewhirst MW. Modulation of murine breast tumor vascularity, hypoxia and chemotherapeutic response by exercise. J Natl Cancer Inst. 2015;107:pii: djv040.
49. Sturgeon K, Schadler K, Muthukumaran G, Ding D, Bajulaiye A, Thomas NJ, Ferrari V, Ryeom S, Libonati JR. Concomitant low-dose doxorubicin treatment and exercise. Am J Physiol Regul Integr Comp Physiol. 2014;307:R685–92.
50. Mills AM, Longacre TA. Endometrial hyperplasia. Semin Diagn Pathol. 2010;27:199–214.
51. Mills AM, Longacre TA. Atypical endometrial hyperplasia and well differentiated endometrioid adenocarcinoma of the uterine corpus. Surg Pathol Clin. 2011;4:149–98.
52. Morice P, Leary A, Creutzberg C, Abu-Rustum N, Darai E. Endometrial cancer. Lancet. 2016;387:1094–108.
53. Sivridis E, Giatromanolaki A. The pathogenesis of endometrial carcinomas at menopause: facts and figures. J Clin Pathol. 2011;64:553–60.
54. Daikoku T, Hirota Y, Tranguch S, Joshi AR, DeMayo FJ, Lydon JP, Ellenson LH, Dey SK. Conditional loss of uterine Pten unfailingly and rapidly induces endometrial cancer in mice. Cancer Res. 2008;68:5619–27.
55. Podsypanina K, Ellenson LH, Nemes A, Gu J, Tamura M, Yamada KM, Cordon-Cardo C, Catoretti G, Fisher PE, Parsons R. Mutation of Pten/Mmac1 in mice causes neoplasia in multiple organ systems. Proc Natl Acad Sci U S A. 1999;96:1563–8.
56. Stambolic V, Tsao MS, Macpherson D, Suzuki A, Chapman WB, Mak TW. High incidence of breast and endometrial neoplasia resembling human Cowden syndrome in pten+/− mice. Cancer Res. 2000;60:3605–11.
57. Yu W, Cline M, Maxwell LG, Berrigan D, Rodriguez G, Warri A, Hilakivi-Clarke L. Dietary vitamin D exposure prevents obesity-induced increase in endometrial cancer in Pten+/− mice. Cancer Prev Res (Phila). 2010;3:1246–58.
58. Iglesias, D.A., Zhang, Q., Celestino, J., Sun, C.C., Yates, M.S., Schmandt, R.E., Lu, K.H. (2017). Lean body weight and metformin are insufficient to prevent endometrial hyperplasia in mice harboring inactivating mutations in PTEN. Oncology 92(2):109-114.
59. Lydon JP, DeMayo FJ, Conneely OM, O'Malley BW. Reproductive phenotpes of the progesterone receptor null mutant mouse. J Steroid Biochem Mol Biol. 1996;56:67–77.
60. Jeong JW, Lee HS, Franco HL, Broaddus RR, Taketo MM, Tsai SY, Lydon JP, DeMayo FJ. Beta-catenin mediates glandular formation and dysregulation of beta-catenin induces hyperplasia formation in the murine uterus. Oncogene. 2009;28:31–40.
61. Kim SS, Cao L, Lim SC, Li C, Wang RH, Xu X, Bachelier R, Deng CX. Hyperplasia and spontaneous tumor development in the gynecologic system in mice lacking the BRCA1-Delta11 isoform. Mol Cell Biol. 2006;26:6983–92.
62. Jin N, Gilbert JL, Broaddus RR, Demayo FJ, Jeong JW. Generation of a Mig-6 conditional null allele. Genesis. 2007;45:716–21.
63. Gonzalez G, Mehra S, Wang Y, Akiyama H, Behringer RR. Sox9 overexpression in uterine epithelia induces endometrial gland hyperplasia. Differentiation. 2016;92(4):204–15.
64. Contreras CM, Akbay EA, Gallardo TD, Haynie JM, Sharma S, Tagao O, Bardeesy N, Takahashi M, Settleman J, Wong KK, et al. Lkb1 inactivation is sufficient to drive endometrial cancers that are aggressive yet highly responsive to mTOR inhibitor monotherapy. Dis Model Mech. 2010;3:181–93.
65. Shorning BY, Clarke AR. Energy sensing and cancer: LKB1 function and lessons learnt from Peutz-Jeghers syndrome. Semin Cell Dev Biol. 2016;52:21–9.
66. Kim TH, Franco HL, Jung SY, Qin J, Broaddus RR, Lydon JP, Jeong JW. The synergistic effect of Mig-6 and Pten ablation on endometrial cancer development and progression. Oncogene. 2010;29:3770–80.
67. Palmer BF, Clegg DJ. The sexual dimorphism of obesity. Mol Cell Endocrinol. 2015;402:113–9.

68. Szmuilowicz ED, Stuenkel CA, Seely EW. Influence of menopause on diabetes and diabetes risk. Nat Rev Endocrinol. 2009;5:553–8.
69. Groothuis PG, Dassen HH, Romano A, Punyadeera C. Estrogen and the endometrium: lessons learned from gene expression profiling in rodents and human. Hum Reprod Update. 2007;13:405–17.
70. Diaz Brinton R. Minireview: translational animal models of human menopause: challenges and emerging opportunities. Endocrinology. 2012;153:3571–8.
71. Danilovich N, Ram Sairam M. Recent female mouse models displaying advanced reproductive aging. Exp Gerontol. 2006;41:117–22.
72. Van Kempen TA, Milner TA, Waters EM. Accelerated ovarian failure: a novel, chemically induced animal model of menopause. Brain Res. 2011;1379:176–87.
73. Brooks HL, Pollow DP, Hoyer PB. The VCD mouse model of menopause and perimenopause for the study of sex differences in cardiovascular disease and the metabolic syndrome. Physiology (Bethesda). 2016;31:250–7.
74. Sairam MR, Danilovich N, Lussier-Cacan S. The FORKO mouse as a genetic model for exploring estrogen replacement therapy. J Reprod Med. 2002;47:412–8.
75. Hariri N, Thibault L. High-fat diet-induced obesity in animal models. Nutr Res Rev. 2010;23:270–99.
76. West DB, York B. Dietary fat, genetic predisposition, and obesity: lessons from animal models. Am J Clin Nutr. 1998;67:505S–12S.
77. Brown NM, Setchell KD. Animal models impacted by phytoestrogens in commercial chow: implications for pathways influenced by hormones. Lab Investig. 2001;81:735–47.
78. Thigpen JE, Setchell KD, Ahlmark KB, Locklear J, Spahr T, Caviness GF, Goelz MF, Haseman JK, Newbold RR, Forsythe DB. Phytoestrogen content of purified, open- and closed-formula laboratory animal diets. Lab Anim Sci. 1999;49:530–6.
79. Mezei O, Banz WJ, Steger RW, Peluso MR, Winters TA, Shay N. Soy isoflavones exert anti-diabetic and hypolipidemic effects through the PPAR pathways in obese Zucker rats and murine RAW 264.7 cells. J Nutr. 2003;133:1238–43.
80. Nickkho-Amiry M, McVey R, Holland C. Peroxisome proliferator-activated receptors modulate proliferation and angiogenesis in human endometrial carcinoma. Mol Cancer Res. 2012;10:441–53.
81. van der Zee M, Jia Y, Wang Y, Heijmans-Antonissen C, Ewing PC, Franken P, DeMayo FJ, Lydon JP, Burger CW, Fodde R, et al. Alterations in Wnt-beta-catenin and Pten signalling play distinct roles in endometrial cancer initiation and progression. J Pathol. 2013;230:48–58.
82. Wu W, Celestino J, Milam MR, Schmeler KM, Broaddus RR, Ellenson LH, Lu KH. Primary chemoprevention of endometrial hyperplasia with the peroxisome proliferator-activated receptor gamma agonist rosiglitazone in the PTEN heterozygote murine model. Int J Gynecol Cancer. 2008;18:329–38.
83. Buettner R, Scholmerich J, Bollheimer LC. High-fat diets: modeling the metabolic disorders of human obesity in rodents. Obesity (Silver Spring). 2007;15:798–808.
84. Cunha TM, Peterson R, Gobbett TA. Conditions of metabolic syndrome (obesity, insulin resistance, dyslipidemia) altered by varied sources of dietary fat in the C57BL/6 mouse. In: Zuberbuehler C, editor. Society for the study of ingestive behavior: annual meeting 2005. Pittsburgh, PA: SSIB; 2005.
85. Kregel KC, editor. Resource book or the design of animal exercise protocols. Washington, DC: American Physiological Society; 2006.
86. Ghosh S, Golbidi S, Werner I, Verchere BC, Laher I. Selecting exercise regimens and strains to modify obesity and diabetes in rodents: an overview. Clin Sci (Lond). 2010;119:57–74.
87. Pedersen L, Christensen JF, Hojman P. Effects of exercise on tumor physiology and metabolism. Cancer J. 2015;21:111–6.
88. Seo DY, Lee SR, Kim N, Ko KS, Rhee BD, Han J. Humanized animal exercise model for clinical implication. Pflugers Arch. 2014;466:1673–87.

89. Fernando P, Bonen A, Hoffman-Goetz L. Predicting submaximal oxygen consumption during treadmill running in mice. Can J Physiol Pharmacol. 1993;71:854–7.
90. Jones LW, Eves ND, Courneya KS, Chiu BK, Baracos VE, Hanson J, Johnson L, Mackey JR. Effects of exercise training on antitumor efficacy of doxorubicin in MDA-MB-231 breast cancer xenografts. Clin Cancer Res. 2005;11:6695–8.
91. Dominoni DM, Borniger JC, Nelson RJ. Light at night, clocks and health: from humans to wild organisms. Biol Lett. 2016;12:20160015.
92. Irwin MR. Why sleep is important for health: a psychoneuroimmunology perspective. Annu Rev Psychol. 2015;66:143–72.
93. Reiche EM, Nunes SO, Morimoto HK. Stress, depression, the immune system, and cancer. Lancet Oncol. 2004;5:617–25.
94. Thaker PH, Sood AK. Neuroendocrine influences on cancer biology. Semin Cancer Biol. 2008;18:164–70.
95. Knab AM, Bowen RS, Moore-Harrison T, Hamilton AT, Turner MJ, Lightfoot JT. Repeatability of exercise behaviors in mice. Physiol Behav. 2009;98:433–40.
96. De Bono JP, Adlam D, Paterson DJ, Channon KM. Novel quantitative phenotypes of exercise training in mouse models. Am J Physiol Regul Integr Comp Physiol. 2006;290:R926–34.
97. Goh J, Ladiges W. Voluntary wheel running in mice. Curr Protoc Mouse Biol. 2015;5:283–90.
98. Betof AS, Dewhirst MW, Jones LW. Effects and potential mechanisms of exercise training on cancer progression: a translational perspective. Brain Behav Immun. 2013;30(Suppl):S75–87.
99. Goh J, Tsai J, Bammler TK, Farin FM, Endicott E, Ladiges WC. Exercise training in transgenic mice is associated with attenuation of early breast cancer growth in a dose-dependent manner. PLoS One. 2013;8:e80123.
100. Notta VF, Aguila MB, Mandarim DELCA. High-intensity interval training (swimming) significantly improves the adverse metabolism and comorbidities in diet-induced obese mice. J Sports Med Phys Fitness. 2016;56:655–63.
101. Wu H, Jin M, Han D, Zhou M, Mei X, Guan Y, Liu C. Protective effects of aerobic swimming training on high-fat diet induced nonalcoholic fatty liver disease: regulation of lipid metabolism via PANDER-AKT pathway. Biochem Biophys Res Commun. 2015;458:862–8.
102. Zhang QB, Zhang BH, Zhang KZ, Meng XT, Jia QA, Zhang QB, Bu Y, Zhu XD, Ma DN, Ye BG, et al. Moderate swimming suppressed the growth and metastasis of the transplanted liver cancer in mice model: with reference to nervous system. Oncogene. 2016;35:4122–31.
103. de Kloet ER, Molendijk ML. Coping with the forced swim stressor: towards understanding an adaptive mechanism. Neural Plast. 2016;2016:6503162.
104. Overstreet DH. Modeling depression in animal models. Methods Mol Biol. 2012;829:125–44.
105. Pollak DD, Rey CE, Monje FJ. Rodent models in depression research: classical strategies and new directions. Ann Med. 2010;42:252–64.
106. Contarteze RV, Manchado Fde B, Gobatto CA, De Mello MA. Stress biomarkers in rats submitted to swimming and treadmill running exercises. Comp Biochem Physiol A Mol Integr Physiol. 2008;151:415–22.
107. Cholewa J, Guimaraes-Ferreira L, da Silva Teixeira T, Naimo MA, Zhi X, de Sa RB, Lodetti A, Cardozo MQ, Zanchi NE. Basic models modeling resistance training: an update for basic scientists interested in study skeletal muscle hypertrophy. J Cell Physiol. 2014;229:1148–56.
108. Lowe DA, Alway SE. Animal models for inducing muscle hypertrophy: are they relevant for clinical applications in humans? J Orthop Sports Phys Ther. 2002;32:36–43.
109. Strickland JC, Smith MA. Animal models of resistance exercise and their application to neuroscience research. J Neurosci Methods. 2016;273:191–200.
110. Mardare C, Kruger K, Liebisch G, Seimetz M, Couturier A, Ringseis R, Wilhelm J, Weissmann N, Eder K, Mooren FC. Endurance and resistance training affect high fat diet-induced increase of ceramides, inflammasome expression, and systemic inflammation in mice. J Diabetes Res. 2016;2016:4536470.

111. Morton GJ, Kaiyala KJ, Fisher JD, Ogimoto K, Schwartz MW, Wisse BE. Identification of a physiological role for leptin in the regulation of ambulatory activity and wheel running in mice. Am J Physiol Endocrinol Metab. 2011;300:E392–401.
112. Lee MC, Inoue K, Okamoto M, Liu YF, Matsui T, Yook JS, Soya H. Voluntary resistance running induces increased hippocampal neurogenesis in rats comparable to load-free running. Neurosci Lett. 2013;537:6–10.
113. Khamoui AV, Park BS, Kim DH, Yeh MC, Oh SL, Elam ML, Jo E, Arjmandi BH, Salazar G, Grant SC, et al. Aerobic and resistance training dependent skeletal muscle plasticity in the colon-26 murine model of cancer cachexia. Metabolism. 2016;65:685–98.
114. Bartling B, Al-Robaiy S, Lehnich H, Binder L, Hiebl B, Simm A. Sex-related differences in the wheel-running activity of mice decline with increasing age. Exp Gerontol. 2017;87(Pt B):139–47.
115. Kullberg J, Brandberg J, Angelhed JE, Frimmel H, Bergelin E, Strid L, Ahlstrom H, Johansson L, Lonn L. Whole-body adipose tissue analysis: comparison of MRI, CT and dual energy X-ray absorptiometry. Br J Radiol. 2009;82:123–30.
116. Naboush A, Hamdy O. Measuring visceral and hepatic fat in clinical practice and clinical research. Endocr Pract. 2013;19:587–9.
117. Brommage R. Validation and calibration of DEXA body composition in mice. Am J Physiol Endocrinol Metab. 2003;285:E454–9.
118. Chen W, Wilson JL, Khaksari M, Cowley MA, Enriori PJ. Abdominal fat analyzed by DEXA scan reflects visceral body fat and improves the phenotype description and the assessment of metabolic risk in mice. Am J Phys Endocrinol Metab. 2012;303:E635–43.
119. Judex S, Luu YK, Ozcivici E, Adler B, Lublinsky S, Rubin CT. Quantification of adiposity in small rodents using micro-CT. Methods. 2010;50:14–9.
120. Luu YK, Lublinsky S, Ozcivici E, Capilla E, Pessin JE, Rubin CT, Judex S. In vivo quantification of subcutaneous and visceral adiposity by micro-computed tomography in a small animal model. Med Eng Phys. 2009;31:34–41.
121. Calderan L, Marzola P, Nicolato E, Fabene PF, Milanese C, Bernardi P, Giordano A, Cinti S, Sbarbati A. In vivo phenotyping of the ob/ob mouse by magnetic resonance imaging and 1H-magnetic resonance spectroscopy. Obesity (Silver Spring). 2006;14:405–14.

Chapter 9
Lifestyle Interventions to Reduce the Risk of Obesity-Associated Gynecologic Malignancies: A Focus on Endometrial Cancer

Faina Linkov, Sharon L. Goughnour, Shalkar Adambekov, Robert P. Edwards, Nicole Donnellan, and Dana H. Bovbjerg

Abstract Obesity is an established risk factor for multiple cancer types, with gynecologic cancers gaining more attention in the past decade. While women with obesity may be at increased risk for ovarian and cervical cancer mortality, yet it is endometrial cancer (EC) that appears to be the most sensitive to obesity. Current adiposity, excess weight at the age of 18, metabolic syndrome, and adult weight gain are all associated with substantial increased lifetime risk of EC risk. The incidence of EC has been gradually increasing in recent years, with approximately 60,050 new cases and 10,470 deaths expected in 2016. A recent publication from our group estimates a 55% increase in the incidence of EC by 2030. Reducing the risk of EC by weight loss is an attractive strategy, as weight loss also improves cardiovascular fitness, reduces/treats type-2 diabetes, and reduces the risk of other obesity-related cancers. A variety of behavioral weight loss options are available to patients who would like to reduce their cancer risk, each with their own advantages and disadvantages. Bariatric surgery is emerging as one of the most effective weight loss options for patients for whom other options have failed. Bariatric surgery

F. Linkov (✉) • S.L. Goughnour • S. Adambekov
Magee-Womens Research Institute, University of Pittsburgh School of Medicine,
3380 Blvd of Allies, Isaly's Building, Suite 307, Pittsburgh, PA 15213, USA
e-mail: Faina.linkov@gmail.com; goughnours@mwri.magee.edu; Sha70@pitt.edu

R.P. Edwards • N. Donnellan
Magee-Womens Hospital of UPMC,
300 Halket Street, Suite 0610, Pittsburgh, PA 15213, USA
e-mail: edwarp@magee.edu; donnellann2@upmc.edu

D.H. Bovbjerg
Hillman Cancer Center, University of Pittsburgh Cancer Institute,
Shadyside Medical Building, Suite 604 & 614 5200 Centre Avenue, 5115 Centre Avenue,
Suite 140, Pittsburgh, PA 15232-1301, USA
e-mail: bovbjergdh@upmc.edu

© Springer International Publishing AG 2018
N.A. Berger et al. (eds.), *Focus on Gynecologic Malignancies*, Energy Balance
and Cancer 13, DOI 10.1007/978-3-319-63483-8_9

patients are an excellent group to explore EC risk reduction as these patients experience a very rapid weight loss in a short period of time. Counseling on obesity prevention, diet, and exercise could potentially play a big role in the prevention of EC and other malignancies.

Keywords Endometrial cancer • Ovarian cancer • Cervical cancer • Gynecologic malignancy • Obesity • Lifestyle • Prevention • Cancer biomarkers • Bariatric surgery

Background: Endometrial Cancer, Ovarian Cancer, Cervical Cancer, and Obesity

Obesity is a worldwide problem, with both developing and developed countries carrying the burden of a large percentage of their population suffering from obesity [1]. The prevalence of obesity has dramatically increased in the last few decades, reaching epidemic proportions in the US with 36.5% of US population being obese [2]. Obesity has been linked to a large number of chronic diseases such as cardiovascular disease, diabetes, and metabolic syndrome; however, the link between obesity and cancer has started to receive attention during the past two decades. While the biological mechanisms underlying the relationship between obesity and cancer are not well understood, published reports include risk factors such as metabolic and growth factors, hormone imbalance, multiple signaling pathways, as well as local and systemic inflammatory processes. Key among the signaling pathways linking obesity and cancer is the PI3K/Akt/mTOR cascade, which is a target of many of the obesity-associated factors. It is also responsible for regulating cell proliferation and survival [3].

Obesity is an established risk factor for multiple cancer types, including colon/rectal, postmenopausal, breast, endometrial, liver, kidney, esophageal, gastric, pancreatic, gallbladder, non-Hodgkin lymphoma, multiple myeloma, and aggressive forms of prostate cancer [4]. In addition, it has been associated with increased morbidity, and increased mortality from several gynecologic cancer types, including cervical, ovarian, and EC. Mortality from cervical cancer appears to be higher for obese women; however, the mechanisms responsible for this association are not well understood. Obese women, especially of European American ancestry, are 40% less likely to undergo cervical cancer screening than their normal weight counterparts, which could contribute to the higher cervical cancer mortality seen in obese white women [5–8]. However, limited screening may not be the full explanation for excess cervical cancer mortality in women with obesity, as hormonal factors may also play a role in cervical cancer development [9].

Incidence of cervical cancer can decrease in the future due to HPV vaccine guidelines implemented in the past decade [10]. These guidelines may be especially relevant for cervical cancer prevention in women with obesity. In particular, Lacey et al. suggests an influence of obesity on the risk of glandular cervical carcinoma

[11]. Based on the literature evidence suggesting that women with obesity may not be meeting recommended screenings guidelines we would like to suggest that:

- Providers need to particularly encourage women with obesity to adhere to established screening guidelines.
- Adherence to HPV vaccine administration needs to be especially encouraged and facilitated among girls and young women with obesity to prevent cervical cancer.
- Special accommodations must be made for women with obesity (and/or mobility limitations) that are unable to lift themselves onto gynecologic chairs or have other barriers to screening.
- Obese women with gynecologic symptoms, such as bleeding, need to be carefully monitored due to increased risk of endometrial cancer. Endometrial sampling through D&C may be recommended for women who cannot be sampled using Pipelle.

Ovarian cancer is the leading cause of gynecologic cancer deaths in the United States. A pooled analysis of 12 cohort studies suggested that body mass index (BMI) of 30 and over was positively associated with ovarian cancer risk in premenopausal women [12]. Recent evidence from the Ovarian Cancer Associated Consortium suggested that high BMI was associated with an increased risk of ovarian cancer for borderline serous, invasive endometrioid, and invasive mucinous tumor subtypes [13]. While obesity appears to increase risk of these less common histological subtypes of ovarian cancer, it does not increase the risk of high-grade invasive serous cancers, and reducing BMI is unlikely to prevent the majority of ovarian cancer deaths [13].

Endometrial cancer (EC) is the most common gynecologic malignancy among American women, with about 60,050 new cases expected to be diagnosed in 2016 [14]. EC incidence is on the rise with 55% increase in the incidence expected by 2030 [15]. As EC is the gynecological cancer most closely associated with obesity, the focus of this chapter will be on EC, with specific discussions highlighting the potential to reduce EC risk through lifestyle interventions (Table 9.1). Age-adjusted

Table 9.1   Which gynecologic cancers may be impacted by lifestyle interventions?

Gynecologic cancer type	Possibility of risk reduction through lifestyle intervention
Endometrial cancer (type I)	Prevention may be possible[a] through • Diet • Exercise • Bariatric surgery
Ovarian cancer	Prevention through lifestyle may not be effective, further research is warranted
Cervical cancer	Intervention may be effective for reducing excess mortality associated with avoidance of cervical cancer screening among obese women of European ancestry

[a]Assuming that significant weight loss is achieved

rates of endometrial cancer are increasing in countries undergoing transition from low- to high-income economies, with EC reported to be the sixth most common cancer in women worldwide [16]. In the context of this chapter, "EC" will be defined as Type I, obesity-associated EC, which accounts for 85–90% of all ECs [17]. Although multiple factors are involved, increasing rates of obesity are thought to be the primary driver of increasing EC incidence [18, 19]. Prospective studies indicate that EC risk increases 1.6-fold with each additional 5 kg/m^2 in BMI, reaching 9.1-fold higher risk at a BMI of 42 kg/m^2 [20]. Onstad et al. examined the association between obesity and EC, highlighting the importance of EC prevention and control in premenopausal women [21]. The international Association for Research and Cancer recently updated findings on body fatness and cancer risk and concluded that the evidence supported "a cancer-preventive effect of the absence of excess body fatness" for many different malignancies, including ovarian and uterine cancers [22]. In addition to obesity, physical inactivity, older age, polycystic ovary syndrome (PCOS), diabetes, metabolic syndrome, and smoking have been shown to be associated with EC [23–32]. Specific to reproductive factors, the risk of endometrial cancer is positively correlated with a younger age at menarche and late age at menopause, infertility, null parity, age of the first child, and long-term use of unopposed estrogens for hormone replacement therapy [33]. Protection against endometrial cancer has been detected with an increase in parity, the use of combined oral contraceptives, and increased age of women at last delivery [33]. Despite the rising incidence and mortality of EC, which coincides with the national epidemic of obesity, no prevention or screening strategy has been proven to be cost-effective. This is largely due to two primary reasons: (1) a relatively low prevalence of endometrial pathology in the asymptomatic general population, and (2) EC is usually detected at early stages due to abnormal bleeding.

EC patients often have a history of irregular or heavy menstrual bleeding prior to diagnosis, symptoms which are also common among women with obesity. In addition, women subsequently found to have EC may also present with abnormal findings during gynecologic exams and ultrasounds (e.g. endometrial thickness >4 mm, associated with EC in postmenopausal women only). In a recent publication, we indicated that increasing BMI is associated with greater risk of endometrial pathology among severely obese (BMI ≥ 35) women [34]. Ideally, it would be very beneficial to identify a systemic biomarker (or panel of biomarkers) that will be able to identify women at high risk of precancerous changes at the time when preventive interventions like weight loss or hormone therapy may still be possible. Since such biomarkers are not yet established, it is advisable to recommend lifestyle interventions to women who are considered to be at high risk for EC development either due to BMI and/or the presence of gynecologic symptoms such as irregular or heavy menstrual bleeding (for women of premenopausal age) and unexplained bleeding or spotting (for women of postmenopausal age). Such preventive strategies are especially beneficial for women with obesity.

Obesity is a growing problem in the US with over one third of adults suffering from obesity. Obesity and physical inactivity have been associated with the development of many cancers including endometrial, postmenopausal breast, and colon, among others. Counseling on obesity prevention, diet, and exercise could potentially play a big role in the prevention of obesity-associated malignancies. However, a number of studies concluded that many physicians are not prepared to provide counseling services on healthy diet, physical activity, and obesity [35, 36]. A survey study of 108 women with EC indicated that only 29% of the women reported being counseled by their health care provider about the link between obesity and EC [37]. Lack of counseling results in low level of awareness among EC patients on the link between obesity and EC. Recent survey study that included 43 women with EC or complex atypical hyperplasia reported that 46.5% of the women were unaware that obesity was a risk for EC or hyperplasia [38]. Future EC prevention efforts need to focus on increasing public awareness on the relationship between obesity and EC.

Mechanisms Linking Endometrial Cancer and Obesity

Obesity increases the risk of EC more than any other cancer [3, 39–41]. Current adiposity, excess weight at the age of 18, metabolic syndrome, and adult weight gain are all associated with substantial increased lifetime risk of EC [42–44]. Physical inactivity has also been found to be an independent risk factor associated with EC development [45]. In a sample of women undergoing hysterectomy, Ward et al. showed a linear increase in the frequency of uterine (mostly EC) cancers associated with increasing BMI [46]. We recently found that up to 20% of severely obese women scheduled for bariatric surgery show histological evidence of endometrial pathologies, including hyperplasia and endometrial polyps [47, 48], which are indicative of possible risks for EC development. Argenta et al. reported resolution of hyperplasia after bariatric surgery in a small sample of bariatric surgery patients [47].

Endometrial proliferation is driven by the cyclic expression of estrogen by the ovaries in premenopausal women and estrogen synthesis in the peripheral tissues (mostly adipose tissues) in the postmenopausal women [21]. The "unopposed estrogen hypothesis" of EC development posits that increased exposure to endogenous or exogenous estrogen that is not opposed by progesterone explains the relationship between obesity and EC risk [49–52]; however, additional factors have been implicated in EC development in recent literature.

In most cases, endometrioid adenocarcinoma of the endometrium is preceded by hyperplasia [53]. Among women with atypical endometrial hyperplasia (AEH), the risk of progression to carcinoma is approximately 30% [54]. Additionally, Trimble et al. reported that the prevalence of endometrial carcinoma in patients who had a community hospital biopsy diagnosis of AEH was high (42.6%) [55]. In recent studies, we and others have found that such preclinical changes in endometrial histology are not uncommon among severely obese women [47, 48, 56]. Accumulating evidence from preclinical research, as well as prospective studies exploring associations between biomarker levels in peripheral blood and the development of EC, strongly implicate three basic biological pathways: heightened inflammatory factors, insulin resistance/ metabolic factors, and steroid hormones (e.g., estradiol) [57–62]. For EC, it is likely that there is more than one system linking obesity and cancer predisposition [63].

Endometrial Thickness

As an additional measure of risk for postmenopausal women, endometrial thickness greater than 4 mm may be indicative of excess estrogen stimulation that is associated with increased risk of EC, estrogen-associated endometrial pathologies, as well as breast cancer [64]. Increased endometrial thickness has been associated with obesity in previous studies [65, 66]. For premenopausal women, an endometrial thickness greater than 6 mm appears to be linked to increased risk of hyperplasia [67], which in most cases precedes endometrioid adenocarcinoma of the endometrium [53]. A recent publication highlighted the importance of evaluating thickened endometria in postmenopausal asymptomatic women due to the high risk of subclinical pathology [68]. Endometrial thickness appears to be linked to a wide range of precancerous endometrial pathologies. Previously published research suggested that in patients with simple endometrial hyperplasia, the endometrium ranged from 6 to 16 mm in thickness, whereas in patients with simple endometrial hyperplasia and metaplasia, the endometrium ranged from 10 to 20 mm. In patients with complex endometrial hyperplasia, the endometrium ranged from 11 to 17 mm; in patients with complex endometrial hyperplasia with atypia, from 8 to 20 mm; and in those with endometrial metaplasia, from 5 to 12 mm [69]. Since endometrial thickness in postmenopausal women appears to be increasing with advancing progression of endometrial pathology from simple hyperplasia to complex hyperplasia with atypia, this risk factor is an important variable to be investigated in studies focusing on EC/EC-precursor risk reduction. Having a better understanding of the high-risk profile would guide the development of better tailored, individualized interventions for high-risk women that include lifestyle interventions.

Need for Investigating Endometrial Cancer Risk Markers

Literature suggests that obesity contributes to the chronic activation of one or more of the three EC risk pathways. The activation of these pathways results in the increased likelihood of preneoplastic changes in endometrial tissue, which can ultimately progress to EC. Early identification of precancerous endometrial changes will have implications for EC prevention programs (e.g., weight loss, hormone-based intervention) and alternative treatment choices for severely obese women (consistent with prevention targets identified by Hursting [70]). Availability of those options will have significant implications for morbidity, mortality, and healthcare expenditures associated with EC, potentially leading to reduction of hysterectomies. While hysterectomy is the traditional treatment for EC, several publications in the past decade suggested that hormonal treatment for EC may be effective for both managing EC and preserving the ability to achieve pregnancy in premenopausal women [71, 72].

Inflammatory Markers

Obesity is associated with a physiological state of chronic, low-grade inflammation characterized by elevated concentrations of circulating inflammatory biomarkers partially mediating the association between obesity and EC [61, 73, 74]. Excess adipose tissue mass may contribute to the development of cancer via increased secretion of pro-inflammatory cytokines and chemokines [24, 75]. A recent study found CRP, an acute-phase reactant protein associated with production of inflammatory cytokines, to be positively related to EC risk [62]. In addition, CRP, IL-6, and IL-1RA have been implicated in EC risk in several prospective investigations [24, 60–62].

Metabolic Factors

Circulating adipokines (small protein molecules produced and secreted by white adipose tissue), such as adiponectin, have systemic immunomodulating effects that have been implicated in the development of several cancers [76]. Insulin, IGFBP-2, leptin, adiponectin, and C-peptide were shown to be associated with EC development in prospective studies [60, 62, 77, 78].

Steroid Hormones

The role of unopposed estrogen in EC development has been reviewed in recent publications, highlighting the importance of increased estrogen levels through the aromatization of the androgens in adipose tissue [49, 79]. Estradiol, the most commonly measured estrogen hormone, has been linked to EC risk in prospective studies [60]. Adipocytes partly contribute to the increased production of estrogen, which is involved in dysregulated cell growth in early endometrial carcinogenesis [80]. Several circulating steroid hormones, including testosterone and sex hormone-binding globulin (SHBG), have also been linked to EC risk in prospective studies [29, 61].

Other Biomarkers

PTEN is one of the most commonly lost tumor suppressors in human EC; its expression is also altered in hyperplastic conditions suggesting a possible role in the development of EC, particularly in the transition from hyperplasia to EC [81]. Although the association between obesity and inflammation is widely recognized [82], there is little published information concerning relationships between weight loss and histological changes in the endometrium, supporting a mechanistic role for inflammation in EC. In addition, concurrent assessment of inflammatory biomarkers in blood, urine, and endometrial tissue will provide evidence as to whether circulating and local biomarker expression levels correlate. Adipose tissue hypoxia may provide cellular mechanistic explanations for chronic inflammation, macrophage infiltration, adiponectin reduction, leptin elevation, adipocyte death, and mitochondrial dysfunction in obese women, which contribute to the risk of cancer development [83]. Regulators of hypoxic responses are likely to play an important role in EC development, with activation of the transcription factor hypoxia-inducible factor 1 (HIF)-1 allowing EC to thrive under conditions of metabolic stress. These regulators of hypoxic responses are detectable in both serum and tissues [84].

Endometrial Cancer Prevention Through Weight Loss

Reducing the risk of EC by weight loss is an attractive strategy, as weight loss also improves cardiovascular fitness, reduces/treats type-2 diabetes, and reduces the risk of other obesity-related cancers [18]. A connection between physical activity and EC risk through hormonal mechanisms, possibly mediated by body weight, is biologically plausible [85]; therefore, it is also important to assess physical activity as a potential preventive strategy for EC. Although some women can effectively lose weight through exercise and diet, literature suggests that diet and exercise programs for morbidly obese individuals result in meaningful weight loss in less than 20% of program participants [86]. While literature suggests that exercise interventions may be feasible in cancer survivors [87], to our knowledge there is no literature exploring diet and exercise interventions to reverse endometrial changes associated with EC onset.

Bariatric Surgery

Recent international cancer prevention guidelines recommend weight loss, where appropriate, for the purpose of cancer risk reduction. Bariatric surgery has demonstrated long-term sustained weight loss, and as a result, patients after bariatric surgery represent an ideal population to explore the relationship between long-term, voluntary weight loss and cancer incidence [88]. The number of bariatric surgeries performed in the past two decades increased from 16,200 in 1992 to 220,000 in 2008 [86]. Bariatric operations are major gastrointestinal procedures, which alter the capacity and/or the anatomy of the digestive system, leading to weight loss. Bariatric surgery has large average effect sizes (e.g., 20–30 kg of weight loss at 1 year of follow-up, maintained for up to 10 years [89]), but entails a risk of serious complications or unpleasant side-effects such as nausea, bloating, diarrhea, and colic [90]. It is only appropriate for individuals who can safely undergo a surgical procedure, and for whom other weight loss options failed. Bariatric surgery is very expensive, although the expense is often covered by health insurance for patients with insurance coverage.

Preliminary research has demonstrated that long-term total mortality after gastric bypass surgery was significantly reduced, particularly deaths from cancer, diabetes, and heart disease [91]. In a prospective Swedish study following a cohort of bariatric surgery patients and obese controls, sustained weight loss was associated with a 38% reduction of cancer incidence in women [92]. In another prospective study, a 24% reduction in incident cancers was seen amongst 6596 women undergoing bariatric surgery in comparison with controls over a 12.5 year follow up period [93]. The most impressive reduction in cancer risk was seen for EC with a sevenfold risk reduction [93]. Taken together, these observations provide proof of principle that EC is preventable through weight loss [18], but the mechanism(s) of risk reduction in the uterus/endometrium have received little research attention.

With the increased numbers of centers performing bariatric surgeries, morbidly obese individuals who cannot lose weight through traditional means resort to this option for reducing their risk of diabetes and other obesity-associated conditions. Previous research demonstrated that even a weight loss of only 5–10% of total weight can provide health benefits [8]. Parker et al. examined the effect of intentional weight loss and found that women who experienced intentional weight loss of 20 or more pounds and were not currently overweight had cancer rates at the level of non-overweight women [11].

Emerging literature suggests that the risk of EC may be particularly responsive to weight loss [18, 19]. Ward et al. recently demonstrated in a large scale study that a history of bariatric surgery is associated with a 71% overall reduced risk for uterine malignancy [94]. A reduction in the incidence of endometrial hyperplasias, which typically precede EC, has also been reported in recent pilot investigations of bariatric surgery patients [47, 48, 94].

Physical Activity

In the United States, inactivity is a serious problem, where in some states (e.g., Alabama, Arkansas, and Mississippi) over 30% of the population does not participate in leisure-time physical activity [95]. Twenty-six percent of adults in Pennsylvania responding to a survey in 2010 indicated that they did not participate in any leisure-time physical activity during the past month [96]. Results of most epidemiological and laboratory studies suggest an inverse relationship between regular exercise and the risk of certain malignancies, such as intestinal, colon, pancreatic, breast, lung, skin, mammary, endometrial, and prostate cancer [97]. High BMI and physical inactivity appear to be strong and independent risk factors for endometrial cancer [98]. Findings from a Swedish mammography cohort suggest that total physical activity has a weak but inverse association with EC risk; however, leisure-time inactivity has a statistically significant association with increased risk for EC [85]. Light and moderate physical activity including daily life activities were associated with lower EC risk (RR = 0.67, 95% CI 0.44–1.03) in the American Cancer Society Cancer Prevention Study II Nutrition Cohort, especially among women who are overweight or obese [99]. Further, preliminary evidence indicates that exercise has a positive effect on the inflammatory biomarkers [100, 101] that have been implicated in cancer development.

A recent systematic review and meta-analysis suggested that recreational physical activity, occupational physical activity, and walking/biking for transportation are related to decreased EC risk [102]. Physical activity seems to be associated with a reduction in the risk of EC independent of body weight [103], especially for those who exercised in adulthood [104].

Myriad of Weight Loss Options: Obese Individuals Need Help in Deciding What Intervention is Best for Them

A variety of weight loss options are available to obese individuals, each with their own advantages and disadvantages. For those who attempt to lose weight through commercial dietary programs, one of the most well-known programs is Weight Watchers® [105]. Weight Watchers® core approach is to assist members to form helpful habits, eat smarter, get more exercise, and have more social support. In a recent prospective study, several other commercial weight loss programs were compared to Weight Watchers® and it was found that most commercial programs result in similar weight loss [106]. In addition to commercial programs, healthy living websites, such as "SparkPeople.com" are gaining popularity [107]. Digital mobile tools can also be helpful for promoting behavior change and weight loss [108]. Behavioral programs attract attention of women who are trying to lose weight. One such intervention, the Diabetes Prevention Program's lifestyle intervention, has been shown to be a cost-effective in research settings [109, 110], and to promote weight loss in community settings for diverse populations [111]. Intensive behavioral programs have modest clinically significant weight loss results, but are sometimes limited by the common phenomenon of weight regain or decreasing program adherence over time.

There are several key issues patients should consider when deciding whether to pursue a lifestyle change. Behavioral programs promoting moderate physical activity and a low-calorie diet have, on average, small yet clinically significant effect sizes (e.g., 3–5 kg at 1 year of follow-up) [112]. These results reflect low levels of intervention adherence [113], with higher levels of adherence shown to be associated with greater weight loss. In addition to just weight loss, evidence-based behavioral weight loss programs can lead to improved physical functioning [114, 115] and entail minimal risk. Improving physical activity for the purpose of weight loss can also provide additional positive health benefits in areas such as increased bone strength and decreased depressive symptoms [116, 117]. However, sustained behavior change requires a difficult and long-term commitment from patients, and the cost of behavioral intervention programs is frequently not covered by health insurance.

Diet

Healthy nutrition is a part of the "CDC's National Prevention Strategy: America's Plan for Better Health and Wellness" [118]. The CDC also suggests that a person's cancer risk can be reduced by eating a diet rich in fruits and vegetables, maintaining a healthy weight, and being physically active [119]. Epidemiological studies suggest that dietary intake of certain vegetables (e.g., cruciferous vegetables) may be protective against the risk of different types of cancers. There is epidemiological, laboratory, and some clinical evidence that certain dietary factors play a role in either promoting or inhibiting cancer development [120]. For example, salt and salted food intake is associated with gastric cancer, while physical activity is protective. A large number of studies identify nutrition and physical activity as key targets for cancer prevention [121–127].

Over the past decade, research on dietary risk factors associated with endometrial cancer development has received attention. However, research publications on the link between EC and dietary factors are limited and inconsistent, with data from large cohort studies becoming available only recently. Nagle et al. reported that diets with high glycemic load significantly increase the risk of EC development [128]. Preliminary evidence was published in a case-control study of 168 cases of EC patients and 334 controls, which demonstrated that more frequent consumption of several vegetables and certain dairy products was associated with a statistically significant decreased risk of EC [129]. Another case control study reported that foods high in fat and cholesterol, such as red meat, margarine, and eggs, were positively associated with EC, whereas cereals, legumes, vegetables, and fruits, particularly those high in lutein, were inversely associated [129]. However, the role of vegetables remains controversial, as it has been suggested that a diet characterized by high fat consumption increased risk, regardless of fruit and vegetable consumption (OR = 1.4, 95% CI: 0.97–2.1 for high fat, low fruit/vegetable intake and OR = 1.4, 95% CI: 0.95–2.1 for high fat, high fruit/vegetable intake compared to low fat, high fruit/vegetable intake [130]).

In addition to exploring large groupings of foods, there is an interest in what specific dietary elements may offer protection or be risk factors for EC development. One study suggested that risk for EC was reduced for women in the highest quartiles of intake of protein (OR 0.4, 95% CI: 0.2–0.9), dietary fiber (OR 0.5, 95% CI: 0.3–1.0), phytosterols (OR 0.6, 95% CI: 0.3–1.0), vitamin C (OR 0.5, 95% CI: 0.3–0.8), folate (OR 0.4, 95% CI: 0.2–0.7), alpha-carotene (OR 0.6, 95% CI: 0.4–1.0), beta-carotene (OR 0.4, 95% CI: 0.2–0.6), lycopene (OR 0.6, 95% CI: 0.4–1.0), lutein + zeaxanthin

(OR 0.3, 95% CI: 0.2–0.5) and vegetables (OR 0.5, 95% CI: 0.3–0.9), but unrelated to energy (OR 0.9, 95% CI: 0.6–1.5) or fat (OR 1.6, 95% CI: 0.7–3.4) [131].

While original data linking dietary patterns and EC has been limited to case-control studies, data from large scale cohort studies became available in the past few years. Specifically, pooled data from three case-control studies provided evidence for a beneficial role of the Mediterranean diet on EC risk, suggesting a favorable effect of a combination of foods rich in antioxidants, dietary fiber, phytochemicals, and unsaturated fatty acids [132]. Merritt et al. evaluated the EC risk associations for dietary intake of 84 foods and nutrients in three prospective studies, the European Prospective Investigation into Cancer and Nutrition (EPIC; N = 1303 cases) followed by validation of nine foods/nutrients (FDR $\leq$ 0.10) in the Nurses' Health Studies (NHS/NHSII; N = 1531 cases). Eight other dietary factors that were associated with EC risk in the EPIC study (total fat, monounsaturated fat, carbohydrates, phosphorus, butter, yogurt, cheese, and potatoes) were not confirmed in the NHS/NHSII. This study suggested that coffee intake may be inversely associated with EC risk [133]. A recent large meta-analysis suggested that increased coffee intake is associated with a reduced risk of EC, and was consistently observed for both cohort and case–control studies [134].

Ollberding et al. suggested that a greater consumption of isoflavone-containing foods is associated with a reduced risk of EC in postmenopausal women [135]. Animal and laboratory studies suggest that long-chain omega-3 (n-3) fatty acids, a type of polyunsaturated fat found in fatty fish, may protect against carcinogenesis, but human studies on dietary intake of polyunsaturated fats and fish with EC risk show mixed results. A case-control study published by Arem et al. suggested that dietary intake of the long-chain polyunsaturated fatty acids EPA and DHA in foods and supplements may have protective associations against the development of EC [136].

Consumption of dairy products also received attention as a risk factor for EC, as it has been suggested that dairy products contain estrogenic compounds that have been implicated in EC development. The association between dairy consumption and EC risk has been investigated in a prospective cohort study with 68,019 female participants in the Nurses' Health Study. Milk and dairy consumption were assessed in 1980, 1984, 1986, 1990, 1994, 1998, and 2002 as servings per day and the follow-up continued through 2006. The association between total dairy intake and EC was significant only among the postmenopausal women (for $\geq$3 svg/day RR = 1.41, 95% CI = 1.01–1.98, p for trend = 0.02) and was evident only among those who were not currently using hormone therapy (RR = 1.58, 95% CI = 1.05–2.36, p for trend = 0.003) [137].

The link between diet and EC deserves further investigation, especially with recent report from Women's Health Initiative and other investigations showing that quality of diet had no impact on EC development or risk [138, 139]. It is possible that EC cannot be prevented through diet modification, unless such diet modification leads to significant weight loss.

Weight Loss Effect on Cancer-Associated Biomarkers

The pro-inflammatory state associated with obesity is thought to play a major role in endothelial cell activation in severely obese individuals [140]. Previous studies demonstrate that long-term weight loss after bariatric surgery is accompanied by a decreased pro-inflammatory state [140]. Bariatric surgery was associated with reduced cancer incidence in obese women in a large scale Swedish investigation [92]. A cancer registry-based study in Utah demonstrated that gastric bypass results in lower cancer risk, supporting recommendations for reducing weight to lower cancer risk [93]. Christou et al. [141] reported that the physician/hospital visits for common cancers such as breast cancer were significantly reduced in the bariatric surgery group; while for all other cancers, the physician/hospital visits showed a trend toward lower risk in the surgery group for all other cancers; however, this was not statistically significant due to low frequency. Similar changes in biomarkers can be achieved with behavioral weight loss interventions [142].

Disparities in the Areas of EC and Circulating Biomarkers: African American and European American Women

An area that has not yet been investigated is the possible difference between African American (AA) and European American (EA) women with regard to EC risk biomarkers or precancerous histological changes in the endometrium. AA women have a 2–2.5 times higher mortality rate from EC than EA women [143, 144]. Oliver et al. reported that AA women have higher grade and stage tumors, with more aggressive histology, suggesting that exploration of possible mechanisms for EC prevention is especially relevant in AA women [145]. Such differences in tumor characteristics also support the possibility of differences in etiological pathways.

It is particularly important to compare biomarker levels between AA and EA women, as AA women have been shown generally to have higher concentrations of inflammatory markers, such as CRP [146] and adipokines, that are not entirely explained by BMI [147]. Demographic and experiential variables may be involved. For example, early life adversity was reported to be predictive of high concentrations of inflammatory markers at midlife for AA women [148]. Higher levels of depressive symptoms associated with obesity are also increasingly recognized to be associated with heightened levels of inflammatory markers [149], which could be another contributor to racial differences among women.

AA women generally have higher rates of obesity and physical inactivity [150], both risk factors for EC development. Previous work published by Park et al. suggests that AA women gain a larger amount of weight in adulthood in comparison to EA women and that they show an increased risk of EC only after reaching a BMI ≥ 42.80 kg/m^2 [151]. However, the literature suggests that the incidence of EC may be underestimated in AA women [152].

Surprisingly, cancer incidence data show no significant differences between AA and EA women with regard to the incidence of EC as reported by national databases

[153]. The similar incidence, despite higher levels of obesity in AA women, could, in part, be due to the underreporting of EC for AA women. However, there is also evidence that AA women may be less sensitive to the negative effects of increasing adiposity on the risk of EC [151], which could reflect qualitative or quantitative differences in the relationships between obesity and EC risk biomarkers in AA women. Behavioral interventions for EC prevention may need to be differentially tailored for AA and EA women.

Survivorship

Population-based epidemiological data indicates that 72% of EC survivors are overweight or obese [154], and do not adopt healthier lifestyles after diagnoses. Obesity increases all cause and EC-specific mortality risk after an EC diagnosis [155, 156], with the majority of these mortality outcomes associated with the extent of obesity. Interventions to reduce weight may improve EC survival [155], as EC is the first obesity-associated morbidity that many women develop, before more chronic and difficult-to-treat conditions occur such as diabetes or heart disease. EC diagnosis is an important marker for the adverse effects of obesity that may effectively be harnessed as a teachable moment to educate patients about prevention of other future morbidities associated with obesity. As noted by McBride et al. [157], the phrase "teachable moment" has been used in the behavioral science literature to describe naturally occurring life transitions or health events that have the potential to motivate individuals to spontaneously adopt risk-reducing or health-protective behaviors. This teachable moment can potentially be used to encourage adoption of a more holistic approach for weight control during survivorship. Considering high obesity rates among EC survivors, incorporating lifestyle changes into their daily lives is very important for this segment of population [158]. Thus lifestyle interventions may not only improve the overall health of these survivors, but may also improve survival and reduce mortality from obesity-associated causes. These interventions may include improving physical activity, losing excess weight, and eating a well-balanced diet. The two published randomized controlled trials evaluating weight loss interventions in EC survivors confirm that recruitment of EC survivors to such interventions is possible [159, 160].

Future Direction: Prevention Counseling

Physician Preparedness in the Area of Cancer Prevention Counseling

Cancer is a growing problem in the US, especially for malignancies associated with excess weight, such as EC. Based on the magnitude of the health problems and our ability to make significant progress in improving outcomes, the Centers for Disease Control and Prevention (CDC) has identified obesity, nutrition, and physical activity as "winnable battles" [161]. It is our belief that with additional effort and support for improving education and counseling skills for obesity, physical activity, and nutrition among healthcare providers (especially early in their career), we will have a significant impact on our nation's health. Preliminary studies of residents, fellows, and physicians managing populations at high risk for cancer development suggest that physicians in training may not receive adequate education in the management of obesity, nutrition, and healthy lifestyles, and may be unprepared to discuss issues related to cancer prevention through risk factor reduction with their patients [162–164].

A number of observers have concluded that many physicians are not well prepared to provide services and manage conditions such as dietary counseling, obesity, and physical activity. Rates of preventive counseling remain below national guidelines. Risk behavior topics were brought up more often for mammography (90%) and smoking (79%) compared to diet (56%) [165]. In the area of cardiovascular disease (CVD), previous research found low counseling rates for CVD prevention, particularly in the areas of diet, exercise, and weight loss among residents and fellows [166], with obesity being the least covered area by physicians' counseling. In previous research, attitudinal survey and knowledge test scores from control PGY-3 residents generally confirmed that their knowledge and counseling skills on obesity prevention and management were well below expectation [167]. Behavioral counseling interventions for nutrition, physical activity, and obesity among primary care patients could be very effective component of a public health approach to reduce the risk of cancer. Patients look to their physician for guidance in disease prevention; however, physicians, especially residents, need to be prepared to provide such services. In the area of nutritional counseling for cancer prevention, it has been reported that physicians who: (a) reported consistently avoiding dietary fat, (b) were more confident in their diet counseling abilities, and (c) were sole owners of their practice were more likely to counsel their patients than physicians who were employees or part owners of the practice [168]. One of the most comprehensive papers in the area of resident readiness to provide preventive services has been published by Blumenthal et al. [169], and suggests that we need to investigate opportunities in improvement of resident training. In a comprehensive multimedia program designed to improve medical students counseling skills in the area of nutrition; however, most students reported that they would not use the program unless it was required that they do so [170].

Counseling on lifestyle factors involves a significant amount of behavior change which physicians may be ill prepared to deliver within the constraints of a short primary care visit. Time constraints limit the ability of physicians to comply with preventive services recommendations [171]. Curricular deficits, in addition to lack of time and administrative barriers, add to the problem. A survey of residency program directors identified deficits in formal childhood obesity curriculum [172]. Despite solid knowledge of the comorbid conditions associated with obesity, residents have a poor grasp of the tools necessary to identify obesity and even fewer skills required for behavioral intervention for prevention. They also have negative opinions about their skills for treating obese patients [173]. Overall, physicians completing residencies in adult primary care did not feel very well prepared to counsel patients about preventive and psychological issues [174]. In previous studies, adding curricula on cancer prevention for residents and nurses improved adherence to cancer prevention counseling recommendations. Specifically, availability of training and tools for residents and community pediatricians improved providers' confidence, ease, and frequency of obesity-related counseling [175].

Future Directions: EC Prevention Guidelines Development?

Various well-known cancer organizations and foundations are actively disseminating nutrition and physical activity cancer prevention recommendations. Thomson et al. recently reported that behaviors concordant with Nutrition and Physical Activity Cancer Prevention Guidelines in the US were associated with lower risk of total, breast, and colorectal cancers, and lower cancer-specific mortality in postmenopausal women [176]. Results from the European Prospective Investigation into Cancer and Nutrition (EPIC) study suggested that adherence to the World Cancer Research Fund (WCRF) and the American Institute of Cancer Research (AICR) recommendations for cancer prevention may lower the risk of developing most types of cancer [177]. In the Cancer Prevention II Nutrition Cohort, adherence to cancer prevention guidelines for obesity, diet, physical activity, and alcohol consumption was associated with lower risk of death from cancer, CVD, and all causes among nonsmokers [178]. These recommendations do not specifically focus on EC, which is a topic on which future policy and cancer prevention research could productively focus. In addition to diet and physical activity, it appears that additional programs, such as bariatric surgery, could be effective in EC risk reduction.

References

1. WHO obesity and overweight 2016. http://www.who.int/mediacentre/factsheets/fs311/en/. Accessed 7 Nov 2016.
2. Centers for Disease Control and Prevention. Adult obesity facts. https://www.cdc.gov/obesity/data/adult.html. Accessed 7 Nov 2016.
3. Vucenik I, Stains JP. Obesity and cancer risk: evidence, mechanisms, and recommendations. Ann N Y Acad Sci. 2012;1271:37–43. Epub 2012/10/12. doi:10.1111/j.1749-6632.2012.06750.x. PubMed PMID: 23050962; PMCID: PMC3476838
4. ACS. Does body weight affect cancer risk? 2016. http://www.cancer.org/cancer/cancer-causes/dietandphysicalactivity/bodyweightandcancerrisk/body-weight-and-cancer-risk-effects. Accessed 8 Nov 2016.
5. Maruthur NM, Bolen SD, Brancati FL, Clark JM. The association of obesity and cervical cancer screening: a systematic review and meta-analysis. Obesity. 2009;17(2):375–81. Epub 2008/11/11. doi:10.1038/oby.2008.480. PubMed PMID: 18997682; PMCID: PMC3008358

6. Fontaine KR, Faith MS, Allison DB, Cheskin LJ. Body weight and health care among women in the general population. Arch Fam Med. 1998;7(4):381–4. Epub 1998/07/31. PubMed PMID: 9682694

7. Adams CH, Smith NJ, Wilbur DC, Grady KE. The relationship of obesity to the frequency of pelvic examinations: do physician and patient attitudes make a difference? Women Health. 1993;20(2):45–57. Epub 1993/01/01. doi:10.1300/J013v20n02_04. PubMed PMID: 8372479

8. Aldrich T, Hackley B. The impact of obesity on gynecologic cancer screening: an integrative literature review. J Midwifery Womens Health. 2010;55(4):344–56. Epub 2010/07/16. doi:10.1016/j.jmwh.2009.10.001. PubMed PMID: 20630361

9. Ursin G, Pike MC, Preston-Martin S, d'Ablaing G 3rd, Peters RK. Sexual, reproductive, and other risk factors for adenocarcinoma of the cervix: results from a population-based case-control study (California, United States). Cancer Causes Control. 1996;7(3):391–401. Epub 1996/05/01. PubMed PMID: 8734834

10. Saslow D, Castle PE, Cox JT, Davey DD, Einstein MH, Ferris DG, Goldie SJ, Harper DM, Kinney W, Moscicki AB, Noller KL, Wheeler CM, Ades T, Andrews KS, Doroshenk MK, Kahn KG, Schmidt C, Shafey O, Smith RA, Partridge EE, Garcia F. American Cancer Society guideline for human papillomavirus (HPV) vaccine use to prevent cervical cancer and its precursors. CA Cancer J Clin. 2007;57(1):7–28. Epub 2007/01/24. PubMed PMID: 17237032.

11. Lacey JV Jr, Swanson CA, Brinton LA, Altekruse SF, Barnes WA, Gravitt PE, Greenberg MD, Hadjimichael OC, McGowan L, Mortel R, Schwartz PE, Kurman RJ, Hildesheim A. Obesity as a potential risk factor for adenocarcinomas and squamous cell carcinomas of the uterine cervix. Cancer. 2003;98(4):814–21. Epub 2003/08/12. doi:10.1002/cncr.11567. PubMed PMID: 12910527

12. Schouten LJ, Rivera C, Hunter DJ, Spiegelman D, Adami HO, Arslan A, Beeson WL, van den Brandt PA, Buring JE, Folsom AR, Fraser GE, Freudenheim JL, Goldbohm RA, Hankinson SE, Lacey JV Jr, Leitzmann M, Lukanova A, Marshall JR, Miller AB, Patel AV, Rodriguez C, Rohan TE, Ross JA, Wolk A, Zhang SM, Smith-Warner SA. Height, body mass index, and ovarian cancer: a pooled analysis of 12 cohort studies. Cancer Epidemiol Biomark Prev. 2008;17(4):902–12. Epub 2008/04/03. doi:10.1158/1055-9965.epi-07-2524. PubMed PMID: 18381473; PMCID: PMC2572258

13. Olsen CM, Nagle CM, Whiteman DC, Ness R, Pearce CL, Pike MC, Rossing MA, Terry KL, Wu AH, Risch HA, Yu H, Doherty JA, Chang-Claude J, Hein R, Nickels S, Wang-Gohrke S, Goodman MT, Carney ME, Matsuno RK, Lurie G, Moysich K, Kjaer SK, Jensen A, Hogdall E, Goode EL, Fridley BL, Vierkant RA, Larson MC, Schildkraut J, Hoyo C, Moorman P, Weber RP, Cramer DW, Vitonis AF, Bandera EV, Olson SH, Rodriguez-Rodriguez L, King M, Brinton LA, Yang H, Garcia-Closas M, Lissowska J, Anton-Culver H, Ziogas A, Gayther SA, Ramus SJ, Menon U, Gentry-Maharaj A, Webb PM. Obesity and risk of ovarian cancer subtypes: evidence from the Ovarian Cancer Association Consortium. Endocr Relat Cancer. 2013;20(2):251–62. Epub 2013/02/14. doi:10.1530/erc-12-0395. PubMed PMID: 23404857; PMCID: PMC3857135

14. Key statistics for endometrial cancer 2016. http://www.cancer.org/cancer/endometrialcancer/detailedguide/endometrial-uterine-cancer-key-statistics. Accessed 2 Dec 2016.

15. Sheikh MA, Althouse AD, Freese KE, Soisson S, Edwards RP, Welburn S, Sukumvanich P, Comerci J, Kelley J, LaPorte RE, Linkov F. USA endometrial cancer projections to 2030: should we be concerned? Future Oncol. 2014;10(16):2561–8. Epub 2014/12/23. doi:10.2217/fon.14.192. PubMed PMID: 25531045.

16. World Cancer Research Fund/American Institute for Cancer Research. 2013. http://wcrf.org/sites/default/files/Endometrial-Cancer-2013-Report.pdf. Accessed 2 Dec 2016.

17. Felix AS, Weissfeld JL, Stone RA, Bowser R, Chivukula M, Edwards RP, Linkov F. Factors associated with type I and type II endometrial cancer. Cancer Causes Control. 2010;21(11):1851–6. Epub 2010/07/16. doi:10.1007/s10552-010-9612-8. PubMed PMID: 20628804; PMCID: Pmc2962676

18. Mackintosh ML, Crosbie EJ. Obesity-driven endometrial cancer: is weight loss the answer? BJOG. 2013;120(7):791–4. Epub 2013/05/11. doi:10.1111/1471-0528.12106. PubMed PMID: 23659328

19. Schmandt RE, Iglesias DA, Co NN, Lu KH. Understanding obesity and endometrial cancer risk: opportunities for prevention. Am J Obstetr Gynecol. 2011;205(6):518–25. Epub 2011/08/02. doi:S0002-9378(11)00727-7 [pii] 10.1016/j.ajog.2011.05.042. PubMed PMID: 21802066

20. Renehan AG, Tyson M, Egger M, Heller RF, Zwahlen M. Body-mass index and incidence of cancer: a systematic review and meta-analysis of prospective observational studies. Lancet. 2008;371(9612):569–78. Epub 2008/02/19. doi:10.1016/s0140-6736(08)60269-x. PubMed PMID: 18280327

21. Onstad MA, Schmandt RE, Lu KH. Addressing the role of obesity in endometrial cancer risk, prevention, and treatment. J Clin Oncol. 2016;34(35):4225–30. Epub 2016/12/03. PubMed PMID: 27903150

22. Lauby-Secretan B, Scoccianti C, Loomis D, Grosse Y, Bianchini F, Straif K. Body fatness and cancer—viewpoint of the IARC Working Group. N Engl J Med. 2016;375(8):794–8. Epub 2016/08/25. doi:10.1056/NEJMsr1606602. PubMed PMID: 27557308

23. Modugno F, Ness RB, Chen C, Weiss NS. Inflammation and endometrial cancer: a hypothesis. Cancer Epidemiol Biomark Prev. 2005;14(12):2840–7. doi:10.1158/1055-9965.EPI-05-0493. PubMed PMID: 16364998

24. Friedenreich CM, Langley AR, Speidel TP, Lau DC, Courneya KS, Csizmadi I, Magliocco AM, Yasui Y, Cook LS. Case-control study of inflammatory markers and the risk of endometrial cancer. Eur J Cancer Prev. 2013;22(4):374–9. Epub 2013/05/25. doi:10.1097/CEJ.0b013e32835b3813. PubMed PMID: 23702681

25. Friedenreich CM, Cook LS, Magliocco AM, Duggan MA, Courneya KS. Case-control study of lifetime total physical activity and endometrial cancer risk. Cancer Causes Control. 2010;21(7):1105–16. doi:10.1007/s10552-010-9538-1. PubMed PMID: 20336482; PMCID: 2883088

26. Lambe M, Wuu J, Weiderpass E, Hsieh CC. Childbearing at older age and endometrial cancer risk (Sweden). Cancer Causes Control. 1999;10(1):43–9. PubMed PMID: 10334641

27. Friberg E, Mantzoros CS, Wolk A. Diabetes and risk of endometrial cancer: a population-based prospective cohort study. Cancer Epidemiol Biomark Prev. 2007;16(2):276–80. Epub 2007/02/16. doi:16/2/276 [pii]. 10.1158/1055-9965.EPI-06-0751. PubMed: 17301260

28. Shoff SM, Newcomb PA. Diabetes, body size, and risk of endometrial cancer. Am J Epidemiol. 1998;148(3):234–40. Epub 1998/08/05. PubMed PMID: 9690359

29. Allen NE, Key TJ, Dossus L, Rinaldi S, Cust A, Lukanova A, Peeters PH, Onland-Moret NC, Lahmann PH, Berrino F, Panico S, Larranaga N, Pera G, Tormo MJ, Sanchez MJ, Ramon Quiros J, Ardanaz E, Tjonneland A, Olsen A, Chang-Claude J, Linseisen J, Schulz M, Boeing H, Lundin E, Palli D, Overvad K, Clavel-Chapelon F, Boutron-Ruault MC, Bingham S, Khaw KT, Bueno-de-Mesquita HB, Trichopoulou A, Trichopoulos D, Naska A, Tumino R, Riboli E, Kaaks R. Endogenous sex hormones and endometrial cancer risk in women in the European Prospective Investigation into Cancer and Nutrition (EPIC). Endocr Relat Cancer. 2008;15(2):485–97. Epub 2008/05/30. doi:10.1677/erc-07-0064. PubMed PMID: 18509001; PMCID: PMC2396334

30. Parazzini F, La Vecchia C, Moroni S, Chatenoud L, Ricci E. Family history and the risk of endometrial cancer. Int J Cancer 1994;59(4):460–462. PubMed.

31. Rosato V, Zucchetto A, Bosetti C, Dal Maso L, Montella M, Pelucchi C, Negri E, Franceschi S, La Vecchia C. Metabolic syndrome and endometrial cancer risk. Ann Oncol. 2011;22(4):884–9. Epub 2010/10/13. doi:mdq464 [pii] 10.1093/annonc/mdq464. PubMed PMID: 20937645

32. Stanford JL, Brinton LA, Berman ML, Mortel R, Twiggs LB, Barrett RJ, Wilbanks GD, Hoover RN. Oral contraceptives and endometrial cancer: do other risk factors modify the association? Int J Cancer. 1993;54(2):243–8. Epub 1993/05/08. PubMed PMID: 8486426

33. Ali AT. Reproductive factors and the risk of endometrial cancer. Int J Gynecol Cancer. 2014;24(3):384–93. Epub 2014/01/28. doi:10.1097/igc.0000000000000075. PubMed PMID: 24463639
34. Kaiyrlykyzy FK, Elishaev E, Bovbjerg DH, Ramanathan R, Hamad G, McCloskey C, Althouse A, Huang M, Edwards RP, Linkov F. Endometrial histology in severely obese bariatric surgery candidates: an exploratory analysis. Surg Obes Relat Dis. 2015;11(3):653–8.
35. Huang J, Yu H, Marin E, Brock S, Carden D, Davis T. Physicians' weight loss counseling in two public hospital primary care clinics. Acad Med. 2004;79(2):156–61. Epub 2004/01/28. PubMed PMID: 14744717
36. Smith S, Seeholzer EL, Gullett H, Jackson B, Antognoli E, Krejci SA, Flocke SA. Primary care residents' knowledge, attitudes, self-efficacy, and perceived professional norms regarding obesity, nutrition, and physical activity counseling. J Grad Med Educ. 2015;7(3):388–94. Epub 2015/10/13. doi:10.4300/jgme-d-14-00710.1. PubMed PMID: 26457144; PMCID: PMC4597949
37. Clark LH, Ko EM, Kernodle A, Harris A, Moore DT, Gehrig PA, Bae-Jump V. Endometrial cancer survivors' perceptions of provider obesity counseling and attempted behavior change: are we seizing the moment? Int J Gynecol Cancer. 2016;26(2):318–24. Epub 2015/11/21. doi:10.1097/igc.0000000000000596. PubMed PMID: 26588234
38. Beavis AL, Cheema S, Holschneider CH, Duffy EL, Amneus MW. Almost half of women with endometrial cancer or hyperplasia do not know that obesity affects their cancer risk. Gynecol Oncol Rep. 2015;13:71–5. Epub 2015/10/02. doi:10.1016/j.gore.2015.07.002. PubMed PMID: 26425728; PMCID: PMC4563798
39. Wang D, Dubois RN. Associations between obesity and cancer: the role of fatty acid synthase. J Natl Cancer Inst. 2012;104(5):343–5. Epub 2012/02/09. doi:djs010 [pii] 10.1093/jnci/djs010. PubMed PMID: 22312133; PMCID: 3295747
40. Wang D, Zheng W, Wang SM, Wang JB, Wei WQ, Liang H, Qiao YL, Boffetta P. Estimation of cancer incidence and mortality attributable to overweight, obesity, and physical inactivity in China. Nutr Cancer. 2012;64(1):48–56. Epub 2011/12/06. doi:10.1080/01635581.2012.63 0166. PubMed PMID: 22136606
41. Calle EE, Rodriguez C, Walker-Thurmond K, Thun MJ. Overweight, obesity, and mortality from cancer in a prospectively studied cohort of U.S. adults. N Engl J Med 2003;348(17):1625–1638. doi:10.1056/NEJMoa021423. PubMed.
42. Chang SC, Lacey JV Jr, Brinton LA, Hartge P, Adams K, Mouw T, Carroll L, Hollenbeck A, Schatzkin A, Leitzmann MF. Lifetime weight history and endometrial cancer risk by type of menopausal hormone use in the NIH-AARP diet and health study. Cancer Epidemiol Biomark Prev. 2007;16(4):723–30. PubMed PMID: 17416763
43. Stevens VL, Jacobs EJ, Patel AV, Sun J, Gapstur SM, McCullough ML. Body weight in early adulthood, adult weight gain, and risk of endometrial cancer in women not using postmenopausal hormones. Cancer Causes Control. 2014;25(3):321–8. doi:10.1007/s10552-013-0333-7. PubMed PMID: 24381074
44. Esposito K, Chiodini P, Capuano A, Bellastella G, Maiorino MI, Giugliano D. Metabolic syndrome and endometrial cancer: a meta-analysis. Endocrine. 2014;45(1):28–36. doi:10.1007/s12020-013-9973-3. PubMed PMID: 23640372
45. Schouten LJ, Goldbohm RA, van den Brandt PA. Anthropometry, physical activity, and endometrial cancer risk: results from the Netherlands cohort study. Int J Gynecol Cancer. 2006;16(Suppl 2):492. doi:10.1111/j.1525-1438.2006.00676.x. PubMed PMID: 17010052
46. Ward KK, Roncancio AM, Shah NR, Davis MA, Saenz CC, McHale MT, Plaxe SC. The risk of uterine malignancy is linearly associated with body mass index in a cohort of US women. Am J Obstet Gynecol. 2013;209(6):579 e1–5. doi:10.1016/j.ajog.2013.08.007. PubMed PMID: 23938608
47. Argenta PA, Kassing M, Truskinovsky AM, Svendsen CA. Bariatric surgery and endometrial pathology in asymptomatic morbidly obese women: a prospective, pilot study. BJOG. 2013;120(7):795–800. Epub 2012/12/13. doi:10.1111/1471-0528.12100. PubMed PMID: 23231632

48. Argenta P, Svendsen C, Elishaev E, Gloyeske N, Geller MA, Edwards R, Linkov F. Hormone receptor expression patterns in teh endometrium of asymptomatic morbidly obese women before and after bariatric surgery. Gynecol Oncol. 2014;133(1):78–82.
49. Ziel HK. Estrogen's role in endometrial cancer. Obstet Gynecol. 1982;60(4):509–15. Epub 1982/10/01. PubMed PMID: 7121937
50. Key TJ, Pike MC. The dose-effect relationship between 'unopposed' oestrogens and endometrial mitotic rate: its central role in explaining and predicting endometrial cancer risk. Br J Cancer. 1988;57(2):205–12. Epub 1988/02/01. PubMed PMID: 3358913; PMCID: 2246441
51. Judd HL, Davidson BJ, Frumar AM, Shamonki IM, Lagasse LD, Ballon SC. Serum androgens and estrogens in postmenopausal women with and without endometrial cancer. Am J Obstet Gynecol. 1980;136(7):859–71. Epub 1980/04/01. PubMed PMID: 7361834
52. Gambrell RD Jr, Bagnell CA, Greenblatt RB. Role of estrogens and progesterone in the etiology and prevention of endometrial cancer: review. Am J Obstet Gynecol. 1983;146(6):696–707. Epub 1983/07/15. PubMed PMID: 6307050
53. Horn LC, Schnurrbusch U, Bilek K, Hentschel B, Einenkel J. Risk of progression in complex and atypical endometrial hyperplasia: clinicopathologic analysis in cases with and without progestogen treatment. Int J Gynecol Cancer. 2004;14(2):348–53. doi:10.1111/j.1048-891x.2004.014220.x. PubMed PMID: 15086736
54. Lacey JV Jr, Chia VM. Endometrial hyperplasia and the risk of progression to carcinoma. Maturitas. 2009;63(1):39–44. doi:10.1016/j.maturitas.2009.02.005. PubMed PMID: 19285814
55. Trimble CL, Kauderer J, Zaino R, Silverberg S, Lim PC, Burke JJ 2nd, Alberts D, Curtin J. Concurrent endometrial carcinoma in women with a biopsy diagnosis of atypical endometrial hyperplasia: a Gynecologic Oncology Group study. Cancer. 2006;106(4):812–9. Epub 2006/01/10. doi:10.1002/cncr.21650. PubMed PMID: 16400639
56. Linkov FEE, Gloyeske N, Edwards RP, Althouse AD, Gller MA, Svendsen C, Argenta PA. Bariatric surgery-induced weight loss changes immune markers in the endometrium of morbidly obese women. Surg Obes Relat Dis. 2014;10(5):921–6.
57. Cust AE, Allen NE, Rinaldi S, Dossus L, Friedenreich C, Olsen A, Tjonneland A, Overvad K, Clavel-Chapelon F, Boutron-Ruault MC, Linseisen J, Chang-Claude J, Boeing H, Schulz M, Benetou V, Trichopoulou A, Trichopoulos D, Palli D, Berrino F, Tumino R, Mattiello A, Vineis P, Quiros JR, Agudo A, Sanchez MJ, Larranaga N, Navarro C, Ardanaz E, Bueno-de-Mesquita HB, Peeters PH, van Gils CH, Bingham S, Khaw KT, Key T, Slimani N, Riboli E, Kaaks R. Serum levels of C-peptide, IGFBP-1 and IGFBP-2 and endometrial cancer risk; results from the European prospective investigation into cancer and nutrition. Int J Cancer. 2007;120(12):2656–64. Epub 2007/02/08. doi:10.1002/ijc.22578. PubMed PMID: 17285578
58. Cust AE, Kaaks R, Friedenreich C, Bonnet F, Laville M, Lukanova A, Rinaldi S, Dossus L, Slimani N, Lundin E, Tjonneland A, Olsen A, Overvad K, Clavel-Chapelon F, Mesrine S, Joulin V, Linseisen J, Rohrmann S, Pischon T, Boeing H, Trichopoulos D, Trichopoulou A, Benetou V, Palli D, Berrino F, Tumino R, Sacerdote C, Mattiello A, Quiros JR, Mendez MA, Sanchez MJ, Larranaga N, Tormo MJ, Ardanaz E, Bueno-de-Mesquita HB, Peeters PH, van Gils CH, Khaw KT, Bingham S, Allen N, Key T, Jenab M, Riboli E. Plasma adiponectin levels and endometrial cancer risk in pre- and postmenopausal women. J Clin Endocrinol Metab. 2007;92(1):255–63. Epub 2006/10/26. doi:10.1210/jc.2006-1371. PubMed PMID: 17062769
59. Dossus L, Becker S, Rinaldi S, Lukanova A, Tjonneland A, Olsen A, Overvad K, Chabbert-Buffet N, Boutron-Ruault MC, Clavel-Chapelon F, Teucher B, Chang-Claude J, Pischon T, Boeing H, Trichopoulou A, Benetou V, Valanou E, Palli D, Sieri S, Tumino R, Sacerdote C, Galasso R, Redondo ML, Bonet CB, Molina-Montes E, Altzibar JM, Chirlaque MD, Ardanaz E, Bueno-de-Mesquita HB, van Duijnhoven FJ, Peeters PH, Onland-Moret NC, Lundin E, Idahl A, Khaw KT, Wareham N, Allen N, Romieu I, Fedirko V, Hainaut P, Romaguera D, Norat T, Riboli E, Kaaks R. Tumor necrosis factor (TNF)-alpha, soluble TNF receptors and endometrial cancer risk: the EPIC study. Int J Cancer. 2011;129(8):2032–7. Epub 2010/12/15. doi:10.1002/ijc.25840. PubMed PMID: 21154749

60. Dossus L, Lukanova A, Rinaldi S, Allen N, Cust AE, Becker S, Tjonneland A, Hansen L, Overvad K, Chabbert-Buffet N, Mesrine S, Clavel-Chapelon F, Teucher B, Chang-Claude J, Boeing H, Drogan D, Trichopoulou A, Benetou V, Bamia C, Palli D, Agnoli C, Galasso R, Tumino R, Sacerdote C, Bueno-de-Mesquita HB, van Duijnhoven FJ, Peeters PH, Onland-Moret NC, Redondo ML, Travier N, Sanchez MJ, Altzibar JM, Chirlaque MD, Barricarte A, Lundin E, Khaw KT, Wareham N, Fedirko V, Romieu I, Romaguera D, Norat T, Riboli E, Kaaks R. Hormonal, metabolic, and inflammatory profiles and endometrial cancer risk within the EPIC cohort—a factor analysis. Am J Epidemiol. 2013;177(8):787–99. Epub 2013/03/16. doi:10.1093/aje/kws309. PubMed PMID: 23492765

61. Dossus L, Rinaldi S, Becker S, Lukanova A, Tjonneland A, Olsen A, Stegger J, Overvad K, Chabbert-Buffet N, Jimenez-Corona A, Clavel-Chapelon F, Rohrmann S, Teucher B, Boeing H, Schutze M, Trichopoulou A, Benetou V, Lagiou P, Palli D, Berrino F, Panico S, Tumino R, Sacerdote C, Redondo ML, Travier N, Sanchez MJ, Altzibar JM, Chirlaque MD, Ardanaz E, Bueno-de-Mesquita HB, van Duijnhoven FJ, Onland-Moret NC, Peeters PH, Hallmans G, Lundin E, Khaw KT, Wareham N, Allen N, Key TJ, Slimani N, Hainaut P, Romaguera D, Norat T, Riboli E, Kaaks R. Obesity, inflammatory markers, and endometrial cancer risk: a prospective case-control study. Endocr Relat Cancer. 2010;17(4):1007–19. Epub 2010/09/17. doi:10.1677/erc-10-0053. PubMed PMID: 20843938; PMCID: Pmc2966326

62. Wang T, Rohan TE, Gunter MJ, Xue X, Wactawski-Wende J, Rajpathak SN, Cushman M, Strickler HD, Kaplan RC, Wassertheil-Smoller S, Scherer PE, Ho GY. A prospective study of inflammation markers and endometrial cancer risk in postmenopausal hormone nonusers. Cancer Epidemiol Biomark Prev. 2011;20(5):971–7. Epub 2011/03/19. doi:10.1158/1055-9965.epi-10-1222. PubMed PMID: 21415362; PMCID: PMC3096873

63. Renehan AG, Roberts DL, Dive C. Obesity and cancer: pathophysiological and biological mechanisms. Arch Physiol Biochem. 2008;114(1):71–83. Epub 2008/05/10. doi:10.1080/13813450801954303 791511691 [pii]. PubMed PMID: 18465361

64. Felix AS, Weissfeld JL, Pfeiffer RM, Modugno F, Black A, Hill LM, Martin J, Sit AS, Sherman ME, Brinton LA. Endometrial thickness and risk of breast and endometrial carcinomas in the prostate, lung, colorectal and ovarian cancer screening trial. Int J Cancer. 2014;134(4):954–60. doi:10.1002/ijc.28404. PubMed PMID: 23907658; PMCID: 3858514

65. Barboza IC, Depes Dde B, Vianna Junior I, Patriarca MT, Arruda RM, Martins JA, Lopes RG. Analysis of endometrial thickness measured by transvaginal ultrasonography in obese patients. Einstein (Sao Paulo). 2014;12(2):164–7. Epub 2014/07/09. PubMed PMID: 25003920; PMCID: PMC4891157

66. Serin IS, Ozcelik B, Basbug M, Ozsahin O, Yilmazsoy A, Erez R. Effects of hypertension and obesity on endometrial thickness. Eur J Obstet Gynecol Reprod Biol. 2003;109(1):72–5. Epub 2003/06/24. PubMed PMID: 12818448

67. Nalaboff KM, Pellerito JS, Ben-Levi E. Imaging the endometrium: disease and normal variants. Radiographics. 2001;21(6):1409–24. doi:10.1148/radiographics.21.6.g01nv211409. PubMed PMID: 11706213

68. Saatli B, Yildirim N, Olgan S, Koyuncuoglu M, Emekci O, Saygili U. The role of endometrial thickness for detecting endometrial pathologies in asymptomatic postmenopausal women. Aust N Z J Obstet Gynaecol. 2014;54(1):36–40. doi:10.1111/ajo.12174. PubMed PMID: 24471845

69. Jorizzo JR, Chen MY, Martin D, Dyer RB, Weber TM. Spectrum of endometrial hyperplasia and its mimics on saline hysterosonography. AJR Am J Roentgenol. 2002;179(2):385–9. doi:10.2214/ajr.179.2.1790385. PubMed PMID: 12130438

70. Hursting SD, Digiovanni J, Dannenberg AJ, Azrad M, Leroith D, Demark-Wahnefried W, Kakarala M, Brodie A, Berger NA. Obesity, energy balance, and cancer: new opportunities for prevention. Cancer Prev Res (Phila). 2012;5(11):1260–72. doi:10.1158/1940-6207.CAPR-12-0140. PubMed PMID: 23034147; PMCID: 3641761

71. Chiva L, Lapuente F, Gonzalez-Cortijo L, Carballo N, Garcia JF, Rojo A, Gonzalez-Martin A. Sparing fertility in young patients with endometrial cancer. Gynecol Oncol. 2008;111(2 Suppl):S101–4. Epub 2008/09/23. doi:10.1016/j.ygyno.2008.07.056. PubMed PMID: 18804267

72. Park JY, Seong SJ, Kim TJ, Kim JW, Kim SM, Bae DS, Nam JH. Pregnancy outcomes after fertility-sparing management in young women with early endometrial cancer. Obstet Gynecol. 2013;121(1):136–42. Epub 2012/12/25. doi:10.1097/AOG.0b013e31827a0643. PubMed PMID: 23262938

73. Balistreri CR, Caruso C, Candore G. The role of adipose tissue and adipokines in obesity-related inflammatory diseases. Mediat Inflamm. 2010;2010:802078. Epub 2010/07/31. doi:10.1155/2010/802078. PubMed PMID: 20671929; PMCID: 2910551

74. Harvey AE, Lashinger LM, Hursting SD. The growing challenge of obesity and cancer: an inflammatory issue. Ann N Y Acad Sci. 2011;1229:45–52. Epub 2011/07/29. doi:10.1111/j.1749-6632.2011.06096.x. PubMed PMID: 21793838

75. Prieto-Hontoria PL, Perez-Matute P, Fernandez-Galilea M, Bustos M, Martinez JA, Moreno-Aliaga MJ. Role of obesity-associated dysfunctional adipose tissue in cancer: a molecular nutrition approach. Biochim Biophys Acta. 2010.; Epub 2010/11/30. doi:S0005-2728(10)00762-0 [pii] 10.1016/j.bbabio.2010.11.004. PubMed PMID: 21111705

76. Cancello R, Clement K. Is obesity an inflammatory illness? Role of low-grade inflammation and macrophage infiltration in human white adipose tissue. BJOG. 2006;113(10):1141–7. Epub 2006/08/15. doi:10.1111/j.1471-0528.2006.01004.x. PubMed PMID: 16903845

77. Dallal CM, Brinton LA, Bauer DC, Buist DS, Cauley JA, Hue TF, Lacroix A, Tice JA, Chia VM, Falk R, Pfeiffer R, Pollak M, Veenstra TD, Xu X, Lacey JV Jr, Group BFR. Obesity-related hormones and endometrial cancer among postmenopausal women: a nested case-control study within the B~FIT cohort. Endocr Relat Cancer. 2013;20(1):151–60. doi:10.1530/ERC-12-0229. PubMed PMID: 23222000; PMCID: 4038326

78. Wang PP, He XY, Wang R, Wang Z, Wang YG. High leptin level is an independent risk factor of endometrial cancer: a meta-analysis. Cell Physiol Biochem. 2014;34(5):1477–84. doi:10.1159/000366352. PubMed PMID: 25322729

79. Kaaks R, Lukanova A, Kurzer MS. Obesity, endogenous hormones, and endometrial cancer risk: a synthetic review. Cancer Epidemiol Biomark Prev. 2002;11(12):1531–43. Epub 2002/12/24. PubMed PMID: 12496040

80. Zhang Z, Zhou D, Lai Y, Liu Y, Tao X, Wang Q, Zhao G, Gu H, Liao H, Zhu Y, Xi X, Feng Y. Estrogen induces endometrial cancer cell proliferation and invasion by regulating the fat mass and obesity-associated gene via PI3K/AKT and MAPK signaling pathways. Cancer Lett. 2012;319(1):89–97. doi:10.1016/j.canlet.2011.12.033. PubMed PMID: 22222214

81. Lacey JV Jr, Mutter GL, Ronnett BM, Ioffe OB, Duggan MA, Rush BB, Glass AG, Richesson DA, Chatterjee N, Langholz B, Sherman ME. PTEN expression in endometrial biopsies as a marker of progression to endometrial carcinoma. Cancer Res. 2008;68(14):6014–20. doi:10.1158/0008-5472.CAN-08-1154. PubMed PMID: 18632658; PMCID: 2493615

82. Dalmas E, Venteclef N, Caer C, Poitou C, Cremer I, Aron-Winewsky J, Lacroix-Desmazes S, Bayry J, Kaveri SV, Clement K, Andre S, Guerre-Millo M. T cell-derived IL-22 amplifies IL-1beta-driven inflammation in human adipose tissue: relevance to obesity and type 2 diabetes. Diabetes. 2014; doi:10.2337/db13-1511. PubMed PMID: 24520123

83. Ye J. Emerging role of adipose tissue hypoxia in obesity and insulin resistance. Int J Obes. 2009;33(1):54–66. Epub 2008/12/04. doi:ijo2008229 [pii] 10.1038/ijo.2008.229. PubMed PMID: 19050672; PMCID: 2650750

84. Yoshida T, Hashimura M, Mastumoto T, Tazo Y, Inoue H, Kuwata T, Saegusa M. Transcriptional upregulation of HIF-1alpha by NF-kappaB/p65 and its associations with beta-catenin/p300 complexes in endometrial carcinoma cells. Lab Investig. 2013;93(11):1184–93. doi:10.1038/labinvest.2013.111. PubMed PMID: 24042437

85. Friberg E, Mantzoros CS, Wolk A. Physical activity and risk of endometrial cancer: a population-based prospective cohort study. Cancer Epidemiol Biomark Prev. 2006;15(11):2136–40. Epub 2006/10/24. doi:10.1158/1055-9965.epi-06-0465. PubMed PMID: 17057024

86. Patterson EJ, Urbach DR, Swanstrom LL. A comparison of diet and exercise therapy versus laparoscopic Roux-en-Y gastric bypass surgery for morbid obesity: a decision analysis model. J Am Coll Surg. 2003;196(3):379–84. Epub 2003/03/22. doi:10.1016/s1072-7515(02)01754-4. PubMed PMID: 12648689

87. von Gruenigen VE, Courneya KS, Gibbons HE, Kavanagh MB, Waggoner SE, Lerner E. Feasibility and effectiveness of a lifestyle intervention program in obese endometrial cancer patients: a randomized trial. Gynecol Oncol. 2008;109(1):19–26. Epub 2008/02/05. doi:10.1016/j.ygyno.2007.12.026. PubMed PMID: 18243282
88. Adams TD, Hunt SC. Cancer and obesity: effect of bariatric surgery. World J Surg. 2009;33(10):2028–33. Epub 2009/08/13. doi:10.1007/s00268-009-0169-1. PubMed PMID: 19672652
89. Maggard MA, Shugarman LR, Suttorp M, Maglione M, Sugerman HJ, Livingston EH, Nguyen NT, Li Z, Mojica WA, Hilton L, Rhodes S, Morton SC, Shekelle PG. Meta-analysis: surgical treatment of obesity. Ann Intern Med. 2005;142(7):547–59. Epub 2005/04/06. doi:142/7/547 [pii]. PubMed PMID: 15809466
90. Brolin RE. Bariatric surgery and long-term control of morbid obesity. JAMA. 2002;288(22):2793–6. Epub 2002/12/11. doi:jct20004 [pii]. PubMed PMID: 12472304
91. Adams TD, Gress RE, Smith SC, Halverson RC, Simper SC, Rosamond WD, Lamonte MJ, Stroup AM, Hunt SC. Long-term mortality after gastric bypass surgery. N Engl J Med. 2007;357(8):753–61. Epub 2007/08/24. doi:10.1056/NEJMoa066603. PubMed PMID: 17715409
92. Sjostrom L, Gummesson A, Sjostrom CD, Narbro K, Peltonen M, Wedel H, Bengtsson C, Bouchard C, Carlsson B, Dahlgren S, Jacobson P, Karason K, Karlsson J, Larsson B, Lindroos AK, Lonroth H, Naslund I, Olbers T, Stenlof K, Torgerson J, Carlsson LM, Swedish Obese Subjects S. Effects of bariatric surgery on cancer incidence in obese patients in Sweden (Swedish Obese Subjects Study): a prospective, controlled intervention trial. Lancet Oncol. 2009;10(7):653–62. doi:10.1016/S1470-2045(09)70159-7. PubMed PMID: 19556163
93. Adams TD, Stroup AM, Gress RE, Adams KF, Calle EE, Smith SC, Halverson RC, Simper SC, Hopkins PN, Hunt SC. Cancer incidence and mortality after gastric bypass surgery. Obesity. 2009;17(4):796–802. Epub 2009/01/17. doi:10.1038/oby.2008.610. PubMed PMID: 19148123; PMCID: PMC2859193
94. Ward KKRA, Shah NR, Davis MA, Saenz CC, McHale MT, Plaxe SC. Bariatric surgery decreases risk of uterine malignancy. Gynecol Oncol. 2014;133(2014):63–6.
95. CDC 2014 state indicator report on physical activity 2014. http://www.cdc.gov/physicalactivity/downloads/pa_state_indicator_report_2014.pdf. Accessed 7 Nov 2016.
96. Behavioral risk of Pennsylvania adults 2014. http://www.statistics.health.pa.gov/HealthStatistics/BehavioralStatistics/BehavioralRiskPAAdults/Pages/BehavioralRisksPAAdults.aspx#.WCIKyTKZN0J. Accessed 8 Nov 2016.
97. Na HK, Oliynyk S. Effects of physical activity on cancer prevention. Ann N Y Acad Sci. 2011;1229:176–83. Epub 2011/07/29. doi:10.1111/j.1749-6632.2011.06105.x. PubMed PMID: 21793853
98. Schouten LJ, Goldbohm RA, van den Brandt PA. Anthropometry, physical activity, and endometrial cancer risk: results from the Netherlands cohort study. J Natl Cancer Inst. 2004;96(21):1635–8. Epub 2004/11/04. doi:96/21/1635 [pii] 10.1093/jnci/djh291. PubMed PMID: 15523093
99. Patel AV, Feigelson HS, Talbot JT, McCullough ML, Rodriguez C, Patel RC, Thun MJ, Calle EE. The role of body weight in the relationship between physical activity and endometrial cancer: results from a large cohort of US women. Int J Cancer. 2008;123(8):1877–82. Epub 2008/07/25. doi:10.1002/ijc.23716. PubMed PMID: 18651569
100. Payne JK, Held J, Thorpe J, Shaw H. Effect of exercise on biomarkers, fatigue, sleep disturbances, and depressive symptoms in older women with breast cancer receiving hormonal therapy. Oncol Nurs Forum. 2008;35(4):635–42. PubMed PMID: 18591167
101. Pullen PR, Nagamia SH, Mehta PK, Thompson WR, Benardot D, Hammoud R, Parrott JM, Sola S, Khan BV. Effects of yoga on inflammation and exercise capacity in patients with chronic heart failure. J Card Fail. 2008;14(5):407–13. PubMed PMID: 18514933
102. Schmid D, Behrens G, Keimling M, Jochem C, Ricci C, Leitzmann M. A systematic review and meta-analysis of physical activity and endometrial cancer risk. Eur J Epidemiol. 2015;30(5):397–412. Epub 2015/03/25. doi:10.1007/s10654-015-0017-6. PubMed PMID: 25800123

103. Voskuil DW, Monninkhof EM, Elias SG, Vlems FA, van Leeuwen FE. Physical activity and endometrial cancer risk, a systematic review of current evidence. Cancer Epidemiol Biomark Prev. 2007;16(4):639–48. Epub 2007/04/10. doi:10.1158/1055-9965.epi-06-0742. PubMed PMID: 17416752

104. Matthews C, Xu W, Zheng W, Gao Y, Ruan Z, Xiang Y, Shu X. Physical activity and endometrial cancer risk. Proc Am Assoc Cancer Res. 2014;64(7):857.

105. Ahern AL, Olson AD, Aston LM, Jebb SA. Weight Watchers on prescription: an observational study of weight change among adults referred to Weight Watchers by the NHS. BMC Public Health. 2011;11:434. Epub 2011/06/08. doi:1471-2458-11-434 [pii] 10.1186/1471-2458-11-434. PubMed PMID: 21645343; PMCID: 3145588

106. Madigan CD, Daley AJ, Lewis AL, Jolly K, Aveyard P. Which weight-loss programmes are as effective as Weight Watchers(R)? Non-inferiority analysis. Br J Gen Pract. 2014;64(620):e128–36. Epub 2014/02/26. doi:10.3399/bjgp14X677491. PubMed PMID: 24567651; PMCID: PMC3933848

107. Hwang KO, Ottenbacher AJ, Green AP, Cannon-Diehl MR, Richardson O, Bernstam EV, Thomas EJ. Social support in an Internet weight loss community. Int J Med Informatics. 2010;79(1):5–13. Epub 2009/12/01. doi:S1386-5056(09)00172-5 [pii] 10.1016/j.ijmedinf.2009.10.003. PubMed PMID: 19945338; PMCID: 3060773

108. Spring B, Duncan JM, Janke EA, Kozak AT, McFadden HG, Demott A, Pictor A, Epstein LH, Siddique J, Pellegrini CA, Buscemi J, Hedeker D. Integrating technology into standard weight loss treatment: a randomized controlled trial. Arch Intern Med. 2012:1–7. Epub 2012/12/12. doi:10.1001/jamainternmed.2013.1221 1485082 [pii]. PubMed PMID: 23229890

109. Eddy DM, Schlessinger L, Kahn R. Clinical outcomes and cost-effectiveness of strategies for managing people at high risk for diabetes. Ann Intern Med. 2005;143(4):251–64. PubMed PMID: 16103469

110. Ratner RE. An update on the diabetes prevention program. Endocr Pract. 2006;12(Suppl 1):20–4. Epub 2006/04/22. doi:DRQH6PD47M6T36KF [pii]. PubMed PMID: 16627375; PMCID: 1762035

111. Ali MK, Echouffo-Tcheugui J, Williamson DF. How effective were lifestyle interventions in real-world settings that were modeled on the diabetes prevention program? Health Aff (Millwood). 2012;31(1):67–75. Epub 2012/01/11. doi:10.1377/hlthaff.2011.1009 31/1/67 [pii]. PubMed PMID: 22232096

112. McTigue KM, Harris R, Hemphill B, Lux L, Sutton S, Bunton AJ, Lohr KN. Screening and interventions for obesity in adults: summary of the evidence for the U.S. Preventive Services Task Force. Ann Intern Med. 2003;139(11):933–49. Epub 2003/12/04. doi:139/11/933 [pii]. PubMed PMID: 14644897

113. Dansinger ML, Gleason JA, Griffith JL, Selker HP, Schaefer EJ. Comparison of the Atkins, Ornish, Weight Watchers, and Zone diets for weight loss and heart disease risk reduction: a randomized trial. JAMA. 2005;293(1):43–53. Epub 2005/01/06. doi:293/1/43 [pii] doi:10.1001/jama.293.1.43. PubMed PMID: 15632335

114. Rejeski WJ, Ip EH, Bertoni AG, Bray GA, Evans G, Gregg EW, Zhang Q. Lifestyle change and mobility in obese adults with type 2 diabetes. N Engl J Med. 2012;366(13):1209–17. Epub 2012/03/30. doi:10.1056/NEJMoa1110294. PubMed PMID: 22455415; PMCID: 3339039

115. Messier SP, Loeser RF, Miller GD, Morgan TM, Rejeski WJ, Sevick MA, Ettinger WH Jr, Pahor M, Williamson JD. Exercise and dietary weight loss in overweight and obese older adults with knee osteoarthritis: the arthritis, diet, and activity promotion trial. Arthritis Rheum. 2004;50(5):1501–10. PubMed PMID: 15146420

116. Eyre HA, Papps E, Baune BT. Treating depression and depression-like behavior with physical activity: an immune perspective. Front Psych. 2013;4:3. Epub 2013/02/06. doi:10.3389/fpsyt.2013.00003. PubMed PMID: 23382717; PMCID: 3562851

117. de Zwaan M, Enderle J, Wagner S, Muhlhans B, Ditzen B, Gefeller O, Mitchell JE, Muller A. Anxiety and depression in bariatric surgery patients: a prospective, follow-

up study using structured clinical interviews. J Affect Disord. 2011.; Epub 2011/04/20. doi:S0165-0327(11)00108-X [pii]. doi:10.1016/j.jad.2011.03.025. PubMed PMID: 21501874

118. National prevention strategy 2011. https://www.surgeongeneral.gov/priorities/prevention/strategy/report.pdf. Accessed 2 Dec 2016.

119. CDC. Cancer prevention 2012. http://www.cdc.gov/cancer/dcpc/prevention/. Accessed 7 Nov 2016.

120. Sanders BG, Kline K. Nutrition, immunology and cancer: an overview. Adv Exp Med Biol. 1995;369:185–94. PubMed PMID: 7598006

121. Thompson R. Preventing cancer: the role of food, nutrition and physical activity. J Fam Health Care. 2010;20(3):100–2. Epub 2010/08/11. PubMed PMID: 20695357

122. Thibault R, Dupertuis YM, Belabed L, Pichard C. Nutrition and physical activity: two targets for cancer prevention. Rev Med Suisse. 2010;6(250):1046–8. 50–2. Epub 2010/06/23. PubMed PMID: 20564863

123. Verma M. Cancer control and prevention by nutrition and epigenetic approaches. Antioxid Redox Signal. 2012.; Epub 2011/11/04. doi:10.1089/ars.2011.4388. PubMed PMID: 22047027

124. Stevens VL, McCullough ML, Sun J, Gapstur SM. Folate and other one-carbon metabolism-related nutrients and risk of postmenopausal breast cancer in the cancer prevention study II nutrition cohort. Am J Clin Nutr. 2010;91(6):1708–15. Epub 2010/04/23. doi:ajcn.2009.28553 [pii] 10.3945/ajcn.2009.28553. PubMed PMID: 20410093

125. Schenk M. Effects of nutrition on the prevention of cancer. Dtsch Med Wochenschr. 2011;136(Suppl 3):S80–4. Epub 2011/10/14. doi:10.1055/s-0031-1292067. PubMed PMID: 21960372.

126. Ross SA, Davis CD. MicroRNA, nutrition, and cancer prevention. Adv Nutr. 2011;2(6):472–85. Epub 2012/02/15. doi:10.3945/an.111.001206 001206 [pii]. PubMed PMID: 22332090; PMCID: 3226385

127. Gonzalez CA, Riboli E. Diet and cancer prevention: contributions from the European Prospective Investigation into Cancer and Nutrition (EPIC) study. Eur J Cancer. 2010;46(14):2555–62. Epub 2010/09/17. doi:S0959-8049(10)00703-3 [pii] 10.1016/j.ejca.2010.07.025. PubMed PMID: 20843485

128. Nagle CM, Olsen CM, Ibiebele TI, Spurdle AB, Webb PM. Glycemic index, glycemic load and endometrial cancer risk: results from the Australian National Endometrial Cancer study and an updated systematic review and meta-analysis. Eur J Nutr. 2013;52(2):705–15. Epub 2012/06/01. doi:10.1007/s00394-012-0376-7. PubMed PMID: 22648201

129. Barbone F, Austin H, Partridge EE. Diet and endometrial cancer: a case-control study. Am J Epidemiol. 1993;137(4):393–403. Epub 1993/02/15. PubMed PMID: 8460621

130. Dalvi TB, Canchola AJ, Horn-Ross PL. Dietary patterns, Mediterranean diet, and endometrial cancer risk. Cancer Causes Control. 2007;18(9):957–66. Epub 2007/07/20. doi:10.1007/s10552-007-9037-1. PubMed PMID: 17638105

131. McCann SE, Freudenheim JL, Marshall JR, Brasure JR, Swanson MK, Graham S. Diet in the epidemiology of endometrial cancer in western New York (United States). Cancer Causes Control. 2000;11(10):965–74. Epub 2001/01/06. PubMed PMID: 11142531

132. Filomeno M, Bosetti C, Bidoli E, Levi F, Serraino D, Montella M, La Vecchia C, Tavani A. Mediterranean diet and risk of endometrial cancer: a pooled analysis of three Italian case-control studies. Br J Cancer. 2015;112(11):1816–21. Epub 2015/05/27. doi:10.1038/bjc.2015.153. PubMed PMID: 26010500; PMCID: PMC4647248

133. Merritt MA, Tzoulaki I, Tworoger SS, De Vivo I, Hankinson SE, Fernandes J, Tsilidis KK, Weiderpass E, Tjonneland A, Petersen KE, Dahm CC, Overvad K, Dossus L, Boutron-Ruault MC, Fagherazzi G, Fortner RT, Kaaks R, Aleksandrova K, Boeing H, Trichopoulou A, Bamia C, Trichopoulos D, Palli D, Grioni S, Tumino R, Sacerdote C, Mattiello A, Bueno-de-Mesquita HB, Onland-Moret NC, Peeters PH, Gram IT, Skeie G, Quiros JR, Duell EJ, Sanchez MJ, Salmeron D, Barricarte A, Chamosa S, Ericson U, Sonestedt E, Nilsson LM,

Idahl A, Khaw KT, Wareham N, Travis RC, Rinaldi S, Romieu I, Patel CJ, Riboli E, Gunter MJ. Investigation of dietary factors and endometrial cancer risk using a nutrient-wide association study approach in the EPIC and Nurses' Health Study (NHS) and NHSII. Cancer Epidemiol Biomark Prev. 2015;24(2):466–71. Epub 2015/02/11. doi:10.1158/1055-9965. epi-14-0970. PubMed PMID: 25662427; PMCID: PMC4324546

134. Je Y, Giovannucci E. Coffee consumption and risk of endometrial cancer: findings from a large up-to-date meta-analysis. Int J Cancer. 2012;131(7):1700–10. Epub 2011/12/23. doi:10.1002/ijc.27408. PubMed PMID: 22190017

135. Ollberding NJ, Lim U, Wilkens LR, Setiawan VW, Shvetsov YB, Henderson BE, Kolonel LN, Goodman MT. Legume, soy, tofu, and isoflavone intake and endometrial cancer risk in postmenopausal women in the multiethnic cohort study. J Natl Cancer Inst. 2012;104(1):67–76. Epub 2011/12/14. doi:10.1093/jnci/djr475. PubMed PMID: 22158125; PMCID: PMC3250383

136. Arem H, Neuhouser ML, Irwin ML, Cartmel B, Lu L, Risch H, Mayne ST, Yu H. Omega-3 and omega-6 fatty acid intakes and endometrial cancer risk in a population-based case-control study. Eur J Nutr. 2013;52(3):1251–60. Epub 2012/08/24. doi:10.1007/s00394-012-0436-z. PubMed PMID: 22915050; PMCID: PMC3548981

137. Ganmaa D, Cui X, Feskanich D, Hankinson SE, Willett WC. Milk, dairy intake and risk of endometrial cancer: a 26-year follow-up. Int J Cancer. 2012;130(11):2664–71. Epub 2011/07/01. doi:10.1002/ijc.26265. PubMed PMID: 21717454; PMCID: PMC3359127

138. George SM, Ballard R, Shikany JM, Crane TE, Neuhouser ML. A prospective analysis of diet quality and endometrial cancer among 84,415 postmenopausal women in the Women's Health Initiative. Ann Epidemiol. 2015;25(10):788–93. Epub 2015/08/12. doi:10.1016/j.annepidem.2015.05.009. PubMed PMID: 26260777

139. Chandran U, Bandera EV, Williams-King MG, Sima C, Bayuga S, Pulick K, Wilcox H, Zauber AG, Olson SH. Adherence to the dietary guidelines for Americans and endometrial cancer risk. Cancer Causes Control. 2010;21(11):1895–904. Epub 2010/07/24. doi:10.1007/s10552-010-9617-3. PubMed PMID: 20652737; PMCID: PMC3065196

140. Nijhuis J, van Dielen FM, Fouraschen SM, van den Broek MA, Rensen SS, Buurman WA, Greve JW. Endothelial activation markers and their key regulators after restrictive bariatric surgery. Obesity (Silver Spring, MD). 2007;15(6):1395–9. PubMed PMID: 17557976

141. Christou NV, Lieberman M, Sampalis F, Sampalis JS. Bariatric surgery reduces cancer risk in morbidly obese patients. Surg Obes Relat Dis. 2008;4(6):691–5. Epub 2008/11/26. doi:S1550-7289(08)00734-X [pii] 10.1016/j.soard.2008.08.025. PubMed PMID: 19026373

142. Linkov F, Maxwell GL, Felix AS, Lin Y, Lenzner D, Bovbjerg DH, Lokshin A, Hennon M, Jakicic JM, Goodpaster BH, DeLany JP. Longitudinal evaluation of cancer-associated biomarkers before and after weight loss in RENEW study participants: implications for cancer risk reduction. Gynecol Oncol. 2012;125(1):114–9. Epub 2011/12/27. doi:10.1016/j.ygyno.2011.12.439. PubMed PMID: 22198242

143. Long B, Liu FW, Bristow RE. Disparities in uterine cancer epidemiology, treatment, and survival among African Americans in the United States. Gynecol Oncol. 2013;130(3):652–9. doi:10.1016/j.ygyno.2013.05.020. PubMed PMID: 23707671; PMCID: 4074587

144. Wright JD, Fiorelli J, Schiff PB, Burke WM, Kansler AL, Cohen CJ, Herzog TJ. Racial disparities for uterine corpus tumors: changes in clinical characteristics and treatment over time. Cancer. 2009;115(6):1276–85. doi:10.1002/cncr.24160. PubMed PMID: 19204905

145. Oliver KE, Enewold LR, Zhu K, Conrads TP, Rose GS, Maxwell GL, Farley JH. Racial disparities in histopathologic characteristics of uterine cancer are present in older, not younger blacks in an equal-access environment. Gynecol Oncol. 2011;123(1):76–81. doi:10.1016/j.ygyno.2011.06.027. PubMed PMID: 21741078

146. Carroll JF, Fulda KG, Chiapa AL, Rodriquez M, Phelps DR, Cardarelli KM, Vishwanatha JK, Cardarelli R. Impact of race/ethnicity on the relationship between visceral fat and inflammatory biomarkers. Obesity. 2009;17(7):1420–7. Epub 2009/02/07. doi:10.1038/oby.2008.657. PubMed PMID: 19197255

147. Azrad M, Gower BA, Hunter GR, Nagy TR. Racial differences in adiponectin and leptin in healthy premenopausal women. Endocrine. 2013;43(3):586–92. Epub 2012/09/18. doi:10.1007/s12020-012-9797-6. PubMed PMID: 22983832; PMCID: PMC3541432

148. Slopen N, Lewis TT, Gruenewald TL, Mujahid MS, Ryff CD, Albert MA, Williams DR. Early life adversity and inflammation in African Americans and whites in the midlife in the United States survey. Psychosom Med. 2010;72(7):694–701. doi:10.1097/PSY.0b013e3181e9c16f. PubMed PMID: 20595419; PMCID: 2939196

149. Castanon N, Lasselin J, Capuron L. Neuropsychiatric comorbidity in obesity: role of inflammatory processes. Front Endocrinol (Lausanne). 2014;5:74. Epub 2014/05/27. doi:10.3389/fendo.2014.00074. PubMed PMID: 24860551; PMCID: PMC4030152

150. DeSantis C, Naishadham D, Jemal A. Cancer statistics for African Americans, 2013. CA Cancer J Clin. 2013;63(3):151–66. doi:10.3322/caac.21173. PubMed PMID: 23386565

151. Park SL, Goodman MT, Zhang ZF, Kolonel LN, Henderson BE, Setiawan VW. Body size, adult BMI gain and endometrial cancer risk: the multiethnic cohort. Int J Cancer. 2010;126(2):490–9. doi:10.1002/ijc.24718. PubMed PMID: 19585578; PMCID: 2795089

152. Allard JE, Maxwell GL. Race disparities between black and white women in the incidence, treatment, and prognosis of endometrial cancer. Cancer Control. 2009;16(1):53–6. PubMed PMID: 19078930

153. Siegel R, Ma J, Zou Z, Jemal A. Cancer statistics, 2014. CA Cancer J Clin. 2014;64(1):9–29. doi:10.3322/caac.21208. PubMed PMID: 24399786

154. Courneya KS, Karvinen KH, Campbell KL, Pearcey RG, Dundas G, Capstick V, Tonkin KS. Associations among exercise, body weight, and quality of life in a population-based sample of endometrial cancer survivors. Gynecol Oncol. 2005;97(2):422–30. Epub 2005/05/03. doi:S0090-8258(05)00033-8 [pii] 10.1016/j.ygyno.2005.01.007. PubMed PMID: 15863140

155. Chia VM, Newcomb PA, Trentham-Dietz A, Hampton JM. Obesity, diabetes, and other factors in relation to survival after endometrial cancer diagnosis. Int J Gynecol Cancer. 2007;17(2):441–6. Epub 2007/03/17. doi:IJG790 [pii] 10.1111/j.1525-1438.2007.00790.x. PubMed PMID: 17362320

156. von Gruenigen VE, Tian C, Frasure H, Waggoner S, Keys H, Barakat RR. Treatment effects, disease recurrence, and survival in obese women with early endometrial carcinoma : a Gynecologic Oncology Group study. Cancer. 2006;107(12):2786–91. Epub 2006/11/11. doi:10.1002/cncr.22351. PubMed PMID: 17096437

157. McBride CM, Emmons KM, Lipkus IM. Understanding the potential of teachable moments: the case of smoking cessation. Health Educ Res. 2003;18(2):156–70. Epub 2003/05/06. PubMed PMID: 12729175

158. Fader AN, Arriba LN, Frasure HE, von Gruenigen VE. Endometrial cancer and obesity: epidemiology, biomarkers, prevention and survivorship. Gynecol Oncol. 2009;114(1):121–7. Epub 2009/05/02. doi:10.1016/j.ygyno.2009.03.039. PubMed PMID: 19406460

159. McCarroll ML, Armbruster S, Frasure HE, Gothard MD, Gil KM, Kavanagh MB, Waggoner S, von Gruenigen VE. Self-efficacy, quality of life, and weight loss in overweight/obese endometrial cancer survivors (SUCCEED): a randomized controlled trial. Gynecol Oncol. 2014;132(2):397–402. Epub 2013/12/27. doi:10.1016/j.ygyno.2013.12.023. PubMed PMID: 24369301

160. Haggerty AF, Huepenbecker S, Sarwer DB, Spitzer J, Raggio G, Chu CS, Ko E, Allison KC. The use of novel technology-based weight loss interventions for obese women with endometrial hyperplasia and cancer. Gynecol Oncol. 2016;140(2):239–44. Epub 2015/12/09. doi:10.1016/j.ygyno.2015.11.033. PubMed PMID: 26644265

161. CDC. Winnable battles 2012. http://www.cdc.gov/WinnableBattles/Obesity/index.html. Accessed 7 Nov 2016.

162. Forman-Hoffman V, Little A, Wahls T. Barriers to obesity management: a pilot study of primary care clinicians. BMC Fam Pract. 2006;7:35. Epub 2006/06/08. doi:10.1186/1471-2296-7-35. PubMed PMID: 16756673; PMCID: PMC1525170

163. Kushner RF. Tackling obesity: is primary care up to the challenge? Arch Intern Med. 2010;170(2):121–3. Epub 2010/01/27. doi:10.1001/archinternmed.2009.479. PubMed PMID: 20101005

164. Kraschnewski JL, Sciamanna CN, Stuckey HL, Chuang CH, Lehman EB, Hwang KO, Sherwood LL, Nembhard HB. A silent response to the obesity epidemic: decline in US physician weight counseling. Med Care. 2013;51(2):186–92. Epub 2012/10/11. doi:10.1097/MLR.0b013e3182726c33. PubMed PMID: 23047128

165. DePue JD, Goldstein MG, Redding CA, Velicer WF, Sun X, Fava JL, Kazura A, Rakowski W. Cancer prevention in primary care: predictors of patient counseling across four risk behaviors over 24 months. Prev Med. 2008;46(3):252–9. Epub 2008/02/01. doi:S0091-7435(07)00509-9 [pii] 10.1016/j.ypmed.2007.11.020. PubMed PMID: 18234324; PMCID: 2408758

166. Tsui JI, Dodson K, Jacobson TA. Cardiovascular disease prevention counseling in residency: resident and attending physician attitudes and practices. J Natl Med Assoc. 2004;96(8):1080–3. 8–91. Epub 2004/08/12. PubMed PMID: 15303414; PMCID: 2568499

167. Gonzalez JL, Gilmer L. Obesity prevention in pediatrics: a pilot pediatric resident curriculum intervention on nutrition and obesity education and counseling. J Natl Med Assoc. 2006;98(9):1483–8. Epub 2006/10/06. PubMed PMID: 17019916; PMCID: 2569712

168. Sciamanna CN, DePue JD, Goldstein MG, Park ER, Gans KM, Monroe AD, Reiss PT. Nutrition counseling in the promoting cancer prevention in primary care study. Prev Med. 2002;35(5):437–46. Epub 2002/11/15. doi:S0091743502910996 [pii]. PubMed PMID: 12431892

169. Blumenthal D, Gokhale M, Campbell EG, Weissman JS. Preparedness for clinical practice: reports of graduating residents at academic health centers. JAMA. 2001;286(9):1027–34. Epub 2001/09/18. doi:joc01827 [pii]. PubMed PMID: 11559286.

170. Kolasa KM, Jobe AC, Miller MG, Clay MC. Teaching medical students cancer risk reduction nutrition counseling using a multimedia program. Fam Med. 1999;31(3):200–4. Epub 1999/03/23. PubMed PMID: 10086257

171. Yarnall KSH, Pollak KI, Østbye T, Krause KM, Michener JL. Primary care: is there enough time for prevention? Am J Public Health. 2003;93(4):635–41. doi:10.2105/ajph.93.4.635.

172. Wolff MS, Rhodes ET, Ludwig DS. Training in childhood obesity management in the United States: a survey of pediatric, internal medicine-pediatrics and family medicine residency program directors. BMC Med Educ. 2010;10:18. Epub 2010/02/19. doi:1472-6920-10-18 [pii] 10.1186/1472-6920-10-18. PubMed PMID: 20163732; PMCID: 2839969

173. Block JP, DeSalvo KB, Fisher WP. Are physicians equipped to address the obesity epidemic? Knowledge and attitudes of internal medicine residents. Prev Med. 2003;36(6):669–75. Epub 2003/05/15. doi:S0091743503000550 [pii]. PubMed PMID: 12744909

174. Park ER, Wolfe TJ, Gokhale M, Winickoff JP, Rigotti NA. Perceived preparedness to provide preventive counseling: reports of graduating primary care residents at academic health centers. J Gen Intern Med. 2005;20(5):386–91. Epub 2005/06/21. doi:JGI40273 [pii] 10.1111/j.1525-1497.2005.0024.x. PubMed PMID: 15963158; PMCID: 1490125

175. Perrin EM, Vann JC, Lazorick S, Ammerman A, Teplin S, Flower K, Wegner SE, Benjamin JT. Bolstering confidence in obesity prevention and treatment counseling for resident and community pediatricians. Patient Educ Couns. 2008;73(2):179–85. Epub 2008/08/30. doi:S0738-3991(08)00377-7 [pii] 10.1016/j.pec.2008.07.025. PubMed PMID: 18755567; PMCID: 2700835.

176. Thomson CA, McCullough ML, Wertheim BC, Chlebowski RT, Martinez ME, Stefanick ML, Rohan TE, Manson JE, Tindle HA, Ockene J, Vitolins MZ, Wactawski-Wende J, Sarto GE, Lane DS, Neuhouser ML. Nutrition and physical activity cancer prevention guidelines, cancer risk, and mortality in the women's health initiative. Cancer Prev Res (Phila). 2014;7(1):42–53. Epub 2014/01/10. doi:10.1158/1940-6207.capr-13-0258. PubMed PMID: 24403289; PMCID: PMC4090781

177. Romaguera D, Vergnaud AC, Peeters PH, van Gils CH, Chan DS, Ferrari P, Romieu I, Jenab M, Slimani N, Clavel-Chapelon F, Fagherazzi G, Perquier F, Kaaks R, Teucher B, Boeing H, von Rusten A, Tjonneland A, Olsen A, Dahm CC, Overvad K, Quiros JR, Gonzalez CA, Sanchez

MJ, Navarro C, Barricarte A, Dorronsoro M, Khaw KT, Wareham NJ, Crowe FL, Key TJ, Trichopoulou A, Lagiou P, Bamia C, Masala G, Vineis P, Tumino R, Sieri S, Panico S, May AM, Bueno-de-Mesquita HB, Buchner FL, Wirfalt E, Manjer J, Johansson I, Hallmans G, Skeie G, Benjaminsen Borch K, Parr CL, Riboli E, Norat T. Is concordance with World Cancer Research Fund/American Institute for Cancer Research guidelines for cancer prevention related to subsequent risk of cancer? Results from the EPIC study. Am J Clin Nutr. 2012;96(1):150–63. Epub 2012/05/18. doi:10.3945/ajcn.111.031674. PubMed PMID: 22592101

178. McCullough ML, Patel AV, Kushi LH, Patel R, Willett WC, Doyle C, Thun MJ, Gapstur SM. Following cancer prevention guidelines reduces risk of cancer, cardiovascular disease, and all-cause mortality. Cancer Epidemiol Biomark Prev. 2011;20(6):1089–97. Epub 2011/04/07. doi:10.1158/1055-9965.epi-10-1173. PubMed PMID: 21467238

Chapter 10
Hormonal and Metabolic Strategies to Overcome Insulin Resistance and Prevent Endometrial Cancer

Sarah Kitson and Emma J. Crosbie

Abstract A role for insulin and its related protein IGF-1 as drivers of endometrial carcinogenesis is now well established, with epidemiological and in vitro evidence demonstrating insulin resistance to be critical to the development of the disease. In addition to a direct effect on the endometrium, stimulating unregulated cell proliferation, insulin also closely interacts with excess adipose tissue, increasing the aromatisation of androgens to oestrogen and decreasing the secretion of the adipokine adiponectin, a major regulator of insulin sensitivity. Interventions aimed at improving the body's response to insulin would, therefore, be expected to have a positive effect on preventing the development of endometrial cancer. Numerous lifestyle, pharmacological and surgical interventions have been shown to influence insulin resistance, either through weight loss, increased insulin secretion or modulation of signalling through the insulin receptor. This review discusses the mechanisms underpinning these strategies and, in particular, the existing data for their role in endometrial cancer prophylaxis.

Keywords Insulin resistance • Insulin sensitizers • Insulin-like growth factor • Sedentary behaviour • Aromatisation • Weight loss drugs • Sibutramine • Orlistat • Bariatric surgery • Sex hormone binding globulin

Introduction

There is increasing evidence to support a causal role for insulin resistance in endometrial carcinogenesis. A recently conducted meta-analysis of observational studies demonstrated higher fasting insulin and C-peptide levels and a greater HOMA-IR (homeostatic model assessment of insulin resistance, a composite measure of insulin

S. Kitson • E.J. Crosbie (✉)
Division of Molecular & Clinical Cancer Sciences, University of Manchester,
5th Floor – Research, St Mary's Hospital, Oxford Road, Manchester M13 9WL, UK
e-mail: sarahkitson@doctors.org.uk; emma.crosbie@manchester.ac.uk

© Springer International Publishing AG 2018   167
N.A. Berger et al. (eds.), *Focus on Gynecologic Malignancies*, Energy Balance
and Cancer 13, DOI 10.1007/978-3-319-63483-8_10

and glucose levels) score in women with endometrial cancer compared with those without the disease [1]. Even allowing for the heterogeneity in study design and inclusion of both fasting and non-fasting results, these findings were consistent across all eligible studies. The effect of insulin resistance on endometrial cancer risk appears to be independent of its association with body mass, as, even accounting for this, genetically predicted higher fasting insulin levels are associated with an elevation in disease risk [2]. Similarly within the SEER database, impaired fasting glucose was associated with a 25% increase in endometrial cancer risk, independent of the other components of the metabolic syndrome, namely obesity, hypertension and hyperlipidaemia [3]. The presence of insulin resistance may well explain the four-fold increased risk of endometrial cancer in women with polycystic ovary syndrome (PCOS) compared with those without the disease and metformin, an insulin sensitising drug, has already shown promise in the treatment of early stage endometrial cancer in this context [4].

In vitro evidence supports a direct effect of insulin, and its related protein insulin-like growth factor-1 (IGF-1), on endometrial cancer cells [5, 6]. Activation of the insulin receptor results in increased cellular proliferation and inhibition of apoptosis, through the MAPK and PI3K/Akt pathways and mTOR activation (Fig. 10.1). Insulin is also able to promote tumour development through the activation of β-catenin, resulting in unregulated cell turnover and the accumulation of genetic alterations. By degrading its binding protein, insulin is able to increase the bioavailability of IGF-1 to enhance its own tumour promoting capacity.

In addition to these direct effects, insulin has been shown to increase local oestrogen synthesis through stimulation of ovarian androgen production and its aromatisation within adipose tissue. This, combined with a reduction in hepatic synthesis of sex hormone binding globulin, contributes to a greater bioavailability of oestrogen, which promotes endometrial cell proliferation as well. Insulin is also responsible for a lowering of adiponectin levels and increase in leptin secretion [6].

Given this weight of evidence, it is logical, therefore, to hypothesise that treatments aimed at improving insulin sensitivity would have a beneficial effect on reducing endometrial cancer risk. To this effect, a number of different strategies have been employed.

Exercise and Avoidance of Sedentary Behaviour

Sedentary behaviour is a risk factor for endometrial cancer, with prolonged periods of sitting (of five or more hours duration each day) being associated with an increased risk of the disease [7, 8]. It is, therefore, not surprising that avoidance of this behaviour is protective against endometrial cancer development. A number of systematic reviews have been undertaken which have consistently shown a benefit from undertaking physical activity, with, on average, a risk reduction of 20–30% [9–12]. There have been no randomised controlled trials (RCTs) of exercise for the prevention of endometrial cancer, meaning that most of the available data has come from case-control studies using self-reported activity levels. Even with this caveat, there is some evidence of a dose-response relationship between exercise and

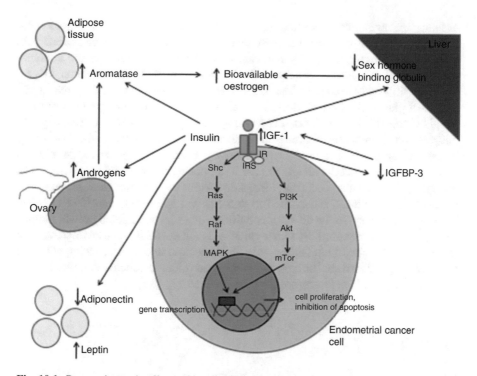

Fig. 10.1 Pro-carcinogenic effects of insulin. Hyperinsulinemia is responsible for increased signalling within endometrial cancer cells through the mTOR and MAPK pathways, resulting in cell proliferation and inhibition of apoptosis. It also acts to promote ovarian androgen production and its aromatisation within adipose tissue. This, alongside a reduction in the hepatic production of sex hormone binding globulin, results in an increase in bioavailable oestrogen, which is able to stimulate endometrial cell turnover, thereby increasing the risk of carcinogenic mutations. Increased serum insulin has also been shown to be associated with a reduction in adiponectin levels and to drive leptin secretion

endometrial cancer risk, though this has only been demonstrated in populations consisting of overweight and obese women [9, 11]. Whilst higher intensity, longer duration exercise would, therefore, be anticipated to be the most beneficial, the available evidence to date suggests that all physical activity reduces endometrial cancer risk to a similar extent [11]. There is no consensus as yet as to at what stage of life exercise participation has the greatest impact on disease risk, suggesting that it can be used as part of a risk reduction strategy at any age [11, 12]. As little as 20 min of moderate intensity exercise sufficient to raise the heart rate on five occasions during the week is sufficient to be beneficial, similar to that recommended for breast cancer reduction [13]. Using the Walter formula, Moore et al. [14] estimated that adherence to such a regime could have prevented up to 22% of endometrial cancers within the NIH-AARP Diet and Health Study.

Physical activity may reduce the risk of endometrial cancer through several different mechanisms, the most apparent being the lowering of body weight. Adipose tissue is the predominant source of oestrogen in postmenopausal women, through the aromatisation of androgens, and postmenopausal women who have high levels of sedentary behaviour have elevated oestradiol and low sex-hormone binding globulin levels. Physical activity reverses these changes, particularly when associated with weight loss, thereby potentially reducing oestrogenic stimulation of the endometrium [15]. It is unclear, however, whether such an effect is also seen in premenopausal women. Exercise also improves insulin sensitivity and increases the uptake of glucose by skeletal muscle, an effect which occurs independent of body weight change [16]. In addition, levels of adiponectin, an adipokine secreted by adipocytes and a regulator of insulin resistance, have been shown to be favourably altered in response to increased physical activity. Long term exercise (6–24 months) appears to be associated with an increase in adiponectin levels and hence improved insulin sensitivity when occurring alongside weight loss; shorter term programmes (4 months), in contrast, have failed to demonstrate any beneficial effect [17–19]. There is no evidence for an effect of activity on other insulin related growth factors, including IGF-1, however [20]. Other potential mechanisms include an improvement in innate and acquired immune response and reduction in oxidative stress, although results from published studies have frequently been either inconclusive or conflicting as to the degree of benefit conferred by physical activity [15].

Weight Loss

Given the close association between excess adiposity, insulin resistance and endometrial cancer [21, 22], interventions designed to promote weight loss might be expected to reduce disease risk. Such interventions can be considered under three separate categories; diet induced weight loss (which may be combined with other lifestyle interventions such as increased physical activity, as discussed above), drug induced weight loss and surgical interventions designed to promote weight reduction.

Diet Induced Weight Loss

Single episodes of intentional weight-loss of 20 pounds or more have been shown to be associated with a 4% reduction in endometrial cancer risk after adjustment for age, body mass index (BMI) and other cancer risk factors [23]. Whilst these findings from the Iowa Women's Health Study were non-significant, the effect of diet induced weight loss on endometrial cancer risk may in fact be greater than that seen in this cohort, which relied upon self-reporting of weight change as either intentional or unintentional. This distinction is notoriously difficult to accurately make and potentially results in disease-related weight loss being inappropriately ascribed as intentional, thereby underestimating the reduction in relative risk.

Only one RCT of the effect of dietary interventions on the risk of endometrial cancer has been completed. The Women's Health Initiative Dietary Modification Randomised Controlled Trial randomised over 48,000 postmenopausal women to either dietary intervention, consisting of an intensive behavioural modification pro-gramme designed to reduce dietary fat intake and increase fruit and vegetable con-sumption, or usual diet [24]. Over a median follow-up period of 8.1 years, there was no difference in the incidence of endometrial cancer between the two groups, although patients in the intervention group, on average, lost only 0.8 kg, potentially explaining the lack of effect seen. A further feasibility study in overweight women with PCOS was undertaken looking at dietary modification, weight loss and endo-metrial cancer risk in this high-risk population; whilst women were agreeable to participation, the inclusion criteria were such that any subsequent RCT would need to recruit women from multiple centres to ensure sufficient numbers to adequately power the study [25].

Low fat diets have been shown to result in reductions in serum oestrone, oestra-diol and testosterone levels and favourable improvements in sex hormone binding globulin to a greater extent than those seen with exercise alone [26]. The magnitude of change in serum hormone levels is proportion to the amount of weight lost, explaining why so many RCTs have failed to show any significant decrease in oes-tradiol levels with dietary intervention when there has been no associated weight reduction [27, 28]. Similar improvements in markers of insulin sensitivity, includ-ing insulin and HOMA-IR, have also been described with calorie restriction [29]. A limitation of dietary intervention studies, however, is that weight loss is frequently also seen in the control arm; women sufficiently motivated to participate in such studies are unlikely to maintain their truly 'normal' diet when requested to do so, even when promised access to the same interventions following completion of the study protocol [26].

Any benefit from diet induced weight loss interventions in terms of normalisa-tion of insulin and hormonal homeostasis is, however, frequently short-lived as the lost body mass is, on the whole, regained at the end of the study period [26]. Long term compliance and permanent weight loss is necessary for such interventions to result in a significant reduction in endometrial cancer risk.

Drug Induced Weight Loss

There have been no studies specifically investigating the effect of weight loss drugs on endometrial cancer prevention. A cost-effectiveness study undertaken in a mod-elled Australian cohort failed to find any cost benefit from prescribing either sibutramine (a centrally acting appetite suppressant and metabolism regulator, which has now been discontinued due to health concerns) or orlistat (an inhibitor of dietary fat absorption) to obese adults with the aim of primary prevention of obe-sity-related conditions [30]. The latter was a composite measure including colorec-tal, breast and endometrial cancer and stroke/ischaemic heart disease. The lack of cost benefit was due to the small amount of anticipated weight loss with the drug (2–5 kg) over the year-long treatment period and, more importantly, the fact that most women would be expected to regain the weight lost within 2 years of discon-tinuing treatment.

Prolonged treatment with Orlistat (6 months) has been shown to reduce serum glucose and insulin levels and improve insulin sensitivity in women with PCOS, whereas short-term treatment has not [31, 32]. As with diet induced weight loss, however, it is the long term adherence to these interventions that is critical for a reduction in endometrial cancer risk to be appreciated.

Bariatric Surgery Induced Weight Loss

More significant, permanent weight loss is seen following bariatric surgical procedures, including intestinal and gastric bypass and gastric banding. Table 10.1 describes the results of four observational studies investigating the effect of surgical induced weight loss on cancer incidence and, in particular, the risk of endometrial cancer. Across all studies, bariatric surgery has been shown to be associated with a significant reduction in the incidence of all and, in particular, obesity-related cancers and this effect appears to be gender-specific, with benefit limited to women [33, 34]. In particular, the risk of developing endometrial cancer for those women undergoing weight loss surgery is 78–81% lower than for their BMI-matched controls. Whilst the greatest risk reduction is seen in women who achieve a normal body weight following surgery, those who remain obese despite intervention still derive significant benefit from undergoing the procedure, signifying that its effect is not simply limited to inducing weight loss [37].

Bariatric surgery is associated with significant improvements in insulin sensitivity and over 75% of diabetic patients will experience resolution of the manifestations of this condition following the procedure, an effect which persists for more than 2 years after surgery [38, 39]. This is supported by biochemical evidence of significantly lower glucose, insulin and HbA1C levels. Whilst undoubtedly weight loss has a role to play in these improvements, the fact that they are seen within days of the procedure being undertaken and before any weight change point to alternative mechanisms of action of bariatric surgery on glucose homeostasis [40]. The highest proportion of patients who benefit from normalisation of their glucose control are those who have undergone biliary pancreatic diversion/duodenal switch, closely followed by gastric bypass and gastroplasty procedures [39]. Only 57% of patients having had gastric banding achieve complete resolution of their diabetes, suggesting that there are fundamental differences between these procedures which are responsible for the profound changes in glucose homeostasis seen [41]. Several potential mechanisms of action have been put forward to explain these findings. The first is the rapid reduction in hepatic fat that occurs following diversion procedures and which coincides with increased hepatic insulin sensitivity and normalisation of glucose levels. This is followed by a slower reduction in pancreatic fat and improved β-cell function, resulting from acute calorie restriction and negative energy balance following surgery. Secondly, rapid delivery of nutrients to the distal gut following gastric bypass results in elevated secretion of glucagon-like peptide-1 (GLP-1) by L cells of the distal intestine, a peptide responsible for increased insulin secretion and action. This is further enhanced by hypertrophy of the alimentary limb (the section

Table 10.1 Results of observational studies investigating the effect of surgical induced weight loss on cancer risk

Reference	Study design	Population	Intervention	Length of follow-up	Cancer risk	Endometrial cancer risk	Limitations
Adams and Hunt [33]	Retrospective cohort study	Intervention group-6596 patients undergoing gastric bypass surgery in Utah, USA Control group-9442 severely obese individuals (BMI $\geq$35 kg/m^2) identified from driver's license or ID cards	Roux-en-Y gastric bypass	12.5 years	Significant decrease in all cancer incidence for women undergoing gastric bypass surgery (HR 0.73, 95% CI 0.62–0.87, $p = 0.0004$). Effect limited to obesity related cancers. No change in men or non-obesity related cancers	Significant decrease in EC incidence (HR 0.22, 95% CI 0.13–0.40, $p < 0.0001$)	Self-reporting of BMI in control group, known to systematically underestimate weight and overestimate height. Attempt made to correct for this by correlating self-reported and measured weight in 500 patients. Control group heavier than surgery group (BMI 47.4 kg/m^2 cf. 44.9 kg/m^2). No data on other risk factors for EC apart from BMI, such as FHx, HRT use etc. Cannot exclude that surgical patients were healthier than controls, history of cancer within the preceding 5 years a contraindication to bypass surgery

(continued)

Table 10.1 (continued)

Reference	Study design	Population	Intervention	Length of follow-up	Cancer risk	Endometrial cancer risk	Limitations
Sjostrom et al. [34]	Prospective controlled intervention study	Intervention group-2010 patients elected to undergo surgery Control group-2037 contemporaneously group matched individuals preferring non-surgical intervention	Surgery-gastric banding, bypass or gastroplasty Control group-varied treatments from nothing to intensive lifestyle intervention	Median 10.9 years	Significant reduction in cancer incidence in women in the surgical intervention arm compared with controls (HR 0.58, 95% CI 0.44–0.77, $p = 0.0001$). No reduction in cancer incidence in men	Effect of surgery on specific cancer types not investigated	No standard treatment in either arm Groups matched for menopausal status, smoking, diabetes, waist: hip ratio, BMI, blood pressure, co-morbidities, cholesterol rather than individual patient matching. Effect of surgery on cancer incidence not specified as secondary outcome measure in original study design

Reference	Study design	Population	Intervention	Length of follow-up	Cancer risk	Endometrial cancer risk	Limitations
Ward et al. [35]	Retrospective cohort study	University Health System Consortium (UHC) database of hospital admissions (USA). A total of 44,345 cases of endometrial cancer analysed	Bariatric surgery (any type) Comparison group-no bariatric surgery Analysed according to current BMI (obese vs. non-obese)	Inpatient admissions from 2009–2013 reviewed	Results only analysed for EC	Previous bariatric surgery associated with a 71% reduction in EC risk (RR 0.29 95% CI 0.26–0.32), compared with obese women who had not undergone bariatric surgery. This increased to an 81% reduction for those women who had achieved a normal weight following surgery	No information on other endometrial cancer risk factors. No detail about the time interval between bariatric surgery and EC diagnosis, to exclude cases of EC being diagnosed at the time of work-up for bariatric surgery. Type, grade, stage and treatment for endometrial cancer not recorded

(continued)

Table 10.1 (continued)

Reference	Study design	Population	Intervention	Length of follow-up	Cancer risk	Endometrial cancer risk	Limitations
Christou et al. [36]	Retrospective cohort study	Intervention group-1035 individuals attending Canadian bariatric surgery centre Comparison group-5746 age, gender matched obese controls from administration database	Bariatric surgery (any type)	Maximum 5 years	Reduction in physician/hospital visits for all cancers (RR 0.22, 95% CI 0.143–0.347, $p = 0.001$) in surgery group compared with control group	Study underpowered to look at specific cancer types, with the exception of breast cancer	No matching of groups for co-morbidities or other risk factors for cancer. BMI not stipulated. Hospital visits rather than cancer diagnoses used as primary outcome

of small intestine directly attached to the newly formed stomach 'pouch') and an increase in the number of GLP-1 secreting cells. Whilst GLP-1 levels are higher in patients who have undergone bypass procedures compared with those undergoing gastric banding, animal experiments in which there has been a genetically induced deficiency of either GLP-1 or its receptor suggest that it may not be critical in determining improvements in glycaemic control following bariatric surgery. Thirdly, these procedures are associated with alterations in the gut microbiome, with an increase in the presence of Bacteroidetes species, which are responsible for bile acid conjugation and the fermentation of complex carbohydrates. This is associated with favourable effects on serum bile acid levels; bile acids inhibit gluconeogenesis and improve insulin signalling, glucose uptake and energy expenditure by peripheral muscle through the farsenoid X receptor [42]. They also stimulate GLP-1 secretion. Fourthly, bariatric surgery is associated with severe calorie restriction in the days and weeks immediately following the procedure and this in itself has been demonstrated to improve insulin sensitivity. Both diabetic and non-diabetic patients respond to a very low calorie diet (200–500 cal/day), mimicking that received after a Roux-en-Y gastric bypass, with lower insulin and glucose levels of a similar magnitude to that seen following surgery [43–45]. This effect is seen after only four days but requires calorific intake to be significantly restricted as less stringent diets, which allow 800–1000 cal/day, do not result in the same beneficial effects on insulin resistance [46, 47]. Intermittent dieting, where calorie restriction of 600-650 cal/day is imposed twice a week, appears to also improve insulin sensitivity, lowering insulin and HOMA-IR levels in obese and normal weight non-diabetic women at high risk of breast cancer [48]. Even though there was no difference in weight at the end of the trial between women receiving the intermittent fasting diet and a standard low calorie continuous diet, those on the intermittent diet had significantly lower body fat and were more likely to adhere to their diet in the longer term, including reducing their calorie intake on non-fasting days as well, a particular problem with other long term diets as highlighted earlier.

Whilst the relative importance of each of these effects is still being debated, it is likely that the exact mechanism is dependent upon the type of surgery undertaken. These findings would, however, support a decision to specifically offer gastric and intestinal bypass surgery to those women with insulin resistance and type 2 diabetes rather than gastric banding as these procedures are more likely to be associated with metabolic improvement and a reduced risk of endometrial cancer above and beyond pure weight loss.

In addition to its effects on insulin resistance, bariatric surgery has also been linked with improvements in other pro-carcinogenic pathways, in particular inflammation and oxidative stress. Higher levels of cytokines, such as IL-6, IL-8 and interferons, have been found in morbidly obese women and precede a diagnosis of endometrial cancer, suggesting a causal link [49, 50]. In line with the resolution of insulin resistance and decrease in adiposity, weight loss procedures have been shown to be associated with a lowering in the levels of these inflammatory mediators and improvements in natural killer activity, which could contribute to an anti-tumour cell immune response [38, 51]. There is also an increase in levels of antioxidants and their activity [38]. Similarly, the release of the adipokines leptin and adiponectin, responsible for increased cancer cell proliferation and insulin sensitivity, respectively, are beneficially influenced by bariatric surgery. Leptin levels are persistently lower and adiponectin secretion chronically elevated following these procedures [38].

The normalisation of the insulin response is also directly linked with the maintenance of sex hormone binding globulin synthesis and lowering of androgen and oestrogen levels, reducing the exaggerated oestrogenic stimulation of the endometrium [38]. This corresponds with the resolution of previously documented endometrial hyperplasia following weight loss, as seen in selected patients in both our own cohort [40] and that of Argenta et al. [52]. It is also supported by favourable changes in hormone receptor expression within the endometrium, with reductions in oestrogen and androgen receptor levels and, somewhat counterintuitively, progesterone receptor expression [52]. We also demonstrated an overall reduction in endometrial proliferation in women following bariatric surgery in our cohort, as measured by Ki-67 immunohistochemistry, when samples were matched for menstrual cycle phase in pre-menopausal women.

The hormonal and metabolic improvements seen with bariatric surgery extend beyond a simple reduction in adiposity and, as can be appreciated from this discussion, when used selectively in women at greatest risk of endometrial cancer, could be an effective strategy for primary prophylaxis.

Insulin and Insulin Sensitisers

Direct pharmacological methods of improving insulin sensitivity and reducing serum insulin levels have also been studied as potential preventive measures to reduce endometrial cancer risk. The majority of this work has been conducted looking specifically at metformin, which is already in widespread use as the first line drug treatment for type 2 diabetes.

Metformin

Metformin, an oral biguanide, was discovered in 1922, although it was not until 1958 that it became available in the UK and had to wait until 1994 for it to receive approval from the US Food and Drug Administration (FDA) for the treatment of type 2 diabetes [53]. The interest in the drug in the primary prevention of malignancy has stemmed from epidemiological evidence demonstrating a 32% reduction in cancer incidence in diabetic patients taking metformin, compared with those exposed to sulphonylureas, insulin or other drug regimes [54]. These results were based on retrospective observations from cohort and case-control studies, but were supported by a later meta-analysis by Noto et al. [55], who included three RCTs and described a similarly lower risk of cancer in metformin treated diabetic patients. A subgroup analysis performed according to study type, however, revealed that this effect was restricted to the observational studies and was not seen in the more methodologically rigorous RCTs.

The heterogeneity within the included populations, though, calls into question the validity of these findings. Many of the studies have failed to collect and analyse data on important cancer risk factors, including smoking and obesity [56]. They have also relied on retrospective patient recall and medical records, without checking the accuracy of entries or taking into account missing records. The generation of prescriptions has been repeatedly used to indicate drug exposure rather than considering patient compliance with treatment, thereby potentially overestimating any benefit. Suissa and Azoulay [57] describe three types of bias frequently seen in these studies; time–lag, immortal time and time-window bias. The former is a reflection of the natural history of diabetes, in that glycaemic control progressively worsens with time as insulin resistance increases and pancreatic β-cell function is lost. Patients initially commenced on metformin will require subsequent modification of their drug treatment to include sulphonylureas and insulin in order to maintain normoglycaemia. Comparisons of metformin with these other drugs in the context of cancer incidence are, therefore, rather superficial, as patients will be at different stages in their disease course. A time-lag is also to be expected between a patient being exposed to a drug and the development of a malignancy, during which time they may well have moved on to second or third line treatment. This results in the erroneous assignation of the cancer diagnosis to the drug currently being used, rather than to those taken 10–15 years earlier. Immortal time bias is introduced by studies failing to account for the time in which a patient was not exposed to the drug if they started therapy only during rather than at the beginning of the follow-up period. The result is the over-exaggeration of the protective effect of metformin, as only those patients who remain alive to be able to receive the treatment are able to be included in the analysis. Time-window bias describes the variations in follow-up periods used for cases and controls, such that one group has a considerably longer period of drug exposure than the other.

More recent meta-analyses have paid heed to these methodological criticisms and have excluded studies with time-lag bias. In so doing, Gandini et al. [56] failed to demonstrate any benefit from exposure to metformin on overall cancer incidence, after adjusting for BMI. This has similarly been the case when endometrial cancer risk has been specifically analysed [58–61]. Any positive effect associated with metformin used in the primary prevention of endometrial cancer may not, however, be seen in the diabetic population, but may instead lie in those with lesser degrees of insulin resistance.

The potential beneficial effects of metformin in terms of endometrial cancer prevention are likely to be mediated by its indirect effects on insulin sensitivity and the lowering of serum insulin levels. Metformin is actively transported into hepatocytes by the organic cation transporter Oct-1 [62]. Here, it inhibits complex 1 of the respiratory electron transport chain resulting in a reduction in ATP generation and a subsequent increase in AMP levels, although the specific details of this interaction are as yet poorly defined [63]. The end result is the activation of AMP-activated protein kinase (AMPK) through the direct binding of AMP to its γ subunit and a conformational change leading to phosphorylation of the catalytic α subunit, and inhibition of gluconeogenesis. Metformin is also able to increase signalling through the insulin receptor and the activity of insulin-receptor substrate 2 (IRS2), enhancing the uptake of glucose into cells through plasma membrane bound transporters such as GLUT-1 [62].

This combined with the counteraction of the gluconeogenic effects of glucagon, results in a lowering of serum glucose and subsequently insulin levels, though only in those whose levels are elevated at baseline. It would be logical to hypothesise that endometrial cancer, whose formation is driven by the mitogenic effects of insulin, could be prevented by lowering insulin levels in those individuals with subclinical insulin resistance. As metformin has no effect on insulin levels in those with normal insulin sensitivity, it is perhaps not surprising that this could be used as a predictive biomarker of metformin response [63, 64].

Whilst not specifically evaluated within the context of endometrial cancer prevention, there is evidence from in vitro studies that metformin also has a direct effect on endometrial cancer cells, affecting those pathways which appear critical to endometrial carcinogenesis, namely mTOR and MAPK/ERK pathways (Fig. 10.2). Through activation of AMPK, metformin is able to inhibit the activation of mTOR at multiple levels, including phosphorylation of tumour sclerosis complex 1 and 2 (TSC1 and 2) and inactivation of signalling through the insulin receptor and IRS1 [65, 66]. Activating mutations within the PI3K/Akt pathway are found in over 90% of endometrioid endometrial cancers, frequently in the form of loss of PTEN protein expression, highlighting the importance of this pathway in disease development [67]. Metformin is also able to act independently of AMPK to reduce signalling through the MAPK/ERK pathway, both in cell culture and in vivo, as demonstrated in response to short term treatment with the drug in a pre-surgical window study [68, 69]. Reducing signalling through these pathways and the corresponding effects on protein synthesis, cell survival and proliferation may be expected, therefore, to translate into a lower incidence of endometrial cancer. Further effects of metformin may also include AMPK induced downregulation of the regulator gene c-myc, a decrease in activity of the transcription regulator nuclear factor kappa B (NF-kB) and reduction in reactive oxygen species production [70–72]. The relative importance of these mechanisms, both in terms of endometrial carcinogenesis and metformin action on the endometrium, is, however, currently unknown.

The only in vivo studies of metformin in the prevention of endometrial cancer have come from animal experiments using the Zucker fa/fa obese rat, itself a model of insulin resistance, which suggest that metformin treatment is associated with a counteraction of the effects of exogenous oestrogen on the endometrium [73]. Treatment resulted in the reversal of hyperplasia and a reduction in mitogenic activity in epithelial, glandular and stromal cells. This was accompanied by a reduction in expression of c-myc and c-fos and inhibition of phosphorylation of both the insulin and IGF-1 receptors and ERK.

Whilst there is limited published data as yet of any clinical benefit in groups at high risk for endometrial cancer, metformin has been used in a small number of women who have developed atypical endometrial hyperplasia and declined surgical intervention for reasons of fertility preservation. Exposure to the drug, both alone and in combination with oral contraceptives, was associated with regression of the endometrial abnormalities, despite previous failed progesterone treatment [74, 75]. Whilst these results are based on only three patients, it is encouraging to note that these findings have been replicated in a small cohort of obese, insulin resistant women with polycys-

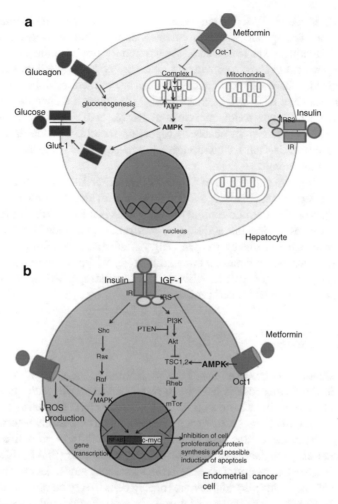

Fig. 10.2 Indirect (**a**) and direct (**b**) mechanisms of action of metformin. (**a**) Metformin enters hepatocytes through its transporter Oct-1, where it inhibits complex I of the respiratory electron transport chain. This has the effect of reducing ATP production by the mitochondria, increasing AMP levels and activating AMPK. The activation of AMPK leads to enhanced signalling through the insulin receptor and IRS2, increased intracellular glucose transport through Glut-1 and inhibition of gluconeogenesis. Metformin is also able to direct suppress glucagon mediated gluconeogenesis. The end result is lowering of serum glucose and subsequently insulin levels. (**b**) Metformin has also been shown to exert direct effects on EC cells. Activation of AMPK is responsible for an increase in TSC1 and 2 signalling and inhibition of mTor activity. This, combined with a reduction in signalling through the insulin receptor and downregulation of c-myc, leads to inhibition of cell proliferation, protein synthesis and a possible increase in apoptosis. Metformin has also been shown to act independently of AMPK within cancer cells to decrease ROS production, inhibit NF-kB activity and inhibit signalling of the MAPK pathway

tic ovary syndrome [76]. Metformin was associated with a lowering in total testosterone, insulin and fasting glucose measurements, but these changes were not statistically significant. Treatment was restricted to six women for three months only and, therefore, underpowered to show a convincing treatment effect. Beyond endometrial cancer, larger studies have been conducted into the use of metformin in primary cancer prevention. A recent RCT by Higurashi et al. [77] reported a decrease in the recurrence of colorectal polyps following year-long treatment of non-diabetic patients with metformin. The authors were unable to report on the effect of the drug on cancer incidence due to their short follow-up time, but these results using surrogate disease markers do show promise.

These findings are supportive of a role for metformin in endometrial cancer prevention, but further mechanistic and clinical trial evidence is clearly warranted before it can be rolled out into routine practice. This is the focus of a currently open clinical trial investigating the addition of metformin alongside lifestyle interventions in obese, insulin resistant women [78]. Although the follow-up period will be too short to report on clinical outcomes, this study will provide novel information on the effect of metformin on tissue biomarkers, including pAMPK and mTOR and genes related to endometrial cell proliferation.

Thiazolidinediones

Whilst evaluating the potential benefit of metformin in the prevention of endometrial cancer, conflicting results have been published in the literature as to whether other diabetic medications have a positive or negative effect on cancer development [79]. The thiazolidinediones are a group of medications commonly referred to as the glitazones, which act to decrease blood glucose levels through activation of the nuclear receptor, peroxisome proliferator-activated receptor (PPAR). The resulting alteration in gene expression indirectly reduces serum glucose levels by increasing the uptake of fatty acids into adipocytes, forcing cells to rely on glucose as their fuel source [80]. Concern over the association between thiazolidinediones and the risk of heart failure and bladder cancer have led to the withdrawal of them from many countries, with the exception of pioglitazone, which continues to be prescribed in the UK and USA [81]. It is used if metformin is not tolerated or to intensify glycaemic control if metformin alone is insufficient and within this context has a beneficial effect on reducing cardiovascular disease, heart failure and all-cause mortality risk within a UK General Practice cohort study [81, 82].

Ever use of pioglitazone has not been shown to be associated with endometrial cancer risk, as demonstrated in a retrospective cohort study conducted using the Kaiser Permanente Northern California Diabetes Registry and its linked cancer registry [79]. Whilst the authors suggested that there was a significant trend between time since initiation of the drug and incidence of endometrial cancer, the duration of time exposed and dose received had no bearing on endometrial cancer risk, calling into doubt the biological relevance of this finding. A nested case-control study from Italy found a similar negative result on reviewing 376 diabetic women with endometrial cancer and matched diabetic controls [83]. Ever use was associated with an odds ratio of 0.77 (95% CI 0.48–1.24) for the disease, after adjusting for co-morbidities and HRT use. The number of patients exposed to these drugs has been relatively small, however, and to date short term use alone has been evaluated as the drug was only licensed for the treatment of type 2 diabetes in 1999.

Sulphonylureas

The sulphonylureas contribute a glucose lowering effect by increasing insulin secretion from the pancreas. By binding to an ATP-sensitive potassium channel on the cell membrane, they induce depolarisation of the cells and the opening of a voltage-gated calcium channel, releasing insulin from its storage granules [84]. They may also reduce hepatic glucose production, inhibit lipolysis and decrease insulin breakdown. Like the thiazolidinediones, they are used as second line drug treatment for type 2 diabetes [82].

Despite concerns that the increased secretion of insulin induced by sulphonylureas may affect cancer risk, the study by Ferrara et al. [79] failed to demonstrate any effect of the drugs on the incidence of endometrial cancer. Similarly, when only new users of the drug were considered alongside those commencing metformin, no effect was observed [59]. This suggests that the relationship between glucose, insulin and endometrial carcinogenesis is a complex one that is yet to be completely understood.

Insulin

Given the compelling evidence linking insulin resistance, high insulin levels and the development of endometrial cancer, treatment of type 2 diabetes with exogenous insulin may be anticipated to result in a higher incidence of the cancer. Epidemiological studies have certainly supported this assumption, with higher risks of malignancy, particularly of breast cancer, being found in patients treated with insulin analogues [85]. This effect appeared to be both dose and treatment duration dependent. More methodologically rigorous RCTs, however, have challenged these findings, noting no increase in cancer risk with glargine use [85]. This difference may well reflect the more advanced stage of diabetes found in patients requiring insulin treatment and the presence of co-morbidities, which are frequently unaccounted or controlled for in large cohort studies. Differences between the body's response to exogenous and endogenous insulin may be of greater important than initially realised.

Conclusion

There is now convincing evidence supporting a critical role for insulin resistance in endometrial carcinogenesis, a theme common to many of the well-established risk factors for the condition, including obesity and diabetes [86]. Interventions associated with improvement in insulin sensitivity have been noted, either incidentally or by design, to be associated with a reduced risk of endometrial cancer, particularly if used long term. The most compelling arguments are for bariatric surgery and metformin, though the specific groups who would benefit most from these interventions have yet to be clearly defined. More accurate models of disease risk prediction are required as a starting point to primary prevention trials and testing for insulin resistance is likely to be central to this.

Conflicts of Interest The authors report no conflicts of interest.

References

1. Hernandez AV, Pasupuleti V, Benites-Zapata VA, Thota P, Deshpande A, Perez-Lopez FR. Insulin resistance and endometrial cancer risk: a systematic review and meta-analysis. Eur J Cancer. 2015;51(18):2747–58.
2. Nead KT, Sharp SJ, Thompson DJ, Painter JN, Savage DB, Semple RK, Barker A, Australian National Endometrial Cancer Study G, Perry JR, Attia J, Dunning AM, Easton DF, Holliday E, Lotta LA, O'Mara T, McEvoy M, Pharoah PD, Scott RJ, Spurdle AB, Langenberg C, Wareham NJ, Scott RA. Evidence of a causal association between insulinemia and endometrial cancer: a Mendelian randomization analysis. J Natl Cancer Inst. 2015;107(9):pii: djv178.
3. Trabert B, Wentzensen N, Felix AS, Yang HP, Sherman ME, Brinton LA. Metabolic syndrome and risk of endometrial cancer in the united states: a study in the SEER-medicare linked database. Cancer Epidemiol Biomark Prev. 2015;24(1):261–7.
4. Li X, Guo YR, Lin JF, Feng Y, Billig H, Shao R. Combination of Diane-35 and metformin to treat early endometrial carcinoma in PCOS women with insulin resistance. J Cancer. 2014;5(3):173–81.
5. Nagamani M, Stuart CA. Specific binding and growth-promoting activity of insulin in endometrial cancer cells in culture. Am J Obstet Gynecol. 1998;179(1):6–12.
6. Renehan AG, Frystyk J, Flyvbjerg A. Obesity and cancer risk: the role of the insulin-IGF axis. Trends Endocrinol Metab. 2006;17(8):328–36.
7. Friberg E, Mantzoros CS, Wolk A. Physical activity and risk of endometrial cancer: a population-based prospective cohort study. Cancer Epidemiol Biomark Prev. 2006;15(11):2136–40.
8. Gierach GL, Chang SC, Brinton LA, Lacey JV Jr, Hollenbeck AR, Schatzkin A, Leitzmann MF. Physical activity, sedentary behavior, and endometrial cancer risk in the NIH-AARP diet and health study. Int J Cancer. 2009;124(9):2139–47.
9. Cust AE, Armstrong BK, Friedenreich CM, Slimani N, Bauman A. Physical activity and endometrial cancer risk: a review of the current evidence, biologic mechanisms and the quality of physical activity assessment methods. Cancer Causes Control. 2007;18(3):243–58.
10. Friedenreich C, Cust A, Lahmann PH, Steindorf K, Boutron-Ruault MC, Clavel-Chapelon F, Mesrine S, Linseisen J, Rohrmann S, Pischon T, Schulz M, Tjonneland A, Johnsen NF, Overvad K, Mendez M, Arguelles MV, Garcia CM, Larranaga N, Chirlaque MD, Ardanaz E, Bingham S, Khaw KT, Allen N, Key T, Trichopoulou A, Dilis V, Trichopoulos D, Pala V, Palli D, Tumino R, Panico S, Vineis P, Bueno-de-Mesquita HB, Peeters PH, Monninkhof E, Berglund G, Manjer J, Slimani N, Ferrari P, Kaaks R, Riboli E. Physical activity and risk of endometrial cancer: the European prospective investigation into cancer and nutrition. Int J Cancer. 2007;121(2):347–55.
11. Schmid D, Behrens G, Keimling M, Jochem C, Ricci C, Leitzmann M. A systematic review and meta-analysis of physical activity and endometrial cancer risk. Eur J Epidemiol. 2015;30(5):397–412.

12. Voskuil DW, Monninkhof EM, Elias SG, Vlems FA, van Leeuwen FE, Task Force Physical, A. & Cancer. Physical activity and endometrial cancer risk, a systematic review of current evidence. Cancer Epidemiol Biomark Prev. 2007;16(4):639–48.
13. Friedenreich CM. The role of physical activity in breast cancer etiology. Semin Oncol. 2010;37(3):297–302.
14. Moore SC, Gierach GL, Schatzkin A, Matthews CE. Physical activity, sedentary behaviours, and the prevention of endometrial cancer. Br J Cancer. 2010;103(7):933–8.
15. McTiernan A. Mechanisms linking physical activity with cancer. Nat Rev Cancer. 2008;8(3):205–11.
16. Boule NG, Haddad E, Kenny GP, Wells GA, Sigal RJ. Effects of exercise on glycemic control and body mass in type 2 diabetes mellitus: a meta-analysis of controlled clinical trials. JAMA. 2001;286(10):1218–27.
17. Campbell KL, McTiernan A. Exercise and biomarkers for cancer prevention studies. J Nutr. 2007;137(1 Suppl):161S–9S.
18. Esposito K, Pontillo A, Di Palo C, Giugliano G, Masella M, Marfella R, Giugliano D. Effect of weight loss and lifestyle changes on vascular inflammatory markers in obese women: a randomized trial. JAMA. 2003;289(14):1799–804.
19. Sturgeon KM, Digiovanni L, Good J, Salvatore D, Fenderson D, Domchek SM, Stopfer JE, Galantino ML, Bryan C, Hwang WT, Schmitz K. Exercise induced dose response alterations in adiponectin and leptin levels are dependent on body fat changes in women at risk for breast cancer. Cancer Epidemiol Biomarkers Prev. 2016;25(8):1195–200.
20. McTiernan A, Sorensen B, Yasui Y, Tworoger SS, Ulrich CM, Irwin ML, Rudolph RE, Stanczyk FZ, Schwartz RS, Potter JD. No effect of exercise on insulin-like growth factor 1 and insulin-like growth factor binding protein 3 in postmenopausal women: a 12-month randomized clinical trial. Cancer Epidemiol Biomark Prev. 2005;14(4):1020–1.
21. Crosbie EJ, Zwahlen M, Kitchener HC, Egger M, Renehan AG. Body mass index, hormone replacement therapy, and endometrial cancer risk: a meta-analysis. Cancer Epidemiol Biomark Prev. 2010;19(12):3119–30.
22. Renehan AG, Tyson M, Egger M, Heller RF, Zwahlen M. Body-mass index and incidence of cancer: a systematic review and meta-analysis of prospective observational studies. Lancet. 2008;371(9612):569–78.
23. Parker ED, Folsom AR. Intentional weight loss and incidence of obesity-related cancers: the Iowa Women's Health Study. Int J Obes Relat Metab Disord. 2003;27(12):1447–52.
24. Prentice RL, Thomson CA, Caan B, Hubbell FA, Anderson GL, Beresford SA, Pettinger M, Lane DS, Lessin L, Yasmeen S, Singh B, Khandekar J, Shikany JM, Satterfield S, Chlebowski RT. Low-fat dietary pattern and cancer incidence in the women's health initiative dietary modification randomized controlled trial. J Natl Cancer Inst. 2007;99(20):1534–43.
25. Atiomo W, Read A, Golding M, Silcocks P, Razali N, Sarkar S, Hardiman P, Thornton J. Local recruitment experience in a study comparing the effectiveness of a low glycaemic index diet with a low calorie healthy eating approach at achieving weight loss and reducing the risk of endometrial cancer in women with polycystic ovary syndrome (PCOS). Contemp Clin Trials. 2009;30(5):451–6.
26. Campbell KL, Foster-Schubert KE, Alfano CM, Wang CC, Wang CY, Duggan CR, Mason C, Imayama I, Kong A, Xiao L, Bain CE, Blackburn GL, Stanczyk FZ, McTiernan A. Reduced-calorie dietary weight loss, exercise, and sex hormones in postmenopausal women: randomized controlled trial. J Clin Oncol. 2012;30(19):2314–26.
27. Crighton IL, Dowsett M, Hunter M, Shaw C, Smith IE. The effect of a low-fat diet on hormone levels in healthy pre- and postmenopausal women: relevance for breast cancer. Eur J Cancer. 1992;28A(12):2024–7.
28. Prentice RL, Caan B, Chlebowski RT, Patterson R, Kuller LH, Ockene JK, Margolis KL, Limacher MC, Manson JE, Parker LM, Paskett E, Phillips L, Robbins J, Rossouw JE, Sarto GE, Shikany JM, Stefanick ML, Thomson CA, Van Horn L, Vitolins MZ, Wactawski-Wende J, Wallace RB, Wassertheil-Smoller S, Whitlock E, Yano K, Adams-Campbell L, Anderson GL,

Assaf AR, Beresford SA, Black HR, Brunner RL, Brzyski RG, Ford L, Gass M, Hays J, Heber D, Heiss G, Hendrix SL, Hsia J, Hubbell FA, Jackson RD, Johnson KC, Kotchen JM, LaCroix AZ, Lane DS, Langer RD, Lasser NL, Henderson MM. Low-fat dietary pattern and risk of invasive breast cancer: the women's health initiative randomized controlled dietary modification trial. JAMA. 2006;295(6):629–42.

29. Soares NP, Santos AC, Costa EC, Azevedo GD, Damasceno DC, Fayh AP, Lemos TM. Diet-induced weight loss reduces DNA damage and cardiometabolic risk factors in overweight/obese women with polycystic ovary syndrome. Ann Nutr Metab. 2016;68(3):220–7.

30. Veerman JL, Barendregt JJ, Forster M, Vos T. Cost-effectiveness of pharmacotherapy to reduce obesity. PLoS One. 2011;6(10):e26051.

31. Kumar P, Arora S. Orlistat in polycystic ovarian syndrome reduces weight with improvement in lipid profile and pregnancy rates. J Hum Reprod Sci. 2014;7(4):255–61.

32. Panidis D, Tziomalos K, Papadakis E, Chatzis P, Kandaraki EA, Tsourdi EA, Katsikis I. The role of orlistat combined with lifestyle changes in the management of overweight and obese patients with polycystic ovary syndrome. Clin Endocrinol. 2014;80(3):432–8.

33. Adams TD, Hunt SC. Cancer and obesity: effect of bariatric surgery. World J Surg. 2009;33(10):2028–33.

34. Sjostrom L, Gummesson A, Sjostrom CD, Narbro K, Peltonen M, Wedel H, Bengtsson C, Bouchard C, Carlsson B, Dahlgren S, Jacobson P, Karason K, Karlsson J, Larsson B, Lindroos AK, Lonroth H, Naslund I, Olbers T, Stenlof K, Torgerson J, Carlsson LM, Swedish Obese Subjects S. Effects of bariatric surgery on cancer incidence in obese patients in Sweden (Swedish Obese Subjects Study): a prospective, controlled intervention trial. Lancet Oncol. 2009;10(7):653–62.

35. Ward KK, Roncancio AM, Shah NR, Davis MA, Saenz CC, McHale MT, et al. Bariatric surgery decreases the risk of uterine malignancy. Gynecol Oncol. 2014;133(1):63–6.

36. Christou NV, Lieberman M, Sampalis F, Sampalis JS. Bariatric surgery reduces cancer risk in morbidly obese patients. Surg Obes Relat Dis. 2008;4(6):691–5.

37. Ward KK, Shah NR, Saenz CC, McHale MT, Alvarez EA, Plaxe SC. Cardiovascular disease is the leading cause of death among endometrial cancer patients. Gynecol Oncol. 2012;126(2):176–9.

38. Ashrafian H, Ahmed K, Rowland SP, Patel VM, Gooderham NJ, Holmes E, Darzi A, Athanasiou T. Metabolic surgery and cancer: protective effects of bariatric procedures. Cancer. 2011;117(9):1788–99.

39. Buchwald H, Estok R, Fahrbach K, Banel D, Jensen MD, Pories WJ, Bantle JP, Sledge I. Weight and type 2 diabetes after bariatric surgery: systematic review and meta-analysis. Am J Med. 2009;122(3):248–56 e5.

40. MacKintosh ML, Crosbie EJ. Obesity-driven endometrial cancer: is weight loss the answer? BJOG. 2013;120:791–4.

41. Batterham RL, Cummings DE. Mechanisms of diabetes improvement following bariatric/metabolic surgery. Diabetes Care. 2016;39(6):893–901.

42. Catoi AF, Parvu A, Muresan A, Busetto L. Metabolic mechanisms in obesity and type 2 diabetes: insights from bariatric/metabolic surgery. Obes Facts. 2015;8(6):350–63.

43. Isbell JM, Tamboli RA, Hansen EN, Saliba J, Dunn JP, Phillips SE, Marks-Shulman PA, Abumrad NN. The importance of caloric restriction in the early improvements in insulin sensitivity after Roux-en-Y gastric bypass surgery. Diabetes Care. 2010;33(7):1438–42.

44. Jackness C, Karmally W, Febres G, Conwell IM, Ahmed L, Bessler M, McMahon DJ, Korner J. Very low-calorie diet mimics the early beneficial effect of Roux-en-Y gastric bypass on insulin sensitivity and beta-cell Function in type 2 diabetic patients. Diabetes. 2013;62(9):3027–32.

45. Lingvay I, Guth E, Islam A, Livingston E. Rapid improvement in diabetes after gastric bypass surgery: is it the diet or surgery? Diabetes Care. 2013;36(9):2741–7.

46. Plum L, Ahmed L, Febres G, Bessler M, Inabnet W, Kunreuther E, McMahon DJ, Korner J. Comparison of glucostatic parameters after hypocaloric diet or bariatric surgery and equivalent weight loss. Obesity (Silver Spring). 2011;19(11):2149–57.

47. Wing RR, Blair EH, Bononi P, Marcus MD, Watanabe R, Bergman RN. Caloric restriction per se is a significant factor in improvements in glycemic control and insulin sensitivity during weight loss in obese NIDDM patients. Diabetes Care. 1994;17(1):30–6.

48. Harvie M, Wright C, Pegington M, McMullan D, Mitchell E, Martin B, Cutler RG, Evans G, Whiteside S, Maudsley S, Camandola S, Wang R, Carlson OD, Egan JM, Mattson MP, Howell A. The effect of intermittent energy and carbohydrate restriction v. daily energy restriction on weight loss and metabolic disease risk markers in overweight women. Br J Nutr. 2013;110(8):1534–47.
49. Dossus L, Rinaldi S, Becker S, Lukanova A, Tjonneland A, Olsen A, Stegger J, Overvad K, Chabbert-Buffet N, Jimenez-Corona A, Clavel-Chapelon F, Rohrmann S, Teucher B, Boeing H, Schutze M, Trichopoulou A, Benetou V, Lagiou P, Palli D, Berrino F, Panico S, Tumino R, Sacerdote C, Redondo ML, Travier N, Sanchez MJ, Altzibar JM, Chirlaque MD, Ardanaz E, Bueno-de-Mesquita HB, van Duijnhoven FJ, Onland-Moret NC, Peeters PH, Hallmans G, Lundin E, Khaw KT, Wareham N, Allen N, Key TJ, Slimani N, Hainaut P, Romaguera D, Norat T, Riboli E, Kaaks R. Obesity, inflammatory markers, and endometrial cancer risk: a prospective case-control study. Endocr Relat Cancer. 2010;17(4):1007–19.
50. Wang T, Rohan TE, Gunter MJ, Xue X, Wactawski-Wende J, Rajpathak SN, Cushman M, Strickler HD, Kaplan RC, Wassertheil-Smoller S, Scherer PE, Ho GY. A prospective study of inflammation markers and endometrial cancer risk in postmenopausal hormone nonusers. Cancer Epidemiol Biomark Prev. 2011;20(5):971–7.
51. Kopp HP, Kopp CW, Festa A, Krzyzanowska K, Kriwanek S, Minar E, Roka R, Schernthaner G. Impact of weight loss on inflammatory proteins and their association with the insulin resistance syndrome in morbidly obese patients. Arterioscler Thromb Vasc Biol. 2003;23(6):1042–7.
52. Argenta P, Svendsen C, Elishaev E, Gloyeske N, Geller MA, Edwards RP, Linkov F. Hormone receptor expression patterns in the endometrium of asymptomatic morbidly obese women before and after bariatric surgery. Gynecol Oncol. 2014;133(1):78–82.
53. Wikipedia. Metformin [Online]. 2016. https://en.wikipedia.org/wiki/Metformin. Accessed 12 Jul 2016.
54. Decensi A, Puntoni M, Goodwin P, Cazzaniga M, Gennari A, Bonanni B, Gandini S. Metformin and cancer risk in diabetic patients: a systematic review and meta-analysis. Cancer Prev Res (Phila). 2010;3(11):1451–61.
55. Noto H, Goto A, Tsujimoto T, Noda M. Cancer risk in diabetic patients treated with metformin: a systematic review and meta-analysis. PLoS One. 2012;7(3):e33411.
56. Gandini S, Puntoni M, Heckman-Stoddard BM, Dunn BK, Ford L, DeCensi A, Szabo E. Metformin and cancer risk and mortality: a systematic review and meta-analysis taking into account biases and confounders. Cancer Prev Res (Phila). 2014;7(9):867–85.
57. Suissa S, Azoulay L. Metformin and the risk of cancer: time-related biases in observational studies. Diabetes Care. 2012;35(12):2665–73.
58. Becker C, Jick SS, Meier CR, Bodmer M. Metformin and the risk of endometrial cancer: a case-control analysis. Gynecol Oncol. 2013;129(3):565–9.
59. Ko EM, Sturmer T, Hong J, Castillo WC, Bae-Jump V, Funk MJ. Metformin and the risk of endometrial cancer: a population-based cohort study. Gynecol Oncol. 2015;136(2):341–7.
60. Luo J, Beresford S, Chen C, Chlebowski R, Garcia L, Kuller L, Regier M, Wactawski-Wende J, Margolis KL. Association between diabetes, diabetes treatment and risk of developing endometrial cancer. Br J Cancer. 2014;111(7):1432–9.
61. Soffer D, Shi J, Chung J, Schottinger JE, Wallner LP, Chlebowski RT, Lentz SE, Haque R. Metformin and breast and gynecological cancer risk among women with diabetes. BMJ Open Diabetes Res Care. 2015;3(1):e000049.
62. Pernicova I, Korbonits M. Metformin—mode of action and clinical implications for diabetes and cancer. Nat Rev Endocrinol. 2014;10(3):143–56.
63. Pollak MN. Investigating metformin for cancer prevention and treatment: the end of the beginning. Cancer Discov. 2012;2(9):778–90.
64. Bonanni B, Puntoni M, Cazzaniga M, Pruneri G, Serrano D, Guerrieri-Gonzaga A, Gennari A, Trabacca MS, Galimberti V, Veronesi P, Johansson H, Aristarco V, Bassi F, Luini A, Lazzeroni M, Varricchio C, Viale G, Bruzzi P, Decensi A. Dual effect of metformin on breast cancer proliferation in a randomized presurgical trial. J Clin Oncol. 2012;30(21):2593–600.
65. Gwinn DM, Shackelford DB, Egan DF, Mihaylova MM, Mery A, Vasquez DS, Turk BE, Shaw RJ. AMPK phosphorylation of raptor mediates a metabolic checkpoint. Mol Cell. 2008;30(2):214–26.

66. Ning J, Clemmons DR. AMP-activated protein kinase inhibits IGF-I signaling and protein synthesis in vascular smooth muscle cells via stimulation of insulin receptor substrate 1 S794 and tuberous sclerosis 2 S1345 phosphorylation. Mol Endocrinol. 2010;24(6):1218–29.
67. Cancer Genome Atlas Research N, Kandoth C, Schultz N, Cherniack AD, Akbani R, Liu Y, Shen H, Robertson AG, Pashtan I, Shen R, Benz CC, Yau C, Laird PW, Ding L, Zhang W, Mills GB, Kucherlapati R, Mardis ER, Levine DA. Integrated genomic characterization of endometrial carcinoma. Nature. 2013;497(7447):67–73.
68. Do MT, Kim HG, Khanal T, Choi JH, Kim DH, Jeong TC, Jeong HG. Metformin inhibits heme oxygenase-1 expression in cancer cells through inactivation of Raf-ERK-Nrf2 signaling and AMPK-independent pathways. Toxicol Appl Pharmacol. 2013;271(2):229–38.
69. Mitsuhashi A, Kiyokawa T, Sato Y, Shozu M. Effects of metformin on endometrial cancer cell growth in vivo: a preoperative prospective trial. Cancer. 2014;120(19):2986–95.
70. Algire C, Moiseeva O, Deschenes-Simard X, Amrein L, Petruccelli L, Birman E, Viollet B, Ferbeyre G, Pollak MN. Metformin reduces endogenous reactive oxygen species and associated DNA damage. Cancer Prev Res (Phila). 2012;5(4):536–43.
71. Blandino G, Valerio M, Cioce M, Mori F, Casadei L, Pulito C, Sacconi A, Biagioni F, Cortese G, Galanti S, Manetti C, Citro G, Muti P, Strano S. Metformin elicits anticancer effects through the sequential modulation of DICER and c-MYC. Nat Commun. 2012;3:865.
72. Tan BK, Adya R, Chen J, Lehnert H, Sant Cassia LJ, Randeva HS. Metformin treatment exerts antiinvasive and antimetastatic effects in human endometrial carcinoma cells. J Clin Endocrinol Metab. 2011;96(3):808–16.
73. Zhang Q, Celestino J, Schmandt R, McCampbell AS, Urbauer DL, Meyer LA, Burzawa JK, Huang M, Yates MS, Iglesias D, Broaddus RR, Lu KH. Chemopreventive effects of metformin on obesity-associated endometrial proliferation. Am J Obstet Gynecol. 2013;209(1):24 e1–24 e12.
74. Session DR, Kalli KR, Tummon IS, Damario MA, Dumesic DA. Treatment of atypical endometrial hyperplasia with an insulin-sensitizing agent. Gynecol Endocrinol. 2003;17(5):405–7.
75. Shen ZQ, Zhu HT, Lin JF. Reverese of progestin-resistant atypical endometrial hyperplasia by metformin and oral contraceptives. Obstet Gynecol. 2008;112(2 Pt 2):465–7.
76. Legro RS, Zaino RJ, Demers LM, Kunselman AR, Gnatuk CL, Williams NI, et al. The effects of metformin and rosiglitazone, alone and in combination, on the ovary and endometrium in polycystic ovary syndrome. Am J Obstet Gynecol. 2007;196(4):402.
77. Higurashi T, Hosono K, Takahashi H, Komiya Y, Umezawa S, Sakai E, et al. Metformin for chemoprevention of metachronous colorectal adenoma or polyps in post-polypectomy patients without diabetes: a multi-centre double-blind, placebo-controlled, randomised phase 3 trial. Lancet Oncol. 2016;17(4):475–83.
78. Clinical Trial.Gov. An endometrial cancer chemoprevention study of metformin [Online]. 2016. https://clinicaltrials.gov/ct2/show/NCT01697566. Accessed 11 Feb 2016.
79. Ferrara A, Lewis JD, Quesenberry CP Jr, Peng T, Strom BL, Van Den Eeden SK, Ehrlich SF, Habel LA. Cohort study of pioglitazone and cancer incidence in patients with diabetes. Diabetes Care. 2011;34(4):923–9.
80. Nickkho-Amiry M, McVey R, Holland C. Peroxisome proliferator-activated receptors modulate proliferation and angiogenesis in human endometrial carcinoma. Mol Cancer Res. 2012;10(3):441–53.
81. Hippisley-Cox J, Coupland C. Diabetes treatments and risk of heart failure, cardiovascular disease, and all cause mortality: cohort study in primary care. BMJ. 2016;354:i3477.
82. NICE. (2014). Type 2 diabetes: the management of type 2 diabetes [Online]. NICE, London. https://www.nice.org.uk/guidance/cg87?unlid=. Accessed 26 Jul 2016.
83. Franchi M, Asciutto R, Nicotra F, Merlino L, La Vecchia C, Corrao G, Bosetti C. Metformin, other antidiabetic drugs, and endometrial cancer risk: a nested case-control study within Italian healthcare utilization databases. Eur J Cancer Prev. 2016;26(3):225–31.
84. Ashcroft FM. Mechanisms of the glycaemic effects of sulfonylureas. Horm Metab Res. 1996;28(9):456–63.
85. Gallagher EJ, LeRoith D. Diabetes, antihyperglycemic medications and cancer risk: smoke or fire? Curr Opin Endocrinol Diabetes Obes. 2013;20(5):485–94.
86. Friberg E, Orsini N, Mantzoros CS, Wolk A. Diabetes mellitus and risk of endometrial cancer: a meta-analysis. Diabetologia. 2007;50(7):1365–74.

Chapter 11
Management of Endometrial Cancer Precursors in Obese Women

Joseph A. Dottino, Karen H. Lu, and Melinda S. Yates

Abstract Endometrial cancer can generally be divided into two clinical subtypes, designated as type I and type II disease, each with different risk factors, histology, genetics, treatment and prognosis. Type I endometrial cancer, or low grade endometrioid adenocarcinoma, accounts for 80–90% of new cases of endometrial cancer. Endometrioid endometrial cancer is strongly associated with unopposed estrogen exposure (such as hormone replacement therapy) and obesity. Type II endometrial cancers, including clear cell carcinoma and uterine papillary serous carcinoma, are relatively rare. While the etiology of these rare tumors is not well understood, type II endometrial cancers are not associated with obesity. As such, this chapter will focus on low grade endometrioid (type I) endometrial cancer and its precursor lesions. Due to the close connection between obesity and endometrioid endometrial cancer, obese women are at increased risk for precancerous lesions and low grade endometrial cancers, and consideration is warranted for management of these conditions in the obese population.

Keywords Endometrial adenocarcinoma • Endometrial intraepithelial neoplasia • Endometrial cancer precursors • Surgical management • Conservative management • Fertility sparing management • Long term management

Introduction

Obesity contributes to endometrioid endometrial cancer development through multiple molecular pathways, as described in detail in previous chapters. Increasing body mass index (BMI), which is calculated by dividing the patient's weight (kg) by

J.A. Dottino • M.S. Yates (✉)
Department of Gynecologic Oncology & Reproductive Medicine, University of Texas MD Anderson Cancer Center, 1155 Pressler Street, Unit 1362, Houston, TX 77030, USA
e-mail: JDottino@mdanderson.org; MSYates@mdanderson.org

K.H. Lu
Department of Gynecologic Oncology and Reproductive Medicine,
MD Anderson Cancer Center, Houston, TX, USA
e-mail: khlu@mdanderson.org

© Springer International Publishing AG 2018
N.A. Berger et al. (eds.), *Focus on Gynecologic Malignancies*, Energy Balance and Cancer 13, DOI 10.1007/978-3-319-63483-8_11

the square of their height (m²), results in a linear increase in risk for endometrial cancer. In a study of 6905 U.S. women undergoing total hysterectomy, Ward et al. found that with each 1 unit increase in BMI, there was a corresponding 11% increase in the proportion of patients diagnosed with endometrial cancer [1]. In the past, obesity (defined as BMI > 30 kg/m²) was believed to contribute to endometrial cancer development primarily through increased estrogen levels from peripheral conversion of androgens to estrone in adipose tissue [2]. However, in addition to pro-proliferative signals from increased estrogen, other signaling pathways, such as mitogen-activated protein kinase (MAPK), are also activated. It is also known that obesity alters adipokine levels and causes hyperactivation of insulin signaling. Other health conditions related to obesity or metabolic syndrome, including type II diabetes and polycystic ovarian syndrome (PCOS), also act on these molecular pathways to increase risk of endometrial hyperplasia and cancer. Features of PCOS include multiple risk factors, such as polycystic ovaries, androgen excess, and anovulation, with resulting reduction in progesterone levels. Also, PCOS is independently associated with insulin resistance, type 2 diabetes, and obesity [3]. Aberrant insulin signaling can result in pro-proliferative signaling via activation of the phosphoinositide kinase 3 (PI3K)/AKT/mTOR (mammalian target of rapamycin) pathway [4–7]. All of the molecular changes described above are important in the progression from normal endometrium to precancerous lesions and then cancer, also making these key targets for the clinical management of precursors and low grade endometrial cancers.

Premalignant Lesions and Progression to Low Grade Endometrial Cancers

The development of endometrioid endometrial cancer occurs following a progression from normal endometrium to a hyperplastic precancerous lesion that then transforms into low grade endometrioid endometrial cancer. Obesity increases the risk of developing precancerous lesions as well as endometrial cancer. Presently, the spectrum of endometrial precancerous lesions are described using two distinct nomenclature schemas. The International Endometrial Collaborative Group utilizes a two-tier quantitative classification system that terms endometrial precancers as "endometrial intraepithelial neoplasia", or EIN. The more widely used 1994 World Health Organization (WHO94) schema is comprised of four classifications of risk based on histologic features of glandular complexity and nuclear atypia: (1) simple hyperplasia, (2) complex hyperplasia, (3) simple hyperplasia with atypia, and (4) complex hyperplasia with atypia [8]. As first described by Kurman and colleagues, risk of progression of endometrial hyperplasia to malignancy is dependent on the histopathologic feature present, namely cytologic and architectural components. The authors describe an increase in the progression to carcinoma associated with degree of glandular complexity and cytologic atypia. In this study, progression to carcinoma occurred in 1% of those women with simple hyperplasia, 3% of women with complex hyperplasia, 8% of women with simple hyperplasia with atypia, and 29% of those women with complex atypical hyperplasia [9]. Mutations accumulate during the development of precursor lesions and the progression to cancer, most commonly including mutations in Phosphatase and Tensin Homolog (*PTEN*), *PIK3CA*, and beta-catenin (*CTNNB1*). *PTEN* is believe to be one of the earliest changes in this continuum, occurring in roughly 70% of complex atypical hyperplasias and low grade endometrial cancers [10].

Incidence varies by age, symptoms, menopausal status, and presence of risk factors (such as PCOS). Using a large integrated health plan in the state of Washington, Reed et al. estimated peak incidence of simple hyperplasia as 142 per 100,000 woman-years, complex hyperplasia as 213 per 100,000 woman-years, and atypical (both simple and complex) of 56 per 100,000 woman-years [11]. While incidence of simple endometrial hyperplasia in asymptomatic premenopausal women is less than 5%, for women with PCOS and abnormal uterine bleeding this incidence may exceed 20% [12]. As in the case of endometrial cancer, endometrial hyperplasia has been demonstrated to be associated with both risk factors for unopposed estrogen exposure and increasing BMI [13]. Compared to the normal BMI population, even asymptomatic morbidly obese patients are at elevated risk of harboring endometrial pathology. One pilot study performed endometrial biopsies in asymptomatic morbidly obese women at the time of roux-en-Y gastric bypass, and found an overall rate of hyperplasia of 6.8%. Amongst those patients who were not receiving anti-estrogen therapy, this rate increased to 9.5% [14]. Obesity also appears to be associated with an earlier age of diagnosis of estrogen-dependent endometrial cancers. A retrospective study of cases of endometrial cancer diagnosed from 1999 to 2009 at a large medical center in New York City found that while the mean age of endometrial cancer diagnosis for those patients with a normal BMI was 67.1 years, the age at diagnosis for women with a BMI greater than 50 was 56.3 years [15]. In addition, awareness of this relationship between obesity and endometrial cancer risk is limited, with one large survey study finding 58% of those responding were not aware that obesity increased risk for endometrial cancer [16].

While the molecular and pathologic progression to endometrial cancer are described as linear with distinct stages, observation of individual tissue specimens shows that these categories are not so clearly delineated in practice. A 2006 Gynecologic Oncology Group study illustrated the subjectivity of rendering a diagnosis of atypical endometrial hyperplasia, and the significant difference in interobserver interpretation. When an independent panel of gynecologic pathologists reviewed slides of atypical endometrial hyperplasia, unanimous agreement for any diagnosis was reached in only 40% of cases [17]. Both under- and overestimation of the severity was present, potentially dramatically impacting management through over- or under-treatment. Additionally, studies have shown that a significant portion of patients who receive a diagnosis of atypical endometrial hyperplasia by biopsy may have an unrecognized concurrent endometrial carcinoma. A study by Trimble et al. reviewed hysterectomy specimens after patients had received a biopsy diagnosis of atypical endometrial hyperplasia, and found that the prevalence of concurrent endometrial carcinoma was 42.6% [18]. Older age, obesity, and presence of diabetes appear to be independently predictive of concurrent carcinoma in endometrial complex atypical hyperplasia patients [19].

Diagnosis of Precursor Lesions and Cancer

Diagnosis of endometrial cancer precursors and endometrial cancers typically occurs via endometrial sampling during clinical evaluation for abnormal uterine bleeding. There are no currently available validated serum biomarkers used for screening or detection of endometrial hyperplasia or endometrial cancer. Evaluation should include detailed history and physical, including a pelvic exam to inform a differential diagnosis and narrow suspicion of endometrial pathology. There are no current recommendations for routine screening for endometrial precancers in the asymptomatic population [20]. However, it is recommended that physicians discuss risks and symptoms of endometrial cancer with patients at the time of menopause to encourage reporting unexpected bleeding or spotting to prompt further work up as indicated [21]. Patients at very high risk, such as those with a predisposing genetic mutation, as in Lynch Syndrome, should receive annual screening with endometrial sampling beginning at age 30–35 or earlier depending on individual family history [22].

As abnormal uterine bleeding may be the result of benign etiologies, including endometrial polyp, fibroid uterus, or dysregulation of the hypothalamic pituitary axis, the extent of a work up should be dictated by clinical suspicion. This may include biopsy of the endometrial cavity especially in those patients with increased risk for hyperplasia or malignancy (increasing age, postmenopausal status, use of hormone replacement therapy). The American College of Obstetricians and Gynecologists (ACOG) recommends performing endometrial sampling in patients younger than 45 with a history of unopposed estrogen exposure, such as in the obese population or patients with PCOS [23]. Other prompts for sampling may include abnormal endometrial glands seen on routine cervical cancer screening with Pap smear [24].

Endometrial sampling is typically performed via pipelle biopsy or dilation and curettage. Pipelle biopsy offers an outpatient method of detection of endometrial cancer that may be performed without anesthesia in the office setting, compared with a dilation and curettage which is typically performed in the operating room. There is some evidence that dilation and curettage may be more likely to diagnose those concurrent cancers only subsequently discovered on hysterectomy specimen [25–27]. Suh-Bermann et al. found those patients who received a diagnosis of atypical endometrial hyperplasia by dilation and curettage preoperatively were less likely to be subsequently diagnosed with endometrial cancer compared with those who received a preoperative diagnosis of atypical endometrial hyperplasia by pipelle biopsy [28].

Negative endometrial pipelle biopsy despite strong clinical suspicion for endometrial pathology, such as abnormal thickening of the endometrium on transvaginal ultrasound in the symptomatic postmenopausal patient, should prompt further work up with dilation and curettage. False negative sampling may be attributed to relatively low percentage of the uterine cavity sampled by either method, and thus focal disease may be missed. Transvaginal ultrasound has been demonstrated to have significant clinical use in the postmenopausal symptomatic patient due to high negative predictive value. A large meta-analysis found that for symptomatic postmenopausal patients (presenting with abnormal uterine bleeding), identification of an endometrial stripe of less than 4 mm carried a 1% risk of malignancy (96% of patients with malignancy had endometrial stripe of >5 mm) [29]. Marked obesity can contribute to difficulty in obtaining reliable transvaginal ultrasound assessment, and the failure to confidently identify and assess endometrial lining should prompt further evaluation [30]. In the premenopausal population, normal fluctuations in endometrial stripe thickness precludes concrete cutoffs to differentiate those at substantial risk of harboring hyperplasia [31, 32].

Considerations for Clinical Management of Precancerous Lesions

Management for precancerous lesions of the endometrium is partially dependent on patient age, desire for future fertility, and medical comorbidities. Regardless of age, for those patients with complex atypical endometrial hyperplasia, consideration should be given to the substantial risk of concurrent cancer. One case control study found significantly decreased likelihood of risk of concurrent cancer for other types of hyperplasia. Approximately 15% of women initially diagnosed with complex hyperplasia without atypia and 4% of those diagnosed with simple hyperplasia (with and without atypia) at preoperative endometrial biopsy were diagnosed with concurrent endometrial cancer at hysterectomy [19]. Further sections in this chapter on management of precancerous complex atypical hyperplasia will also include discussion of low grade, early stage cancers due to the risk of concurrent cancer. Given the relatively poor preoperative ability to diagnose concurrent cancer that would only be detected on hysterectomy specimen, all management strategies should incorporate counseling about the potential for delay in diagnosis of malignancy if surgical management is not pursued.

Surgical Management

Total hysterectomy (removal of the uterus and cervix) provides definitive treatment for atypical endometrial hyperplasia. Simple dilation and curettage may aid in diagnosis, but is not by itself considered therapeutic. Options for surgical approach include abdominal via laparotomy, and vaginal or minimally invasive through laparoscopic or robotic-assisted laparoscopic techniques. Choice may be influenced by the surgeon's comfort or skill set, in combination with individual patient factors. Vaginal surgery, for example, may limit ability to visually evaluate ovaries. Patient body habitus, surgical history, or uterine size may influence decision to pursue laparotomy versus a minimally invasive approach.

The risk of concurrent cancer and the importance of adequate pathology specimens makes some surgical procedures inadequate for surgical management of endometrial precancers. Supracervical hysterectomy, or amputation of the uterine corpus above the level of the cervix is not a recommended strategy as this procedure creates the potential for residual disease remaining post-procedure, transection of undiagnosed concurrent malignancy, and obscuring the specimen such that pathologic staging could be inaccurate [31]. In addition, if a minimally invasive surgical approach is pursued, morcellation of the surgical specimen is not recommended due to risk of spread of malignancy and the subsequent inability to perform an adequate pathology assessment of the surgical specimen.

Bilateral salpingo-oophorectomy, or removal of the fallopian tubes and ovaries, allows for formal gross pathologic and histologic assessment of these organs in the case of concurrent malignancy. In the case of purely premalignant endometrial conditions there is no clear benefit of performing this additional procedure. Consideration should be given to adverse effects of surgical menopause in premenopausal women, where oophorectomy is associated with increased risk of osteoporosis, cardiovascular disease, cognitive impairment, and also overall mortality [33].

Currently, expert consensus recommends intraoperative assessment of the uterine specimen for occult carcinoma if hysterectomy is performed for complex atypical endometrial hyperplasia [31]. While intraoperative pathologic assessment with frozen section analysis may determine the need for comprehensive surgical staging with lymphadenectomy, an ability to perform this procedure is limited to surgeons with specialized training in gynecologic oncology. If a general obstetrician gynecologist is performing a hysterectomy for atypical endometrial hyperplasia, intraoperative frozen section may only be beneficial in the case where a gynecologic oncologist is available for intraoperative consultation. Furthermore, intraoperative pathologic assessment has moderate sensitivity for diagnosis of concurrent malignant in the complex atypical hyperplasia population and may result in false reassurance, which underscores the importance of follow up with final pathologic assessment [34, 35]. Routine lymphadenectomy for atypical endometrial hyperplasia is not recommended. The probability of concurrent diagnosis of an endometrial cancer with features considered high-risk for lymphatic spread outside the uterus is overall low, and routine lymphadenectomy would therefore lead to overtreatment. Lymphadenectomy also has the potential for morbidity, including lymphedema [36].

Surgical management of endometrial cancer precursors can also be complicated by risks imparted by obesity on surgical outcomes [37]. Increasing BMI is associated with an increased risk of venous thromboembolism for patients undergoing surgery [38]. Previous reports have shown that obesity is a risk factor for adverse surgical events in endometrial cancer patients [39–41]. For those patients undergoing abdominal hysterectomy via laparotomy, risks of surgical site infection and wound complication risks are increased with increasing BMI [42, 43]. Patients with type 2 diabetes should be counseled that glycemic control is critical for improved postoperative wound healing. In those patients who are morbidly obese (BMI > 40 kg/m^2) or suffer from multiple medical comorbidities, including hypertension or diabetes, adverse surgical events are not uncommon [44]. When needed, dosing of prophylactic antibiotics may need to be modified for obese patients. A previous study of prophylactic antibiotic usage in obese women undergoing cesarean delivery has shown decreased tissue drug levels [45]. Due to the potential impact on surgical site infections, some guidelines suggest increasing dose of prophylactic antibiotics based on body weight [46].

A minimally invasive approach, such as laparoscopic or robotic-assisted laparoscopic hysterectomy, provides the patient with benefits of earlier hospital discharge and quicker overall recovery from surgery. In the morbidly obese patient, minimally invasive or laparoscopic surgeries have been associated with fewer complications relative to open surgery [47]. Unfortunately, intraoperative conversion from minimally invasive surgery to larger open incisions occurs more frequently with increasing BMI [48]. Obesity brings additional considerations to surgical planning, including the need for preoperative anesthesia consultation for risks associated with airway complication, ensuring availability of bariatric equipment, and longer operative times [49].

Conservative Management

Despite the high risk of concurrent malignancy with complex atypical endometrial hyperplasia, nonsurgical options, often called "conservative management", may be considered for two particular patient populations. If the patient's general health or medical comorbidities prevent her from safely undergoing surgery, hysterectomy is not a viable option due to potential for severe morbidity or mortality (such as in the case of the most extremes of obesity, or severe cardiovascular or pulmonary disease). Another population for whom conservative management should be considered is the premenopausal patient desiring fertility. Between 5 and 30% of endometrial cancer patients and patients with complex atypical hyperplasia are diagnosed younger than age 50 [11, 50]. To date, conservative management for both populations has typically utilized similar approaches, described in more detail below. However, some unique issues should be considered in these two very different conservative management scenarios.

As women increasingly delay childbearing to later in life, premenopausal patients desiring future fertility may represent a growing demographic of patients with premalignant conditions of the endometrium [51]. Pretreatment counseling for patients desiring to preserve fertility should include discussion of the potential for conservative management leading to delay in diagnosis of concurrent malignancy. Definitive surgical treatment should be offered after completion of childbearing. Reproductive endocrinology referral is a critical consideration in this patient population because risk factors for atypical endometrial hyperplasia (such as obesity and metabolic syndrome) also impact fertility [52]. For those patients who choose conservative medical management with uterine preservation, further significant delay in definitive treatment may result from low chance of conception per cycle and delay in achieving pregnancy. An alternative surgical strategy could include hysterectomy with ovarian preservation to allow for oocyte retrieval and use of gestational carrier to achieve pregnancy, while providing definitive treatment of hyperplasia.

Conservative Management Using Progestins

Conservative management using synthetic progestogens (progestins) to mimic the action of progesterone has been the most commonly used strategy for treatment of endometrial cancer precursors in both women desiring future fertility and women who are not surgical candidates due to multiple medical comorbidities. In addition, it is important to consider the risk of adverse events when choosing a specific progestin agent for morbidly obese women with multiple medical comorbidities. Risk of adverse events will be described later with specific treatment regimens. Given the high overall response to progestins, other agents under evaluation have been typically studied as an addition to progestin therapy.

The use of progestins as a method of treatment for precancerous lesions of the endometrium has strong biologic basis. Progesterone is often described as the "brakes" for estrogen-induced proliferation in the endometrium. Stimulation of the endometrium by estrogen in the absence of progesterone as counterbalance promotes transformation to hyperplasia and ultimately cancer. Progesterone counters the mitogenic effect of estrogen on the endometrium through multiple mechanisms. Progesterone reduces local levels of estradiol by promoting the conversion of estradiol to the less potent estrone and other metabolites that are more readily cleared from cells; this is accomplished by upregulating 17β-hydroxysteroid hydrogenase and estrogen sulfotransferase [53]. In addition, progesterone induces expression of IGFBP1 (insulin like growth factor binding protein 1), which reduces the activity of estrogen-induced mitogenic factor, IGF-I (insulin like growth factor 1). The therapeutic effect of progestins in hyperplasia is also mediated by the induction of apoptosis [54].

Use of progestins has been studied as treatment for both atypical endometrial hyperplasia and early stage endometrial cancer, but ongoing surveillance following progestin therapy is needed to ensure regression and rule out progression. This is performed with serial sampling via endometrial biopsy or curettage, typically every 3 months. For patients with hyperplasia without atypia, progestin therapy is commonly used as first line therapy given the low risk of concurrent malignancy [55].

There is little consensus regarding optimal type of progestin, dose, and duration of treatment for treatment of endometrial hyperplasia patients (Table 11.1). Various

Table 11.1 Selected publications of outcomes of progestin therapy for complex atypical hyperplasia[a]

Type of progestin therapy	No. of patients with CAH	Response rate (%)	No. of patients achieving pregnancy	Live births	Median follow-up (months)	References
Oral MPA, megace or hydroxy-progesterone caproate	17	82	4	2	18	Yu et al. [56]
Oral MPA	17	82	7	5	47.9	Ushijima et al. [57]
Oral progestins and levonorgestrel IUD	18	67	n/a	n/a	11	Wheeler and Bristow [58]
Oral MPA	12	58	5	4	42	Minaguhi et al. [59]
Levonorgestrel IUD	6	100	n/a	n/a	6	Orbo et al. [60]
Oral MPA	8	88	n/a	n/a	6	Orbo et al. [60]
MPA or MA, or oral progestins + GnRH agonist or IUD	16	75	9	6	6	Chen et al. [61]
MPA and/or levonorgestrel IUD	13	54	5[b]	4[b]	13	Kudesia et al. [62]
MPA	11	82	4	7	39.2	Ohyagi-Hara et al. [63]
MPA and metformin	17	94	n/a	n/a	38	Mitsuhashi et al. [64]
Levonorgestrel IUD	8	88	n/a	n/a	32	Wildemeersch [65]
Levonorgestrel IUD	8	88	n/a	n/a	29	Tjalma [66]

Abbreviations: *CAH* complex atypical hyperplasia, *MPA* medroxyprogesterone acetate, *IUD* intrauterine device, *GnRH* Gonadotropin-releasing hormone
[a]Adapted and updated from Gunderson et al. [67]
[b]Includes those patients with endometrial cancer who attempted pregnancy after resolution following progestin therapy

progestin formulations are available, including those administered orally, by injection, vaginal application, or via intrauterine device. The most commonly used oral progestins for complex atypical hyperplasia are medroxyprogesterone acetate and megestrol acetate. Dose ranges and duration exceed those typically used in progestin-containing contraceptive pills or to treat heavy abnormal uterine bleeding. For example, medroxyprogesterone dosing ranges from 10 to 100 mg daily, and megestrol dosing ranges from 40 to 200 mg/day or higher [12, 31, 68]. In one systematic review, median time to complete response of hyperplasia was 6 months [67]. Ongoing therapy may be utilized in the absence of progression. If progression is apparent on repeat endometrial sampling, hysterectomy should be performed, if possible.

The levonorgestrel containing intrauterine device (IUD) provides an alternative to oral progestin formulations that result in systemic progestin exposure. The levonorgestrel-containing intrauterine device is inserted into the uterine cavity through the cervix in an office procedure. One benefit of the intrauterine delivery method is that higher levels of progestin are delivered to the endometrium with relatively low systemic exposure or adverse side effects. For example, an IUD that contains 52 mg levonorgestrel has an initial release rate of 20 μg daily, with plasma concentrations plateauing at 100–200 pg/mL. While levonorgestrel concentration within the myometrium and fallopian tubes are within comparable range as that found following oral administration of 30 μg levonorgestrel, concentrations within the endometrium are 200–800 times higher [69]. Only 15% of patients using the device have complete inhibition of ovulation [70]. While oral formations require the patient to remember to take one or more tablets at what may be multiple dosing intervals, the intrauterine device ensures compliance with therapy and can remain in the uterus for up to 5 years.

Risk of adverse events is an important consideration for choice of progestin therapy. Adverse effects associated with systemic progestin therapy include hypertension, gastrointestinal upset, fatigue, and weight gain [71–73]. Reducing systemic exposures through the use of the levonorgestrel intrauterine device and local delivery of progestins also has the benefit of minimizing adverse effects. When comparing different formulations of progestins for the indication of treatment of complex atypical hyperplasia and endometrial cancer, oral progestin therapy appears to be associated with increased weight gain compared with the levonorgestrel IUD [74]. This weight gain appears to be greater in those patients with BMI < 35 compared with BMI > 35. Excess adiposity may pose a risk to not only overall patient health in the long term, but also compromise the potential goal of achieving a healthy pregnancy after regression of hyperplasia. Even more concerning is the potential risk of venous thromboembolism, and this risk may differ from dosing utilized for contraceptive purposes. In a recent systematic review by Tepper et al., there was evidence of association with VTE when progestins were used for therapeutic indications, although progestin-only contraception was not suggestive of an increase in odds for venous or arterial events [75]. Adverse events of levonorgestrel IUDs are primarily related to changes in bleeding patterns and abdominal or pelvic pain, and are not influenced by BMI.

Review of Outcomes for Conservative Management Using Progestins

While direct comparison of efficacy against endometrial hyperplasia and low grade cancers is difficult because studies include a mix of prospective and retrospective analyses and often include heterogeneous patient populations (normal weight, obese, morbidly obese, patients seeking fertility preservation, etc.), there is some evidence that the intrauterine device may be superior in achieving regression of hyperplasia. A systematic review and meta-analysis found a statistically significant difference in regression rate of 66–69% vs. 90–92% for oral progestins versus the levonorgestrel IUD in complex and atypical hyperplasia [76]. A large retrospective cohort study of 344 women compared the levonorgestrel IUD with oral progestins (norethisterone 5 mg three times daily or medroxyprogesterone 10 mg twice daily) and found high overall regression rates with a median follow up of 58.8 months. For patients treated with the levonorgestrel IUD, there was a 96.5% regression of complex hyperplasia without atypia and 76.2% regression of complex atypical hyperplasia compared to regression rates for oral progestins of 90.1% for complex hyperplasia without atypia and 46.2% for complex atypical hyperplasia patients. Interestingly, one study showed that in patients treated with the levonorgestrel IUD, BMI was a strong independent predictor of both rates of regression and relapse. Only 3.3% of patients with complex hyperplasia and BMI < 35 recurred compared with 32.6% of women with a BMI of 35 or higher [77]. However, other studies have not demonstrated this effect of BMI [78]. The levonorgestrel IUD has also been compared with oral progestins in randomized controlled trials. After 6 months of treatment, patients with simple, complex, and complex atypical hyperplasia who received the levonorgestrel IUD had 100% regression rate compared with 96% regression rate for patients on continuous daily progestins and 69% for those receiving cyclic progestins, with IUD and continuous daily progestins shown to be significantly superior to the cyclic oral progestins (P = 0.01). In this study, BMI did not influence rates of regression. The majority of women experienced some adverse events, with more women in the IUD arm experiencing irregular bleeding. Pain or nausea was not significantly different between groups [60]. The same authors reported long term follow-up on these patients at 24 months. This follow-up study showed that histologic relapse was observed for 41% of women who had demonstrated initial complete response, with relapse rates similar between the three treatment arms, and most relapses occurred during the first 6 months after withdrawal of therapy. Relapse rates were independent of BMI [79].

Several reviews include both oncologic and pregnancy outcomes. One systematic review of 45 studies with 391 study subjects included a wide range of progestin types and varying doses, but showed that patients with complex atypical hyperplasia had a higher complete response rate compared to patients with low grade endometrial cancer (65.8 vs. 48.2% p = 0.002), with a median time to complete response of 6 months. Recurrence rates after complete response were 23% in those patients with complex atypical hyperplasia, which suggests the need for ongoing surveillance and consideration of definitive surgical management after childbearing [67]. A separate 2012 meta-analysis evaluated the rates of regression, relapse and live births in both endometrial cancer and complex atypical hyperplasia patients. Again, studies included a heterogeneous collection of treatment regimens, with medroxyprogesterone most common but included other oral progestins and the levonorgestrel IUD. They found a pooled regression rate for complex atypical hyperplasia of 85.6%, with a relapse rate of 26% [80]. This study did not stratify rates of regression or recurrence by BMI. Park et al. published pregnancy outcomes of young women with early stage endometrial cancer treated with progestins. Of those who attempted to conceive, 73% were successful and 66% had live births, with a median interval to attempted pregnancy after treatment of 5 months [81]. Data in the endometrial cancer population suggests that assisted reproductive technology (ART) is associated with higher live birth rate in young women compared with spontaneous conception following conservative management [82]. A 2014 meta-analysis and systematic review evaluating possible prognostic factors on fertility-sparing management found that neither prior pregnancy, obesity, nor prior infertility appeared to be associated with pregnancy probability on multivariate analysis [83].

Conservative Management Using Non-progestin Hormonal Agents

Gonadotropin-releasing hormone (GnRH) therapy has also been explored as an additional potential therapy for conservative management of endometrial hyperplasia. GnRH therapy employs GnRH agonists to suppress the hypothalamic pituitary axis, suppressing estrogen production to generate an anti-proliferative effect on the endometrium [68]. This approach uses a direct effect to mitigate proliferative signals by decreasing estrogen levels, instead of using progestins to counteract the action of estrogen in the endometrium. Specific GnRH therapies include triptorelin and leuprolide acetate (both administered as an injection). GnRH agonists were evaluated as single agents in a study of 42 women with hyperplasia (30 women with simple hyperplasia, 10 with complex hyperplasia without atypia, and 2 women with complex hyperplasia with atypia) treated with leuprolide acetate or triptorelin monthly for 6 months [84]. Treatment showed significant decrease in proliferative activity and regression of hyperplasia was seen by 3 months of treatment for all women except one (a case of simple hyperplasia). Seven women (24%) had a recurrence of simple hyperplasia. Interestingly, recurrence was not seen in patients initially diagnosed with complex hyperplasia. A study by Perez-Medina et al. included patients with atypical endometrial hyperplasia desiring conservative management (n = 22) who were treated with combination norethisterone acetate (a progestin) and GnRH agonist (triptorelin) injections every 6 months. At 5 year follow up, regression was seen in 84% of patients with a recurrence rate of 5% [85]. Another combination study evaluating a GnRH agonist therapy (leuprolide acetate) with tibolone (a synthetic hormonal therapy with both estrogenic and progestagenic effects) found regression in all 26 women treated after 12 months of treatment but with nearly 20% recurrence rate over first 2 years of follow up [86].

Conservative Management Using Non-hormonal Agents

Metformin, a biguanide used as treatment for type 2 diabetes, is a well-tolerated oral medication that has demonstrated promising results in preclinical in vivo models and is under evaluation as combination therapy for endometrial hyperplasia. Epidemiologic studies provided the first evidence that patients taking metformin had a reduced risk of developing cancer [87, 88]. There is also molecular evidence for anti-cancer properties of metformin, including action on AMPK/mTOR pathway [89]. A recent prospective observational study of fertility-sparing treatment of atypical endometrial hyperplasia and early stage endometrial cancer using combined metformin and medroxyprogesterone found an 81% complete response at 36 weeks. A 10% relapse rate was seen during a median follow up of 38 months after remission [64]. Rates of regression and relapse were not stratified by BMI. A small pilot study compared combination metformin with megestrol acetate or megestrol acetate monotherapy for patients with atypical endometrial hyperplasia, which showed a nonsignificant increase in response rate in the combination therapy arm [90]. Additional clinical studies are ongoing, including combinations with weight loss and the levonorgestrel IUD [91].

The mTOR inhibitor, everolimus (previously called RAD001), is currently under investigation for treatment of grade 1 endometrial cancers or complex atypical hyperplasia in combination with the levonorgestrel IUD at The University of Texas MD Anderson Cancer Center (Clinicaltrials.gov identifier: NCT02397083). Patients diagnosed with progestin-resistant disease at 3 months after initiating the levonorgestrel IUD, will then be randomized to continue with the levonorgestrel IUD alone for an additional 3 months or add daily oral everolimus (10 mg/day) in combination with the levonorgestrel IUD. Response to combination of oral everolimus and the levonorgestrel IUD will be compared to response following treatment with the levonorgestrel IUD alone, with biopsies obtained every 3 months. While this study is ongoing, previous studies have shown promising activity against endometrial hyperplasia and cancer. Everolimus showed significant efficacy in a preclinical model of endometrial hyperplasia [92] and has proven anti-cancer activity in combination with an anti-estrogen agent in advanced and recurrent endometrial cancer [93].

Long-Term Management Strategies

After primary treatment, women have a variety of available strategies for reducing the risk for relapse of endometrial cancer precursors and cancer. As discussed in more detail elsewhere in this book volume, lifestyle interventions and weight loss play a key role in reducing endometrial cancer risk and can still provide benefit after initial treatment has been completed [94]. Effective treatment of type 2 diabetes is essential for overall reduction in morbidity and mortality, and specific use of metformin appears to improve long-term endometrial cancer survivor outcomes, possibly reducing risk of recurrence in obese women with Type I endometrial cancer [95, 96]. While no strict surveillance consensus is available, for those women who are unable to undergo hysterectomy, long-term surveillance is necessary as the underlying etiology causing endometrial pathology is likely unchanged. One protocol for surveillance involves endometrial sampling at 3–6 month intervals until three negative biopsies, after which sampling frequency may be reduced. For those patients who retain their uterus, they remain at risk for endometrial precancerous lesions.

Other Management Strategies Currently Under Clinical Investigation

Bariatric surgery has been proposed as a procedure that could reverse endometrial pathology through rapid weight loss and resulting improvements in hormone levels, metabolic syndrome, and insulin signaling. A pilot study by Argenta et al. evaluated endometrial pathology in asymptomatic morbidly obese women before surgery and at 1 year after bariatric surgery. While there was no statistically significant reduction in the overall prevalence of endometrial pathology after bariatric surgery, a post hoc analysis including only women who were not receiving hormonal agents showed a significant decrease in endometrial hyperplasia after bariatric surgery [14]. Metabolic profiles, including insulin sensitivity and glucose homeostasis, are significantly improved after bariatric surgery [97]. Additional studies are needed to better understand how bariatric surgery impacts endometrial pathology both as a standalone and in combination with medical therapy.

Hysteroscopic resection of early stage cancers followed by treatment with progestins has shown promising results, and while this is not standard of care, may represent a future direction in conservative surgical management of endometrial cancer precursors [98, 99]. A study of 23 women with CAH or low grade endometrial cancer seeking to preserve fertility evaluated hysteroscopic resection followed by progestin therapy [100]. At the first follow-up after hysteroscopic resection, 13 women (56.6%) showed a complete response, while 6 patients underwent a second hysteroscopic resection. By 9 months, all women achieved a complete response, with one relapse reported at 6 months after completing progestin therapy. Obstetrical outcomes showed that 6 women achieved pregnancy and 15 women were trying to conceive at the time of the report [100].

Photodynamic therapy could be an alternative treatment strategy for precursor lesions and endometrial cancer in obese women with high surgical risk or who wish to maintain fertility. Photodynamic therapy is conducted by administering a photosensitizing agent and then targeting light of a specific wavelength to the lesion. This results in a photodynamic reaction that generates oxidative stress and causes cancer cell death. This approach has only recently been reported in the primary treatment of endometrial cancer, but there is a longer history of successful treatment in recurrent gynecologic cancers [101]. A retrospective study was conducted by Choi et al., evaluating outcomes for young women with low grade endometrioid endometrial cancer that received photodynamic therapy for fertility preservation. Intravenous photosensitizer (Photogem) was administered followed by photoillumination with red laser (630 nm) applied to the endometrial cavity and endocervical canal 48 h later [102]. Of 16 patients assessed, 12 women had a complete response as determined at follow-up dilation & curettage. Four of these patients later had recurrence. Adverse events for photodynamic therapy are mild, including facial angioedema. In this study, seven women later attempted pregnancy and four (57%) had successful pregnancies resulting in a live birth. Given the limited adverse events, this approach could be further evaluated in the future for women seeking conservative management of endometrial precursor lesions or low grade, early stage cancers.

Future Directions to Improve Conservative Management Outcomes for Obese Women

As obesity rates remain high, we expect that the number of women requiring conservative management for endometrial cancer and endometrial cancer precursors will continue to rise. As such, it is critical to continue to develop therapeutic strategies with improved response rates, lower risk of adverse events, and additional opportunities for therapeutic tailoring. Individualized conservative management strategies are necessary for co-existing conditions such as PCOS or co-morbidities resulting from obesity, as well as individual circumstances such as desire for maintaining fertility, molecular heterogeneity that contributes to response/non-response to hormonal agents and targeted therapeutics, and finally, altered pharmacokinetics (drug absorption, distribution, or metabolism) related to obesity.

Biomarkers and Identifying New Molecular Targets

While biomarkers have not been established in endometrial hyperplasia screening, there have been studies to evaluate potential markers of both cancer risk and response to progestin therapy. For example, loss of p27 has been shown to occur early in the progression to endometrial cancer [103] with studies showing that this aberration is intensified in obese women [104]. Parallel animal studies suggested that this aberrant loss of p27 might be correlated with increased risk of endometrial cancer in the context of obesity, even in histologically normal endometrium, as p27 loss occurred concurrently with loss of the tumor suppressor Tsc2 [104]. When stratified by BMI, PTEN loss was associated with improved progression-free survival in endometrial cancer, suggesting that biomarkers may differ in the context of obesity [105]. In the setting of treatment response, further biomarker studies are needed to identify patients who are unlikely to respond to progestin therapy. Poor expression of estrogen receptor (ER) and progesterone receptor (PR) is weakly associated with persistent hyperplasia after progestin therapy with the levonorgestrel IUD [106]. Within endometrial cancer, loss of PR is associated with increased proliferation, and poor survival [107]. Multiple molecular studies are ongoing to identify targets for progestin-resistant precursor lesions and low grade endometrial cancers. As these studies continue to advance, an improved understanding of the molecular aberrations that play a role in progression of precancerous lesions to cancer or contribute to therapeutic resistance will provide avenues for further research to improve outcomes for these patients.

Pharmacologic Issues of Obesity and Related Conditions

The obese patient population presents unique challenges for successfully delivering hormonal and pharmacologic agents at appropriate therapeutic levels for multiple reasons. Obesity-related changes in pharmacokinetics of orally administered hormonal contraceptives have received significant attention due to concerns that obese women may have higher rates of contraceptive failure [108–110]. Most studies show lower systemic blood levels of contraceptive hormones in obese women, but maintain levels above the minimum required to suppress ovulation and thus, provide comparable contraceptive efficacy rates. Oral emergency contraceptives that rely on levonorgestrel also result in lower serum concentrations in obese women and may have lower efficacy. In the context of contraception, it is necessary to stay above a minimum level to prevent ovulation; however, use of these hormones for treating low grade endometrial cancer or complex atypical hyperplasia likely relies on total dose delivered to the lesion. For this reason, alterations in synthetic hormone metabolism after oral administration is of significant concern in the management of endometrial cancer precursor lesions and low grade cancers in obese women. As discussed previously in this book volume, bariatric surgery procedures can be utilized by some obese women to achieve substantial weight loss, improve related medical co-morbidities, and reduce the risk of endometrial cancer. Yet, this can present new uncertainties in medical treatment for women with endometrial cancer or precursor lesions, as bariatric surgery can significantly change oral drug absorption due to altered gastrointestinal tract anatomy and function [111]. In achieving improved therapeutic outcomes for obese women, research must focus not only on developing effective therapeutic agents to eliminate or reverse endometrial lesions, but also on developing methods to effectively deliver these agents at required levels to endometrial tissue in obese women.

In addition to concerns of altered systemic hormone and drug metabolism, adverse effects related to systemic exposure to hormonal agents and/or molecularly targeted therapeutics can be particularly problematic in obese women with multiple co-morbidities. Additional research that focuses on restricting drug exposure to only the target tissue will be critical to reducing systemic side effects. Local drug delivery could be an ideal strategy for these patients because of the ability to potentially achieve higher drug exposure levels at the target lesion, which could increase treatment efficacy.

Drug Delivery Strategies

In our efforts to improve treatment efficacy and reduce side effects, our own research has recently focused on local intrauterine drug delivery. Localized delivery of hormonal agents has a long history in clinical use; however, intrauterine delivery of anti-cancer agents is a novel approach. Given the proven anti-cancer activity of intrauterine progestin via the levonorgestrel IUD, improved therapies can build from a combinatorial approach adding to the existing progestin intrauterine delivery strategies. While the levonorgestrel IUD has been fine-tuned for delivering levonorgestrel for up to 5 years for contraceptive purposes, this "T" scaffold is an ideal platform for further modification and optimization. Multiple minor variations of the structure are already in use, including those for shorter delivery time periods (3 years) and a smaller device designed for use in both nulliparous and parous patients [65, 112]. The center stem of these intrauterine devices contains a polymer cylinder impregnated with hormone and is surrounded by a polymer membrane that controls long-term hormone release. Our initial studies are focused on local intrauterine delivery of everolimus due to the known efficacy of everolimus in combination with an anti-estrogen treatment (letrozole) in advanced/recurrent endometrioid endometrial cancer [93]. In addition, localized delivery of everolimus has been in use clinically in the form of drug-eluting coronary stents for many years [113], providing some proof of principal towards the feasibility of formulating everolimus to be delivered through a polymer-based system. Our studies are currently focused on preclinical models providing long-term intrauterine delivery of everolimus. The T-shaped intrauterine device can be readily modified to support various polymer cylinders containing therapeutic agents of choice and can be tuned to provide different tissue doses. The history of extensive preclinical and clinical studies with these agents should support the rapid evaluation of safety and efficacy for intrauterine delivery.

Vaginal drug delivery strategies have been employed in cervical cancer studies, and combination with a levonorgestrel IUD could also provide opportunities for rapidly adaptable localized drug delivery for conservative management strategies for low grade endometrial cancers and precursors. Again, localized uterine exposure via vaginal drug delivery strategies have largely focused on hormonal agents used for contraception or other reproductive health applications. Yet, pharmacokinetic studies of vaginally administered progesterone or estrogen show a preferential delivery to the uterus, dubbed the "first uterine pass effect" [114, 115]. Vaginal administration can be achieved using a variety of approaches, including gels, hydrogel formulations, and intravaginal ring devices. These local delivery systems could be readily modifiable during the course of treatment, providing opportunities for the treating physician to alter the drug amount dosed, frequency of administration, or easily change therapeutic agents depending on treatment response or side effects. While management of endometrial cancers and precursor lesions have not been evaluated using these approaches, further consideration could provide significant benefit for obese women.

Conclusions/Summary

As rates of obesity continue to increase, the prevalence of women at increased risk for either endometrial cancers or their precursor lesions will continue to rise. Many factors, including health status and desire for fertility must be considered for treatment of precursor lesions in obese women. It is paramount that management of atypical endometrial hyperplasia involves the consideration of the substantial risk of progression to endometrial cancer as well as the risk of yet undiagnosed, concurrent endometrial cancer. In the case of definitive surgical management, obese patients should be counseled on potential for higher rate of complications compared to their lower BMI counterparts. For those patients undergoing conservative management for fertility or medical indications, pretreatment discussion with obese patients should include caution that oncologic risk may remain increased as long as the underlying mechanism for endometrial pathology is unchanged. As research continues into conservative management for cancer precursors, pharmacologic implications in the obese population should be included in study design. Novel approaches to conservative management, including local intrauterine drug delivery and identification of biomarkers for cancer risk or likelihood of progestin response, will significantly improve treatment planning and outcomes for these women.

References

1. Ward KK, Roncancio AM, Shah NR, Davis MA, Saenz CC, McHale MT, et al. The risk of uterine malignancy is linearly associated with body mass index in a cohort of US women. Am J Obstet Gynecol. 2013;209(6):579 e1–5.
2. Sivridis E, Giatromanolaki A. The pathogenesis of endometrial carcinomas at menopause: facts and figures. J Clin Pathol. 2011;64(7):553–60.
3. Charalampakis V, Tahrani AA, Helmy A, Gupta JK, Singhal R. Polycystic ovary syndrome and endometrial hyperplasia: an overview of the role of bariatric surgery in female fertility. Eur J Obstet Gynecol Reprod Biol. 2016;207:220–6.
4. Burzawa JK, Schmeler KM, Soliman PT, Meyer LA, Bevers MW, Pustilnik TL, et al. Prospective evaluation of insulin resistance among endometrial cancer patients. Am J Obstet Gynecol. 2011;204(4):355 e1–7.
5. Friberg E, Mantzoros CS, Wolk A. Diabetes and risk of endometrial cancer: a population-based prospective cohort study. Cancer Epidemiol Biomark Prev. 2007;16(2):276–80.
6. Mu N, Zhu Y, Wang Y, Zhang H, Xue F. Insulin resistance: a significant risk factor of endometrial cancer. Gynecol Oncol. 2012;125(3):751–7.
7. Schmandt RE, Iglesias DA, Co NN, Lu KH. Understanding obesity and endometrial cancer risk: opportunities for prevention. Am J Obstet Gynecol. 2011;205(6):518–25.
8. Parkash V, Fadare O, Tornos C, WG MC, Committee Opinion No. 631. Endometrial Intraepithelial Neoplasia. Obstet Gynecol. 2015;126(4):897.
9. Kurman RJ, Kaminski PF, Norris HJ. The behavior of endometrial hyperplasia. A long-term study of "untreated" hyperplasia in 170 patients. Cancer. 1985;56(2):403–12.
10. Huang M, Djordjevic B, Yates MS, Urbauer D, Sun C, Burzawa J, et al. Molecular pathogenesis of endometrial cancers in patients with Lynch syndrome. Cancer. 2013;119(16):3027–33.
11. Reed SD, Newton KM, Clinton WL, Epplein M, Garcia R, Allison K, et al. Incidence of endometrial hyperplasia. Am J Obstet Gynecol. 2009;200(6):678 e1–6.
12. Armstrong AJ, Hurd WW, Elguero S, Barker NM, Zanotti KM. Diagnosis and management of endometrial hyperplasia. J Minim Invasive Gynecol. 2012;19(5):562–71.
13. Epplein M, Reed SD, Voigt LF, Newton KM, Holt VL, Weiss NS. Risk of complex and atypical endometrial hyperplasia in relation to anthropometric measures and reproductive history. Am J Epidemiol. 2008;168(6):563–70. discussion 71–6

14. Argenta PA, Kassing M, Truskinovsky AM, Svendsen CA. Bariatric surgery and endometrial pathology in asymptomatic morbidly obese women: a prospective, pilot study. BJOG. 2013;120(7):795–800.
15. Nevadunsky NS, Van Arsdale A, Strickler HD, Moadel A, Kaur G, Levitt J, et al. Obesity and age at diagnosis of endometrial cancer. Obstet Gynecol. 2014;124(2 Pt 1):300–6.
16. Soliman PT, Bassett RL Jr, Wilson EB, Boyd-Rogers S, Schmeler KM, Milam MR, et al. Limited public knowledge of obesity and endometrial cancer risk: what women know. Obstet Gynecol. 2008;112(4):835–42.
17. Zaino RJ, Kauderer J, Trimble CL, Silverberg SG, Curtin JP, Lim PC, et al. Reproducibility of the diagnosis of atypical endometrial hyperplasia: a Gynecologic Oncology Group study. Cancer. 2006;106(4):804–11.
18. Trimble CL, Kauderer J, Zaino R, Silverberg S, Lim PC, Burke JJ 2nd, et al. Concurrent endometrial carcinoma in women with a biopsy diagnosis of atypical endometrial hyperplasia: a Gynecologic Oncology Group study. Cancer. 2006;106(4):812–9.
19. Matsuo K, Ramzan AA, Gualtieri MR, Mhawech-Fauceglia P, Machida H, Moeini A, et al. Prediction of concurrent endometrial carcinoma in women with endometrial hyperplasia. Gynecol Oncol. 2015;139(2):261–7.
20. Practice Bulletin No. 149. Endometrial cancer. Obstet Gynecol. 2015;125(4):1006–26.
21. Smith RA, Brooks D, Cokkinides V, Saslow D, Brawley OW. Cancer screening in the United States, 2013: a review of current American Cancer Society guidelines, current issues in cancer screening, and new guidance on cervical cancer screening and lung cancer screening. CA Cancer J Clin. 2013;63(2):88–105.
22. Meyer LA, Broaddus RR, Lu KH. Endometrial cancer and Lynch syndrome: clinical and pathologic considerations. Cancer Control. 2009;16(1):14–22.
23. American College of O, Gynecologists. ACOG committee opinion no. 557. Management of acute abnormal uterine bleeding in nonpregnant reproductive-aged women. Obstet Gynecol. 2013;121(4):891–6.
24. Massad LS, Einstein MH, Huh WK, Katki HA, Kinney WK, Schiffman M, et al. 2012 updated consensus guidelines for the management of abnormal cervical cancer screening tests and cancer precursors. Obstet Gynecol. 2013;121(4):829–46.
25. Ben-Baruch G, Seidman DS, Schiff E, Moran O, Menczer J. Outpatient endometrial sampling with the Pipelle curette. Gynecol Obstet Investig. 1994;37(4):260–2.
26. Leitao MM Jr, Kehoe S, Barakat RR, Alektiar K, Rabbitt C, Chi DS, et al. Endometrial sampling diagnosis of FIGO grade 1 endometrial adenocarcinoma with a background of complex atypical hyperplasia and final hysterectomy pathology. Am J Obstet Gynecol. 2010;202(3):278 e1–6.
27. Costales AB, Schmeler KM, Broaddus R, Soliman PT, Westin SN, Ramirez PT, et al. Clinically significant endometrial cancer risk following a diagnosis of complex atypical hyperplasia. Gynecol Oncol. 2014;135(3):451–4.
28. Suh-Burgmann E, Hung YY, Armstrong MA. Complex atypical endometrial hyperplasia: the risk of unrecognized adenocarcinoma and value of preoperative dilation and curettage. Obstet Gynecol. 2009;114(3):523–9.
29. Smith-Bindman R, Kerlikowske K, Feldstein VA, Subak L, Scheidler J, Segal M, et al. Endovaginal ultrasound to exclude endometrial cancer and other endometrial abnormalities. JAMA. 1998;280(17):1510–7.
30. American College of O, Gynecologists. ACOG Committee Opinion No. 440. The role of Transvaginal ultrasonography in the evaluation of postmenopausal bleeding. Obstet Gynecol. 2009;114(2 Pt 1):409–11.
31. Trimble CL, Method M, Leitao M, Lu K, Ioffe O, Hampton M, et al. Management of endometrial precancers. Obstet Gynecol. 2012;120(5):1160–75.
32. Kim MJ, Kim JJ, Kim SM. Endometrial evaluation with transvaginal ultrasonography for the screening of endometrial hyperplasia or cancer in premenopausal and perimenopausal women. Obstet Gynecol Sci. 2016;59(3):192–200.

33. Holman LL, Friedman S, Daniels MS, Sun CC, Lu KH. Acceptability of prophylactic sal-pingectomy with delayed oophorectomy as risk-reducing surgery among BRCA mutation carriers. Gynecol Oncol. 2014;133(2):283–6.
34. Stephan JM, Hansen J, Samuelson M, McDonald M, Chin Y, Bender D, et al. Intra-operative frozen section results reliably predict final pathology in endometrial cancer. Gynecol Oncol. 2014;133(3):499–505.
35. Morotti M, Menada MV, Moioli M, Sala P, Maffeo I, Abete L, et al. Frozen section pathology at time of hysterectomy accurately predicts endometrial cancer in patients with preoperative diagnosis of atypical endometrial hyperplasia. Gynecol Oncol. 2012;125(3):536–40.
36. Hareyama H, Hada K, Goto K, Watanabe S, Hakoyama M, Oku K, et al. Prevalence, clas-sification, and risk factors for postoperative lower extremity lymphedema in women with gynecologic malignancies: a retrospective study. Int J Gynecol Cancer. 2015;25(4):751–7.
37. Orekoya O, Samson ME, Trivedi T, Vyas S, Steck SE. The impact of obesity on surgical out-come in endometrial cancer patients: a systematic review. J Gynecol Surg. 2016;32(3):149–57.
38. Parkin L, Sweetland S, Balkwill A, Green J, Reeves G, Beral V, et al. Body mass index, surgery, and risk of venous thromboembolism in middle-aged women: a cohort study. Circulation. 2012;125(15):1897–904.
39. Bouwman F, Smits A, Lopes A, Das N, Pollard A, Massuger L, et al. The impact of BMI on surgical complications and outcomes in endometrial cancer surgery–an institutional study and systematic review of the literature. Gynecol Oncol. 2015;139(2):369–76.
40. Kondalsamy-Chennakesavan S, Janda M, Gebski V, Baker J, Brand A, Hogg R, et al. Risk factors to predict the incidence of surgical adverse events following open or laparoscopic surgery for apparent early stage endometrial cancer: results from a randomised controlled trial. Eur J Cancer. 2012;48(14):2155–62.
41. Walker JL, Piedmonte MR, Spirtos NM, Eisenkop SM, Schlaerth JB, Mannel RS, et al. Laparoscopy compared with laparotomy for comprehensive surgical staging of uterine can-cer: Gynecologic Oncology Group Study LAP2. J Clin Oncol. 2009;27(32):5331–6.
42. Olsen MA, Higham-Kessler J, Yokoe DS, Butler AM, Vostok J, Stevenson KB, et al. Developing a risk stratification model for surgical site infection after abdominal hysterec-tomy. Infect Control Hosp Epidemiol. 2009;30(11):1077–83.
43. Nugent EK, Hoff JT, Gao F, Massad LS, Case A, Zighelboim I, et al. Wound complications after gynecologic cancer surgery. Gynecol Oncol. 2011;121(2):347–52.
44. Obermair A, Brennan DJ, Baxter E, Armes JE, Gebski V, Janda M. Surgical safety and per-sonal costs in morbidly obese, multimorbid patients diagnosed with early-stage endometrial cancer having a hysterectomy. Gynecol Oncol Res Pract. 2016;3:1.
45. Pevzner L, Swank M, Krepel C, Wing DA, Chan K, Edmiston CE Jr. Effects of maternal obesity on tissue concentrations of prophylactic cefazolin during cesarean delivery. Obstet Gynecol. 2011;117(4):877–82.
46. Bratzler DW, Dellinger EP, Olsen KM, Perl TM, Auwaerter PG, Bolon MK, et al. Clinical practice guidelines for antimicrobial prophylaxis in surgery. Surg Infect. 2013;14(1):73–156.
47. Chan JK, Gardner AB, Taylor K, Thompson CA, Blansit K, Yu X, et al. Robotic versus lapa-roscopic versus open surgery in morbidly obese endometrial cancer patients - a comparative analysis of total charges and complication rates. Gynecol Oncol. 2015;139(2):300–5.
48. Cosin JA, Brett Sutherland MA, Westgate CT, Fang H. Complications of robotic gynecologic surgery in the severely morbidly obese. Ann Surg Oncol. 2016;23(12):4035–41.
49. Committee on Gynecologic P. Committee opinion no. 619. Gynecologic surgery in the obese woman. Obstet Gynecol. 2015;125(1):274–8.
50. Soliman PT, Oh JC, Schmeler KM, Sun CC, Slomovitz BM, Gershenson DM, et al. Risk factors for young premenopausal women with endometrial cancer. Obstet Gynecol. 2005;105(3):575–80.
51. Matthews TJ, Hamilton BE. Delayed childbearing: more women are having their first child later in life. NCHS Data Brief. 2009;21:1–8.

52. Wise MR, Jordan V, Lagas A, Showell M, Wong N, Lensen S, et al. Obesity and endometrial hyperplasia and cancer in premenopausal women: A systematic review. Am J Obstet Gynecol. 2016;214(6):689 e1–e17.
53. Kaaks R, Lukanova A, Kurzer MS. Obesity, endogenous hormones, and endometrial cancer risk: a synthetic review. Cancer Epidemiol Biomark Prev. 2002;11(12):1531–43.
54. Wang S, Pudney J, Song J, Mor G, Schwartz PE, Zheng W. Mechanisms involved in the evolution of progestin resistance in human endometrial hyperplasia–precursor of endometrial cancer. Gynecol Oncol. 2003;88(2):108–17.
55. Salman MC, Usubutun A, Boynukalin K, Yuce K. Comparison of WHO and endometrial intraepithelial neoplasia classifications in predicting the presence of coexistent malignancy in endometrial hyperplasia. J Gynecol Oncol. 2010;21(2):97–101.
56. Yu M, Yang JX, Wu M, Lang JH, Huo Z, Shen K. Fertility-preserving treatment in young women with well-differentiated endometrial carcinoma and severe atypical hyperplasia of endometrium. Fertil Steril. 2009;92:2122–4.
57. Ushijima K, Yahata H, Yoshikawa H, Konishi I, Yasugi T, Saito T, et al. Multicenter phase II study of fertility-sparing treatment with medroxyprogesterone acetate for endometrial carcinoma and atypical hyperplasia in young women. J Clin Oncol. 2007;25:2798–803.
58. Wheeler DT, Bristow RE, Kurman RJ. Histologic alterations in endometrial hyperplasia and well-differentiated carcinoma treated with progestins. Am J Surg Pathol. 2007;31:988–98.
59. Minaguchi T, Nakagawa S, Takazawa Y, Nei T, Horie K, Fujiwara T, et al. Combined phospho-Akt and PTEN expressions associated with post-treatment hysterectomy after conservative progestin therapy in complex atypical hyperplasia and stage Ia, G1 adenocarcinoma of the endometrium. Cancer Lett. 2007;248:112–22.
60. Orbo A, Vereide A, Arnes M, Pettersen I, Straume B. Levonorgestrel-impregnated intrauterine device as treatment for endometrial hyperplasia: a national multicentre randomised trial. BJOG. 2014;121(4):477–86.
61. Chen M, Jin Y, Li Y, Bi Y, Shan Y, Pan L. Oncologic and reproductive outcomes after fertility-sparing management with oral progestin for women with complex endometrial hyperplasia and endometrial cancer. Int J Gynaecol Obstet. 2016;132:34–8.
62. Kudesia R, Singer T, Caputo TA, Holcomb KM, Kligman I, Rosenwaks Z, Gupta D. Reproductive and oncologic outcomes after progestin therapy for endometrial complex atypical hyperplasia or carcinoma. Am J Obstet Gynecol. 2014;210:1–4.
63. Ohyagi-Hara C, Sawada K, Aki I, Mabuchi S, Kobayashi E, Ueda Y, Yoshino K, Fujita M, Tsutsui T, Kimura T. Efficacies and pregnant outcomes of fertility-sparing treatment with medroxyprogesterone acetate for endometrioid adenocarcinoma and complex atypical hyperplasia: our experience and a review of the literature. Arch Gynecol Obstet. 2015;291:151–7.
64. Mitsuhashi A, Sato Y, Kiyokawa T, Koshizaka M, Hanaoka H, Shozu M. Phase II study of medroxyprogesterone acetate plus metformin as a fertility-sparing treatment for atypical endometrial hyperplasia and endometrial cancer. Ann Oncol. 2016;27(2):262–6.
65. Wildemeersch D, Janssens D, Vrijens M, Weyers S. Ease of insertion, contraceptive efficacy and safety of new T-shaped levonorgestrel-releasing intrauterine systems. Contraception. 2005;71(6):465–9.
66. Tjalma WAA, Janssens D, Wildemeersch D, Colpaert C, Watty K. Conservative management of atypical endometrial hyperplasia and early invasive carcinoma with intrauterine levonorgestrel: a progesterone receptor study. EJC Suppl. 2004;2:93–4.
67. Gunderson CC, Fader AN, Carson KA, Bristow RE. Oncologic and reproductive outcomes with progestin therapy in women with endometrial hyperplasia and grade 1 adenocarcinoma: a systematic review. Gynecol Oncol. 2012;125(2):477–82.
68. Chandra V, Kim JJ, Benbrook DM, Dwivedi A, Rai R. Therapeutic options for management of endometrial hyperplasia. J Gynecol Oncol. 2016;27(1):e8.
69. Nilsson CG, Luukkainen T, Diaz J, Allonen H. Clinical performance of a new levonorgestrel-releasing intrauterine device. A randomized comparison with a nova-T-copper device. Contraception. 1982;25(4):345–56.

70. Lahteenmaki P, Rauramo I, Backman T. The levonorgestrel intrauterine system in contraception. Steroids. 2000;65(10-11):693–7.
71. Bafaloukos D, Aravantinos G, Samonis G, Katsifis G, Bakoyiannis C, Skarlos D, et al. Carboplatin, methotrexate and 5-fluorouracil in combination with medroxyprogesterone acetate (JMF-M) in the treatment of advanced or recurrent endometrial carcinoma: A Hellenic cooperative oncology group study. Oncology. 1999;56(3):198–201.
72. Kaku T, Yoshikawa H, Tsuda H, Sakamoto A, Fukunaga M, Kuwabara Y, et al. Conservative therapy for adenocarcinoma and atypical endometrial hyperplasia of the endometrium in young women: central pathologic review and treatment outcome. Cancer Lett. 2001;167(1):39–48.
73. Thigpen JT, Brady MF, Alvarez RD, Adelson MD, Homesley HD, Manetta A, et al. Oral medroxyprogesterone acetate in the treatment of advanced or recurrent endometrial carcinoma: a dose-response study by the Gynecologic Oncology Group. J Clin Oncol. 1999;17(6):1736–44.
74. Cholakian D, Hacker K, Fader AN, Gehrig PA, Tanner EJ 3rd. Effect of oral versus intrauterine progestins on weight in women undergoing fertility preserving therapy for complex atypical hyperplasia or endometrial cancer. Gynecol Oncol. 2016;140(2):234–8.
75. Tepper NK, Whiteman MK, Marchbanks PA, James AH, Curtis KM. Progestin-only contraception and thromboembolism: A systematic review. Contraception. 2016;94(6):678–700.
76. Gallos ID, Shehmar M, Thangaratinam S, Papapostolou TK, Coomarasamy A, Gupta JK. Oral progestogens vs levonorgestrel-releasing intrauterine system for endometrial hyperplasia: a systematic review and metaanalysis. Am J Obstet Gynecol. 2010;203(6):547 e1–10.
77. Gallos ID, Ganesan R, Gupta JK. Prediction of regression and relapse of endometrial hyperplasia with conservative therapy. Obstet Gynecol. 2013;121(6):1165–71.
78. Varma R, Soneja H, Bhatia K, Ganesan R, Rollason T, Clark TJ, et al. The effectiveness of a levonorgestrel-releasing intrauterine system (LNG-IUS) in the treatment of endometrial hyperplasia–a long-term follow-up study. Eur J Obstet Gynecol Reprod Biol. 2008;139(2):169–75.
79. Orbo A, Arnes M, Vereide AB, Straume B. Relapse risk of endometrial hyperplasia after treatment with the levonorgestrel-impregnated intrauterine system or oral progestogens. BJOG. 2016;123(9):1512–9.
80. Gallos ID, Yap J, Rajkhowa M, Luesley DM, Coomarasamy A, Gupta JK. Regression, relapse, and live birth rates with fertility-sparing therapy for endometrial cancer and atypical complex endometrial hyperplasia: a systematic review and metaanalysis. Am J Obstet Gynecol. 2012;207(4):266 e1–12.
81. Park JY, Seong SJ, Kim TJ, Kim JW, Kim SM, Bae DS, et al. Pregnancy outcomes after fertility-sparing management in young women with early endometrial cancer. Obstet Gynecol. 2013;121(1):136–42.
82. Kalogera E, Dowdy SC, Bakkum-Gamez JN. Preserving fertility in young patients with endometrial cancer: current perspectives. Int J Womens Health. 2014;6:691–701.
83. Koskas M, Uzan J, Luton D, Rouzier R, Darai E. Prognostic factors of oncologic and reproductive outcomes in fertility-sparing management of endometrial atypical hyperplasia and adenocarcinoma: systematic review and meta-analysis. Fertil Steril. 2014;101(3):785–94.
84. Agorastos T, Bontis J, Vakiani A, Vavilis D, Constantinidis T. Treatment of endometrial hyperplasias with gonadotropin-releasing hormone agonists: pathological, clinical, morphometric, and DNA-cytometric data. Gynecol Oncol. 1997;65(1):102–14.
85. Perez-Medina T, Bajo J, Folgueira G, Haya J, Ortega P. Atypical endometrial hyperplasia treatment with progestogens and gonadotropin-releasing hormone analogues: long-term follow-up. Gynecol Oncol. 1999;73(2):299–304.
86. Agorastos T, Vaitsi V, Paschopoulos M, Vakiani A, Zournatzi-Koiou V, Saravelos H, et al. Prolonged use of gonadotropin-releasing hormone agonist and tibolone as add-back therapy for the treatment of endometrial hyperplasia. Maturitas. 2004;48(2):125–32.

87. Decensi A, Puntoni M, Goodwin P, Cazzaniga M, Gennari A, Bonanni B, et al. Metformin and cancer risk in diabetic patients: a systematic review and meta-analysis. Cancer Prev Res. 2010;3(11):1451–61.
88. Libby G, Donnelly LA, Donnan PT, Alessi DR, Morris AD, Evans JM. New users of metformin are at low risk of incident cancer: a cohort study among people with type 2 diabetes. Diabetes Care. 2009;32(9):1620–5.
89. Chae YK, Arya A, Malecek MK, Shin DS, Carneiro B, Chandra S, et al. Repurposing metformin for cancer treatment: current clinical studies. Oncotarget. 2016;7(26):40767–80.
90. Shan W, Wang C, Zhang Z, Gu C, Ning C, Luo X, et al. Conservative therapy with metformin plus megestrol acetate for endometrial atypical hyperplasia. J Gynecol Oncol. 2014;25(3):214–20.
91. Hawkes AL, Quinn M, Gebski V, Armes J, Brennan D, Janda M, et al. Improving treatment for obese women with early stage cancer of the uterus: rationale and design of the levonorgestrel intrauterine device +/− metformin +/− weight loss in endometrial cancer (feMME) trial. Contemp Clin Trials. 2014;39(1):14–21.
92. Milam MR, Celestino J, Wu W, Broaddus RR, Schmeler KM, Slomovitz BM, et al. Reduced progression of endometrial hyperplasia with oral mTOR inhibition in the Pten heterozygote murine model. Am J Obstet Gynecol. 2007;196(3):247 e1–5.
93. Slomovitz BM, Jiang Y, Yates MS, Soliman PT, Johnston T, Nowakowski M, et al. Phase II study of everolimus and letrozole in patients with recurrent endometrial carcinoma. J Clin Oncol. 2015;33(8):930–6.
94. Smits A, Lopes A, Das N, Bekkers R, Massuger L, Galaal K. The effect of lifestyle interventions on the quality of life of gynaecological cancer survivors: A systematic review and meta-analysis. Gynecol Oncol. 2015;139(3):546–52.
95. Hall C, Stone RL, Gehlot A, Zorn KK, Burnett AF. Use of metformin in obese women with type I endometrial cancer is associated with a reduced incidence of cancer recurrence. Int J Gynecol Cancer. 2016;26(2):313–7.
96. Tancredi M, Rosengren A, Svensson AM, Kosiborod M, Pivodic A, Gudbjornsdottir S, et al. Excess mortality among persons with type 2 diabetes. N Engl J Med. 2015;373(18):1720–32.
97. Modesitt SC, Hallowell PT, Slack-Davis JK, Michalek RD, Atkins KA, Kelley SL, et al. Women at extreme risk for obesity-related carcinogenesis: Baseline endometrial pathology and impact of bariatric surgery on weight, metabolic profiles and quality of life. Gynecol Oncol. 2015;138(2):238–45.
98. Laurelli G, Di Vagno G, Scaffa C, Losito S, Del Giudice M, Greggi S. Conservative treatment of early endometrial cancer: preliminary results of a pilot study. Gynecol Oncol. 2011;120(1):43–6.
99. Mazzon I, Corrado G, Morricone D, Scambia G. Reproductive preservation for treatment of stage IA endometrial cancer in a young woman: hysteroscopic resection. Int J Gynecol Cancer. 2005;15(5):974–8.
100. De Marzi P, Bergamini A, Luchini S, Petrone M, Taccagni GL, Mangili G, et al. Hysteroscopic resection in fertility-sparing surgery for atypical hyperplasia and endometrial cancer: safety and efficacy. J Minim Invasive Gynecol. 2015;22(7):1178–82.
101. Mayor PC, Lele S. Photodynamic therapy in gynecologic malignancies: a review of the Roswell Park Cancer Institute experience. Cancers (Basel). 2016;8(10):E88.
102. Choi MC, Jung SG, Park H, Cho YH, Lee C, Kim SJ. Fertility preservation via photodynamic therapy in young patients with early-stage uterine endometrial cancer: a long-term follow-up study. Int J Gynecol Cancer. 2013;23(4):698–704.
103. Gezginc ST, Celik C, Dogan NU, Toy H, Tazegul A, Colakoglu MC. Expression of cyclin A, cyclin E and p27 in normal, hyperplastic and frankly malignant endometrial samples. J Obstet Gynaecol. 2013;33(5):508–11.
104. McCampbell AS, Mittelstadt ML, Dere R, Kim S, Zhou L, Djordjevic B, et al. Loss of p27 associated with risk for endometrial carcinoma arising in the setting of obesity. Curr Mol Med. 2016;16(3):252–65.

105. Westin SN, Ju Z, Broaddus RR, Krakstad C, Li J, Pal N, et al. PTEN loss is a context-dependent outcome determinant in obese and non-obese endometrioid endometrial cancer patients. Mol Oncol. 2015;9(8):1694–703.
106. Gallos ID, Devey J, Ganesan R, Gupta JK. Predictive ability of estrogen receptor (ER), progesterone receptor (PR), COX-2, Mlh1, and Bcl-2 expressions for regression and relapse of endometrial hyperplasia treated with LNG-IUS: a prospective cohort study. Gynecol Oncol. 2013;130(1):58–63.
107. Tangen IL, Werner HM, Berg A, Halle MK, Kusonmano K, Trovik J, et al. Loss of progesterone receptor links to high proliferation and increases from primary to metastatic endometrial cancer lesions. Eur J Cancer. 2014;50(17):3003–10.
108. Abkevich V, Timms KM, Hennessy BT, Potter J, Carey MS, Meyer LA, et al. Patterns of genomic loss of heterozygosity predict homologous recombination repair defects in epithelial ovarian cancer. Br J Cancer. 2012;107(10):1776–82.
109. Jusko WJ. Clarification of contraceptive drug pharmacokinetics in obesity. Contraception. 2016;95(1):10–6.
110. Simmons KB, Edelman AB. Hormonal contraception and obesity. Fertil Steril. 2016;106(6): 1282–8.
111. Azran C, Wolk O, Zur M, Fine-Shamir N, Shaked G, Czeiger D, et al. Oral drug therapy following bariatric surgery: an overview of fundamentals, literature and clinical recommendations. Obes Rev. 2016;17(11):1050–66.
112. Nelson A, Apter D, Hauck B, Schmelter T, Rybowski S, Rosen K, et al. Two low-dose levonorgestrel intrauterine contraceptive systems: a randomized controlled trial. Obstet Gynecol. 2013;122(6):1205–13.
113. Panoulas VF, Mastoris I, Konstantinou K, Tespili M, Ielasi A. Everolimus-eluting stent platforms in percutaneous coronary intervention: comparative effectiveness and outcomes. Med Devices (Auckl). 2015;8:317–29.
114. Bulletti C, de Ziegler D, Flamigni C, Giacomucci E, Polli V, Bolelli G, et al. Targeted drug delivery in gynaecology: the first uterine pass effect. Hum Reprod. 1997;12(5):1073–9.
115. Ficicioglu C, Gurbuz B, Tasdemir S, Yalti S, Canova H. High local endometrial effect of vaginal progesterone gel. Gynecol Endocrinol. 2004;18(5):240–3.

Chapter 12
Exercise and Lifestyle Interventions in Gynecologic Cancer Survivors

Nora L. Nock

Abstract In this chapter, we review trials (randomized and non-randomized) involving exercise and other lifestyle components (dietary counseling) in gynecological cancer survivors. In particular, we focus on endometrial and ovarian cancer survivor trials since the majority of studies have been conducted in these cancer populations. To date, only two randomized controlled trials (RCTs) and two non-randomized trials have been completed in ovarian cancer survivors. In addition, there have been three RCTs and two non-randomized trials in endometrial cancer and two other RCTs are currently underway. There has also been a RCT involving a mixed population of ovarian and endometrial cancer survivors and a RCT involving a mixed population of endometrial cancer survivors and women with endometrial hyperplasia, a precursor to endometrial cancer. Most of the RCTs have involved lifestyle counseling and home-based exercise with walking programs, predominantly.; and, most studies have examined changes in physical activity using self-reported measures. Several, but not all, trials have shown some improvement in quality of life with exercise in gynecologic cancer survivors. Given the limited number of RCTs, there is clearly a need for more lifestyle interventions in gynecological survivors. However, future studies should evaluate supervised exercise programs that include objective measures for evaluating changes in physical activity, cardiopulmonary fitness, physical function and body composition. Given the rising rates of uterine cancer incidence and mortality coupled with the strong associations between obesity and endometrial cancer incidence and mortality, as well as the poor fitness levels in endometrial cancer survivors, there should be a particular focus on providing these programs to endometrial cancer survivors and women with endometrial hyperplasia.

Keywords Exercise • Quality of life • Ovarian cancer • Endometrial cancer

N.L. Nock, Ph.D. (✉)
Department of Epidemiology and Biostatistics, Case Western Reserve University School of Medicine, 10900 Euclid Avenue, Cleveland, OH 44106, USA
e-mail: nln@case.edu

© Springer International Publishing AG 2018
N.A. Berger et al. (eds.), *Focus on Gynecologic Malignancies*, Energy Balance and Cancer 13, DOI 10.1007/978-3-319-63483-8_12

Introduction

Uterine cancer is the most common gynecological cancer and fourth leading cause of cancer in females in the U.S. with 60,050 new cases and 10,470 deaths estimated in 2016 [1]. Ovarian cancer is less prevalent, with an estimated 22,280 new cases in 2016, but is the leading cause of death from gynecological cancer and fifth leading cause of death from any cancer in females with 14,240 deaths estimated in 2016 [1]. The 5 year survival rate for endometrial cancer exceeds 80% but is only approximately 46% for ovarian cancer [1].

Worldwide, endometrial cancer is the sixth leading cancer in women and higher rates of endometrial cancer and ovarian cancer are observed in more developed nations (13.0 per 100,000 and 9.3 per 100,000, respectively) compared to less developed nations (5.9 per 100,000 and 5.0 per 100,000, respectively) [2]. Mortality rates worldwide are higher for ovarian cancer compared to endometrial cancer in both more developed (5.1 per 100,000 and 3.1 per 100,000, respectively) and less developed countries (2.3 and 1.7 per 100,000, respectively) [2].

Rates of uterine cancer incidence and mortality are increasing while rates for ovarian cancer have been fairly stable. A 2.3% increase per year in prevalence and a 2.0% increase per year in deaths was estimated during the period from 2008–2013 for uterine cancer [1]. An estimated increase to 42.1 cases per 100,000 is expected in 2030, which represents an a 55% increase over 2010 rates [3]. Obesity, which is also rising in our nation, is a leading risk factor for endometrial cancer [4, 5]; and, Type I (endometrioid) cancer, which represents about 85% of all endometrial cancers [6, 7], appears to be the specific type of endometrial cancer driving the increased rates of uterine cancer in the U.S [8].

Epidemiological evidence suggests that cancer survivors, in general, are less active than their non-cancer counterparts. One study reported that cancer survivors were less physically active on an 'at least weekly' basis than their non-cancer counterparts (45.3% vs. 53.0%) [9]. In particular, endometrial cancer survivors were found, on average, to conduct approximately 10 min less moderate intensity exercise per week compared to similar aged non-cancer females using 2009 Behavioral Risk Factor Surveillance System (BRFSS) data [10]. However, means of moderate intensity exercise were not found to be statistically significantly different between ovarian cancer survivors and non-cancer females of similar age using the 2009 BRFSS data [10].

Furthermore, endometrial cancer patients have been found to have poorer fitness and physical function than women of similar age without cancer. In one study involving obese women, endometrial cancer survivors had a significantly lower fitness level compared to women of similar age without cancer ($VO_{2\ peak}$: 15.0 vs. 17.9 mL/kg/min) [11]. Another study showed that endometrial cancer patients (<75 years old) had lower physical function (as measured using the physical component of the Short-Form Health Survey, SF-12) compared to population-based age-standardized normative values [12]. In addition, peak METs during a maximal exercise tolerance test (treadmill) were 8.4 ± 1.9 and 8.9 ± 2.2 for endometrial and ovarian cancer patients, respectively, and were approximately one MET lower than age-, gender- and BMI-matched controls [13].

Epidemiological evidence suggests that physical activity may improve survival and quality of life in gynecological cancer survivors. Physical activity levels exceeding 7 h/week compared to never/rarely was shown to decrease all-cause 5-year mortality by 43% in endometrial cancer survivors using data from the National Institutes of Health–AARP Diet and Health Study [14]. Vigorous intensity physical activity was associated with a 26% lower risk of ovarian cancer specific mortality and a 24% lower risk of all-cause mortality compared to conducting no vigorous intensity physical activity using data from the Women's Health Initiative (WHI) study [15]. Furthermore, endometrial cancer survivors who perform 150 min/week or more of physical activity may be potentially protected from the negative effects of having a higher body mass index (BMI) on quality of life [16]. Similarly, ovarian cancer survivors meeting public health activity guidelines (at least 60 min of strenuous or 150 min of moderate/strenuous physical activity per week) reported significantly better quality of life than those not meeting the physical activity guidelines [17].

Taken together, there is a need to provide exercise and overall wellness programs to gynecological cancer survivors to improve their quality of life and overall survival. There is a particular need for programs in endometrial cancer survivors who have higher BMIs that increase their mortality rates [18], who are less active [10] and less functionally fit [11, 13], and desire to receive advice on exercise and healthy eating in-person [19]. However, only a limited number of randomized clinical trials (RCTs) involving an exercise or physical activity component in gynecologic cancer survivors have been conducted. In the sections that follow, we will review the completed RCTs as well as the RCTs that are currently underway (based upon published protocol papers) in endometrial (three RCTs completed, two RCTs ongoing) and ovarian (two RCTs completed) and combined endometrial and ovarian (one RCT) cancer survivors. We will also discuss the non-randomized single arm trials that included endometrial [4] and ovarian [2] cancer survivors.

Endometrial Cancer Survivors: Completed RCTs Involving Exercise

The first RCT conducted in endometrial cancer survivors was a large pilot study conducted by von Gruenigen et al. [20], which involved randomizing 45 Stage I or II, overweight or obese (BMI $\geq$ 25 kg/m^2) endometrial cancer survivors to 6 months of group and individual based behavioral counseling that encouraged home-based walking or usual care ($N_{intervention}$ = 23; $N_{control}$ = 22) [20]. They reported that "the intervention group lost 3.5 kg compared to a 1.4 kg gain in the control group" and, that "the intervention group had a significant increase in their self-reported physical activity score at 12 months compared to baseline" [20]. In addition, they reported "no statistically significant change in quality of life" (using the Functional Assessment of Cancer Therapy-General, FACT-G) [21].

von Gruenigen et al. [22] followed up this pilot study with a similar but larger RCT entitled "Survivors of Uterine Cancer Empowered by Exercise and Healthy Diet (SUCCEED)" that involved 6 months of behavioral counseling in 75 Stage I or II, overweight or obese (BMI ≥ 25 kg/m²) endometrial cancer survivors [22]. In the SUCCEED trial, the weight loss goal was 5% at 6 months and patients were encouraged to conduct physical activity at 150 min/week during months 1–2, 225 min/week during months 3–4, and 300 min/week during months 5–6 [22]. Participants were also given pedometers (with the goal of 10,000 steps/day or an increase of 2000 steps/day from baseline levels) and 3 lb hand and ankle weights with instructions for performing resistance exercises (specific exercises not denoted) [22]. They reported that "the mean [and 95% C.I.] difference in weight change between treatment and control groups was −4.4 kg [−5.3, −3.5] at 6 months and −4.6 kg [−5.8, −3.5] at 12 months" and, that "the mean difference in self-reported physical activity minutes between groups was 100 [6, 194] at 6 months and 89 [14, 163] at 12 months" [22]. In addition, they reported "a significant between-group difference in quality of life (using the FACT-G) from baseline to 6 months in the physical domain" [23].

Rossi et al. [24] evaluated a 12-week intervention involving behavioral counseling (1, 30 min session/week), supervised exercise (2, 60 min moderate-to-vigorous intensity group sessions per week) and a home-based walking program (90 min/week of moderate intensity) compared to a wait-list control in 28 obese (BMI ≥ 30 kg/m²) Stage I–IV endometrial cancer survivors [24]. They evaluated the intensity level of the exercise using ratings of perceived exertion (RPE) and evaluated fitness at baseline and after the 12 week program using the Six Minute Walk Test (6 MWT) [24]. Rossi et al. [24] reported that the intervention group significantly increased the distance walked in the 6MWT by 22.0 ± 16.7 m compared to 1.1 ± 22.0 m in the control group [24]. In addition, they reported a significant difference between groups after compared to before the program for FACT-En but the difference between groups was not statistically significant for the FACT-G [24], which suggests the significant difference may be driven by the endometrial subdomain scale.

Endometrial Cancer Survivors: Ongoing (Not Completed) RCTs Involving Exercise

We are currently conducting a RCT entitled "Revving-Up Exercise for Sustained Weight Loss by Altering Neurological Reward and Drive (REWARD)" that is recruiting 120 obese (BMI ≥ 30 kg/m²) Stage I endometrial cancer survivors, whereby patients are being randomized to receive either 'assisted' or voluntary rate cycling (3 days/week, ~1 h sessions, 60–80% of maximal heart rate) and group-based behavioral counseling intervention (1 day/week, 1–1.5 h sessions) for 16 weeks [25]. Exercise intensity is being measured using heart rate monitors (and

RPE) by exercise physiologists during the 16-week intervention period and tracked using accelerometers equipped with heart rate monitors during the 6-month follow up period. The 'assisted' exercise on a stationary bike provides mechanical assistance to enable the patients to pedal up to 35% faster than their voluntary/preferred rates, which has been shown previously to provide global improvements in motor function and increased activity in cortical and subcortical regions, consistent with activation patterns after applying a dopamine agonist, suggesting that 'assisted' exercise may modulate dopamine levels in the brain [26–28]. Thus, we hypothesize that patients performing 'assisted' exercise will have improved neurological stimulus in reward and motivation brain regions in response to exercise, potentially leading to enhanced and/or sustained weight loss. The primary outcome of the REWARD trial is change in weight from baseline to 16 weeks and 24 weeks after completion of the 16 week program and, secondary outcomes include changes in fitness (cardiopulmonary exercise test), exercise motivation and appetitive behavior as measured using questionnaires and functional magnetic resonance imaging (MRI) tasks as well as other physiological and behavioral outcomes including quality of life (FACT-G, FACT-En) [25].

Koutoukidis et al. [29] are currently conducting a RCT entitled "Shape-up following cancer treatment" in 64 endometrial cancer survivors randomized to an 8 week group-based behavior counseling program (1, 90 min session/week) or usual care [29]. The physical activity goal in this trial is to encourage patients to aim for 30 min of moderate intensity activity per day and resistance training exercises twice a week [29]. Physical activity will be assessed using a questionnaire and a 15-min interview administered tool, strength via a hand grip device and quality of life using a questionnaire (EORTC Quality of Life Questionnaire, QLQ-C-30) [29].

Endometrial Cancer Survivors: Completed and Ongoing Non-randomized Trials Involving Exercise

A large single-arm non-randomized trial entitled "Steps to Health" was conducted by Basen-Engquist et al. [30] in 100 Stage I–III endometrial cancer survivors receiving a 6-month behavioral counseling program involving print materials and telephone counseling (20–30-min calls: weekly in months 1–2, 2 times a month in months 3–4 and 1 time a month in months 5–6) and an exercise prescription with a physical activity goal of ultimately achieving at least 150 min of moderate intensity physical activity per week [30]. Physical activity was measured using an accelerometer and, fitness was evaluated using a submaximal exercise test on an ergometer at baseline and after the 6-month program [30]. They reported significant differences in physical activity minutes at 6 months compared to baseline in obese (15.88 ± 10.64 vs. 13.64 ± 12.48) and non-obese (19.80 ± 10.14 vs. 16.35 ± 9.90) patients but no significant changes in fitness at 6 months compared to baseline [31]. In addition, they reported significant improvements in quality of life (SF-36 and QLACS measures) at 6 months compared to baseline [31].

Smits et al. [32] is currently conducting a single-arm trial evaluating a 10-week individually supervised exercise program (1, 60 min sessions of combined aerobic/cardiovascular at 40–60% maximum heart rate and resistance training 40–60% with one repetition maximum per week) [32]. Exercise intensity will be measured using heart rate monitors and physical fitness will be evaluated using the 6 MWT at baseline and after the 10 week program [32].

Ovarian Cancer Survivors: Completed RCTs Involving Exercise

Hwang et al. [33] conducted a RCT in 40 Stage I–III ovarian cancer survivors randomized to an 8-week group-based behavioral counseling (1, 60 min sessions/week) with patients being encouraged to conduct exercise and relaxation therapy at home (3 times/week, relaxation therapy (3, 15 min sessions/week), 50 min of combined aerobic and resistance exercise, medium intensity, 40–60% maximum heart rate) [33]. They found that fitness as measured by the 12 MWT was significantly improved between treatment and control groups (239.12 vs. 12.57 m) [33]. They also reported a significant improvement in quality of life scores (using the FACT-G) [33].

The Women's Activity in Lifestyle Study in Connecticut (WALC), led by Dr. Melinda Irwin, is currently evaluating the effects of a six-month RCT of home-based exercise (goal: moderate intensity, 150 min/week, facilitated using weekly phone calls) versus attention control in Stage I–IV ovarian cancer survivors (n = 144). Preliminary results suggest that ovarian cancer survivors in the exercise arm compared to the attention control arm had improved quality of life in the physical domain (using the SF-36) at 6 months compared to baseline (3.7 (0.7–6.8); p = 0.02) (personal communication, 3/5/2017).

Ovarian Cancer Survivors: Non-randomized Trials Involving Exercise

Von Gruenigen et al. [21] evaluated a single arm trial in 27 Stage I–IV ovarian cancer patients undergoing chemotherapy (6 cycles) that received a behavioral counseling program (30 min sessions during each chemotherapy cycle) [34]. They reported "an increase in mean (95% C.I.) minutes of physical activity from cycle #3 to after cycle #6 (61 (−3, 120) min) and from baseline to after cycle #6 (73 (−10, 15) min)" [34]. A significant increase in quality of life (FACT-G measure) was reported from baseline to cycle #6 [34].

Moonsammy et al. [35] single-arm non-randomized trial in 19 Stage I–III ovarian cancer survivors (seven undergoing adjuvant chemotherapy) involving a 24-week home-based exercise intervention (combined aerobic (60–70% of maximum heart rate) and resistance training, 30–60 min/session, 3–5 times/week) with 12 weeks of cognitive behavioral therapy (2 sessions/month) [35]. They found a significant improvement in fitness from baseline to 6 months in the treatment group (VO_2 peak (mL/kg/min): 30.0 ± 8.0 vs. 38.3 ± 2.9) compared to the control group (VO_2 peak (mL/kg/min): 29.1 ± 7.7 vs. 33.0 ± 3.1) [35]. No statistically significant differences were reported for quality of life (including the FACT-G and FACT-O) measures.

Combined Cancer Survivor and/or Cancer Precursor Conditions: RCTs and Non-randomized Trials Involving Exercise

Donnelly et al. [36] conducted a RCT in 33 sedentary Stage I–III gynecological cancer survivors (Endometrial Cancer = 11, Ovarian Cancer = 12) randomized to a 12-week, telephone-based behavioral counseling intervention (home-based moderate intensity physical activity (150 min/week), n = 16) or a contact control (n = 17) [36]. Using the 12 MWT, they found that fitness improved at 12 weeks compared to baseline but the difference between groups was not statistically significant (adjusted mean difference: 10.84 (−59.74–81.44) m). The improvements in quality of life (using the FACT-G) were also not statistically significant between treatment and control groups.

Haggerty et al. [37] conducted a RCT in obese Type 1 endometrial cancer survivors (n = 16) and obese women with endometrial hyperplasia (n = 4) randomized to a 6-month behavioral counseling program delivered via telephone (weekly phone calls) or text (3–5 personalized messages daily via Text4Diet™) [37]. They found greater weight loss in the telemedicine compared to the Text4Diet arm (median loss: 9.7 kg (range: 1.6–22.9 kg) vs. 3.9 kg (0.3–11.4 kg)) [37]. There was no discussion regarding potential changes in physical activity and quality of life.

A non-randomized single-arm trial conducted by McCarroll et al. [38] in overweight and obese (BMI ≥ 25 kg/m^2) breast (n = 26) and endometrial (n = 24, five with breast and endometrial) cancer survivors evaluated a 1 month web- and mobile-based exercise and nutritional counseling program using the LoseIt!® app [38]. No significant differences were noted for physical activity or quality of life (using the FACT-G) but they reported post-intervention weight was significantly lower than baseline (105.0 ± 21.8 kg vs. 98.6 ± 22.5 kg) [38].

Conclusions and Proposed Future Directions

Most RCTs conducted to date have involved lifestyle counseling and home-based exercise, with walking programs, predominantly; and, most studies have examined changes in physical activity using self-reported measures. Several, but not all, trials have shown an improvement in quality of life with exercise in gynecologic cancer survivors. Future studies should evaluate supervised exercise programs that include objective measures for evaluating changes in physical activity, cardiopulmonary fitness, physical function and body composition. Given the rising rates of uterine cancer incidence and mortality coupled with the strong associations between obesity and endometrial cancer incidence and mortality, as well as the poor fitness levels in endometrial cancer survivors, there should be a particular focus on providing lifestyle programs to endometrial cancer survivors and women with precursor conditions including endometrial hyperplasia.

Acknowledgement This work was supported, in part, by NIH NCI grant R01CA175100 [to N. L. N.].

References

1. Siegel RL, Miller KD, Jemal A. Cancer statistics, 2016. CA Cancer J Clin. 2016;66(1):7–30.
2. Ferlay J, Parkin DM, Steliarova-Foucher E. Estimates of cancer incidence and mortality in Europe in 2008. Eur J Cancer. 2010;46(4):765–81.
3. Sheikh MA, Althouse AD, Freese KE, et al. USA endometrial cancer projections to 2030: should we be concerned? Future Oncol. 2014;10(16):2561–8.
4. Renehan AG, Tyson M, Egger M, Heller RF, Zwahlen M. Body-mass index and incidence of cancer: a systematic review and meta-analysis of prospective observational studies. Lancet. 2008;371(9612):569–78.
5. Schmandt RE, Iglesias DA, Co NN, Lu KH. Understanding obesity and endometrial cancer risk: opportunities for prevention. Am J Obstet Gynecol. 2011;205(6):518–25.
6. Calle EE, Kaaks R. Overweight, obesity and cancer: epidemiological evidence and proposed mechanisms. Nat Rev Cancer. 2004;4(8):579–91.
7. Kaaks R, Lukanova A, Kurzer MS. Obesity, endogenous hormones, and endometrial cancer risk: a synthetic review. Cancer Epidemiol Biomark Prev. 2002;11(12):1531–43.
8. Duong LM, Wilson RJ, Ajani UA, Singh SD, Eheman CR. Trends in endometrial cancer incidence rates in the United States, 1999-2006. J Womens Health (Larchmt). 2011;20(8):1157–63.
9. Mayer DK, Terrin NC, Menon U, et al. Health behaviors in cancer survivors. Oncol Nurs Forum. 2007;34(3):643–51.
10. Kwon S, Hou N, Wang M. Comparison of physical activity levels between cancer survivors and non-cancer participants in the 2009 BRFSS. J Cancer Surviv. 2012;6(1):54–62.
11. Modesitt SC, Geffel DL, Via J, Weltman L. Morbidly obese women with and without endometrial cancer: are there differences in measured physical fitness, body composition, or hormones? Gynecol Oncol. 2012;124(3):431–6.
12. Zhang X, Brown JC, Schmitz KH. Association between body mass index and physical function among endometrial cancer survivors. PLoS One. 2016;11(8):e0160954.

13. Peel AB, Barlow CE, Leonard D, et al. Cardiorespiratory fitness in survivors of cervical, endometrial, and ovarian cancers: The Cooper Center Longitudinal Study. Gynecol Oncol. 2015;138(2):394–7.
14. Arem H, Park Y, Pelser C, et al. Prediagnosis body mass index, physical activity, and mortality in endometrial cancer patients. J Natl Cancer Inst. 2013;105(5):342–9.
15. Zhou Y, Chlebowski R, Lamonte MJ, et al. Body mass index, physical activity, and mortality in women diagnosed with ovarian cancer: results from the Women's Health Initiative. Gynecol Oncol. 2014;133(1):4–10.
16. Lin LL, Brown JC, Segal S, Schmitz KH. Quality of life, body mass index, and physical activity among uterine cancer patients. Int J Gynecol Cancer. 2014;24(6):1027–32.
17. Stevinson C, Faught W, Steed H, et al. Associations between physical activity and quality of life in ovarian cancer survivors. Gynecol Oncol. 2007;106(1):244–50.
18. Secord AA, Hasselblad V, von Gruenigen VE, et al. Body mass index and mortality in endometrial cancer: A systematic review and meta-analysis. Gynecol Oncol. 2016;140(1):184–90.
19. Koutoukidis DA, Beeken RJ, Lopes S, Knobf MT, Lanceley A. Attitudes, challenges and needs about diet and physical activity in endometrial cancer survivors: a qualitative study. Eur J Cancer Care (Engl). 2016.
20. von Gruenigen VE, Courneya KS, Gibbons HE, et al. Feasibility and effectiveness of a lifestyle intervention program in obese endometrial cancer patients: a randomized trial. Gynecol Oncol. 2008;109(1):19–26.
21. von Gruenigen VE, Gibbons HE, Kavanagh MB, et al. A randomized trial of a lifestyle intervention in obese endometrial cancer survivors: quality of life outcomes and mediators of behavior change. Health Qual Life Outcomes. 2009;7:17.
22. von Gruenigen VE, Frasure H, Kavanagh MB, et al. Survivors of uterine cancer empowered by exercise and healthy diet (SUCCEED): A randomized controlled trial. Gynecol Oncol. 2012;125(3):699–704.
23. McCarroll ML, Armbruster S, Frasure HE, et al. Self-efficacy, quality of life, and weight loss in overweight/obese endometrial cancer survivors (SUCCEED): a randomized controlled trial. Gynecol Oncol. 2014;132(2):397–402.
24. Rossi A, Garber CE, Ortiz M, et al. Feasibility of a physical activity intervention for obese, socioculturally diverse endometrial cancer survivors. Gynecol Oncol. 2016;142(2):304–10.
25. Nock NL, Dimitropoulos A, Rao SM, et al. Rationale and design of REWARD (revving-up exercise for sustained weight loss by altering neurological reward and drive): a randomized trial in obese endometrial cancer survivors. Contemp Clin Trials. 2014;39(2):236–45.
26. Alberts JL, Linder SM, Penko AL, Lowe MJ, Phillips M. It is not about the bike, it is about the pedaling: forced exercise and Parkinson's disease. Exerc Sport Sci Rev. 2011;39(4):177–86.
27. Alberts JL, Phillips M, Lowe MJ, et al. Cortical and motor responses to acute forced exercise in Parkinson's disease. Parkinsonism Relat Disord. 2016;24:56–62.
28. Ridgel AL, Vitek JL, Alberts JL. Forced, not voluntary, exercise improves motor function in Parkinson's disease patients. Neurorehabil Neural Repair. 2009;23(6):600–8.
29. Koutoukidis DA, Beeken RJ, Manchanda R, et al. Diet and exercise in uterine cancer survivors (DEUS pilot) - piloting a healthy eating and physical activity program: study protocol for a randomized controlled trial. Trials. 2016;17(1):130.
30. Basen-Engquist K, Carmack CL, Perkins H, et al. Design of the steps to health study of physical activity in survivors of endometrial cancer: testing a social cognitive theory model. Psychol Sport Exerc. 2011;12(1):27–35.
31. Basen-Engquist K, Carmack C, Brown J, et al. Response to an exercise intervention after endometrial cancer: differences between obese and non-obese survivors. Gynecol Oncol. 2014;133(1):48–55.
32. Smits A, Lopes A, Das N, et al. The effect of lifestyle interventions on the quality of life of gynaecological cancer survivors: A systematic review and meta-analysis. Gynecol Oncol. 2015;139(3):546–52.

33. Hwang KH, Cho OH, Yoo YS. The effect of comprehensive care program for ovarian cancer survivors. Clin Nurs Res. 2016;25(2):192–208.
34. von Gruenigen VE, Frasure HE, Kavanagh MB, et al. Feasibility of a lifestyle intervention for ovarian cancer patients receiving adjuvant chemotherapy. Gynecol Oncol. 2011;122(2):328–33.
35. Moonsammy SH, Guglietti CL, Santa MD, et al. A pilot study of an exercise & cognitive behavioral therapy intervention for epithelial ovarian cancer patients. J Ovarian Res. 2013;6(1):21.
36. Donnelly CM, Blaney JM, Lowe-Strong A, et al. A randomised controlled trial testing the feasibility and efficacy of a physical activity behavioural change intervention in managing fatigue with gynaecological cancer survivors. Gynecol Oncol. 2011;122(3):618–24.
37. Haggerty AF, Huepenbecker S, Sarwer DB, et al. The use of novel technology-based weight loss interventions for obese women with endometrial hyperplasia and cancer. Gynecol Oncol. 2016;140(2):239–44.
38. McCarroll ML, Armbruster S, Pohle-Krauza RJ, et al. Feasibility of a lifestyle intervention for overweight/obese endometrial and breast cancer survivors using an interactive mobile application. Gynecol Oncol. 2015;137(3):508–15.

Chapter 13
Physical Activity as a Risk Factor for Ovarian Cancer

Tianyi Huang and Shelley S. Tworoger

Abstract Ovarian cancer is a highly fatal gynecologic malignancy that is the fifth leading cause of cancer death among women in the United States. Most known risk factors are not easily modifiable, necessitating examination of modifiable lifestyle factors, such as physical activity and sedentary behavior, with risk. While putative biologic mechanisms of action, such as reduced adiposity, sex hormones, and inflammation, suggest that physical activity should lower ovarian cancer risk, results from epidemiologic studies have been less clear. In general, case-control studies have shown an inverse association, however potential recall bias and reverse causation may play a role in this relationship. Conversely, prospective studies generally have observed either a positive association or null results. This may be due to influences of moderate to vigorous activity on increasing ovulatory function compared to physical inactivity. Little research is available regarding associations with survival or the role of sedentary behavior. Clearly, additional research in cohort-based consortia with harmonized physical activity data is needed to further understand the complex role of physical activity with ovarian cancer risk and survival, overall and by tumor subtype.

Keywords Physical activity • Ovulatory function • Ovarian cancer risk • Ovarian cancer risk • Exercise • Sedentary behavior • Obesity

T. Huang
Department of Epidemiology, Harvard University,
677 Huntington Avenue, Boston, MA 02115, USA
e-mail: thuang@hsph.harvard.edu

S.S. Tworoger (✉)
Department of Epidemiology, Harvard University,
181 Longwood Ave., 3rd Floor, Channing Laboratory, Boston, MA 02115, USA
e-mail: stworoge@hsph.harvard.edu

© Springer International Publishing AG 2018   223
N.A. Berger et al. (eds.), *Focus on Gynecologic Malignancies*, Energy Balance
and Cancer 13, DOI 10.1007/978-3-319-63483-8_13

Introduction

Regular physical activity exerts general beneficial effects on various health outcomes. It has been estimated that 9% of premature deaths worldwide in 2008 were attributed to physical inactivity [1]. The World Health Organization recommends a minimum of 150-min moderate-intensity or 75-min vigorous-intensity leisure-time physical activity per week for maintaining and promoting health among individuals aged 18–64; a doubled physical activity level was recommended to achieve additional health benefits [2]. Particularly, the protective effects of physical activity have been well established for several types of cancer. For example, physical inactivity accounted for 10% of breast cancer and 10% of colon cancer incidence worldwide in 2008 [1]. Higher levels of physical activity have been consistently and strongly associated with lower risk of endometrial cancer in a linear dose-response pattern [3, 4]. As a result, the US National Cancer Institute has identified physical activity as an important risk factor for preventing breast, colon and endometrial cancers [5]. However, despite a growing body of evidence from more than 20 epidemiologic studies, the potential benefits of physical activity on ovarian cancer prevention remains unclear. Physical activity is a modifiable lifestyle risk factor hypothesized to have the potential to reduce risk of ovarian cancer.

In 2012, approximately 238,700 new cases of ovarian cancer were diagnosed globally and about 151,900 women died from the disease, with higher incidence and mortality in more developed regions including US and European countries [6]. Ovarian cancer ranks as the fifth leading cause of cancer death among US women [7]. It is the most fatal gynecologic malignancy due to lack of early detection modality that leads to clinical presentation at an advanced stage (e.g., 85% of diagnosed cases) and poor prognosis following diagnosis and treatment (e.g., 5-year survival rate <45%) [7]. Recently, two large randomized controlled trials evaluated the effect of annual ovarian cancer screening, reporting no overall benefits on mortality [8, 9]. This underscores the importance of primary prevention for reducing incidence and mortality of this highly fatal disease. Yet, current prevention recommendations for ovarian cancer are limited, because most confirmed risk factors for ovarian cancer, such as age, family history, parity and oral contraceptive use, are not easily modifiable [10]. Thus, physical activity, a behavioral risk factor that is modifiable at the population level with established health benefits for other diseases, has attracted considerable research interest and may have high potential to improve prevention strategies for ovarian cancer.

Another challenge to identifying modifiable risk factors for ovarian cancer is the heterogeneous nature of ovarian tumors. As common histologic subtypes of ovarian cancer, such as high-grade serous, endometrioid, mucinous, and clear cell tumors, may originate through different etiologic pathways, ovarian cancer has a high level of heterogeneity with regard to its relations with established reproductive and hormonal risk factors [11–13]. For example, a recent study from the Ovarian Cancer Cohort Consortium suggested that most reproductive and hormonal factors show stronger associations with nonserous ovarian cancers vs. the serous subtype [11]; serous tumors are the most common and most aggressive tumor subtype. Similarly, it is important to consider such etiologic heterogeneity to fully understand the association between physical activity and ovarian cancer.

The goal of this chapter is to present the current state of evidence-based knowledge for the relationship between physical activity and ovarian cancer, and provide a discussion of the implications in these research findings that may be conducive to future studies. The chapter begins with a brief review of potential biological mechanisms linking physical activity with the carcinogenic process, in general and specific to ovarian cancer. Next, we focus on population-based, epidemiological studies, particularly those with prospective design, to shed light on the mixed but intriguing associations between physical activity and ovarian cancer. Interpretation of these findings is discussed in some detail from both methodological and biological perspectives. We further set our discussion into a broader context by briefly summarizing the associations of ovarian cancer with sedentary behavior, which appears to have independent effects on health from physical activity. The relationship between obesity and ovarian cancer is covered in Chap. 2. We conclude the chapter with prospects for future research on physical activity and ovarian cancer.

Potential Mechanisms

Physical activity may reduce cancer risk through multiple mechanisms. Most notably, maintaining a physically active lifestyle has a strong effect on reducing obesity and long-term weight gain [14–16], which results in reduced inflammation, higher insulin sensitivity, and decreased sex hormones [17, 18]. These biological alterations have been implicated as general mechanisms for carcinogenesis [19]. Most studies reported that the impact of physical activity on these carcinogenic pathways persisted after accounting for anthropometric measures, suggesting additional anti-cancer benefits of physical activity independent of its effects on adiposity [19]. In addition, immune function may act as another possible mediator of the association between physical activity and cancer [20]. For example, physical activity may strengthen the immune system by boosting number or function of natural killer cells [21, 22], which have a role in tumor development and progression [23].

These mechanisms can be directly translated to imply potential beneficial effects of physical activity on ovarian cancer. First, obesity, particularly increased adiposity during premenopausal periods, is moderately associated higher risk of ovarian cancer [24]. Higher physical activity, which helps reduce obesity, is therefore hypothesized to lower ovarian cancer risk. Second, physical activity is inversely associated with circulating estrogen concentrations, particularly among postmenopausal women [25–29]. Experimental evidence demonstrates that exposure to estrogen promotes the growth of ovarian epithelial cells positive for estrogen receptors and may increase ovarian cancer risk [30]. Higher ovarian cancer risk has been consistently observed among postmenopausal women with regular use of estrogen-only hormone therapy [31–33], although studies that focused on the direct associations between circulating sex hormone concentrations and ovarian cancer risk do not provide conclusive evidence [34–36]. Interestingly, analyses by histologic subtypes suggest a positive association between estradiol and endometrioid tumors, which have higher expression of estrogen receptor and progesterone receptor than other tumor subtypes [37]. Physical activity also induces a significant decrease in circulating androgen levels [29]. Polycystic ovarian syndrome (PCOS), a predominantly hyperandrogenic syndrome common in women of reproductive age, is associated with a 2.5-fold increased risk of ovarian cancer among women younger than 54 years of age [38]. However, similar to the findings on estrogen, epidemiologic evidence has been mixed regarding the association between androgen and ovarian cancer risk. While some observational studies provide evidence for a positive relationship between circulating androgen concentrations and ovarian cancer risk [34–36], other studies of small sample size do not support this hypothesis [39–41]. Of note, recent findings from two larger studies suggest that an increase in androgens is only associated with higher risk of low-grade serous and mucinous ovarian cancers [35, 42].

Third, physical activity also has well-documented anti-inflammatory effects, and chronic inflammation has been suggested as an important carcinogenic pathway for ovarian cancer. Systemic inflammation, as measure by circulating levels of C-reactive protein (CRP), has been consistently associated with increased ovarian cancer risk [43–46]. Inflammatory cytokines, such as interleukin (IL)-6 and tumor necrosis factor (TNF)-α, are significantly elevated in ovarian tumors [47–49], and may predict prognosis and survival in ovarian cancer patients [50, 51]. Finally, participation in regular physical activity improves insulin sensitivity, and prevents or delays development of hyperinsulinemia and insulin resistance [52, 53]. Insulin resistance and type 2 diabetes have been associated with an increased risk of ovarian cancer in some, but not all, studies [54–57]. Other biomarkers involved in the insulin-related pathways and insulin-like growth factor (IGF) axis, such as IGF-1 and IGF-1 receptor, has been shown experimentally to stimulate the proliferation and inhibit apoptosis of ovarian carcinoma cells [58, 59]. While some studies reported a significant positive association between IGF-1 and ovarian cancer risk [60, 61], other studies found no compelling evidence for this association [62–65], including a recent meta-analysis [66].

There are additional exercise-induced mechanisms that have been proposed with specific relevance to ovarian cancer development. According to the 'incessant ovulation' hypothesis [67, 68], the accumulation of deleterious mutations from the ovulation-induced wounds on the ovarian surface can lead to neoplasia and ovarian tumors [68–70]. Factors that result in fewer ovulations, such as higher parity and longer use of oral contraceptive use, have been consistently associated with lower risk of ovarian cancer [10]. Physical activity, particularly at very vigorous and strenuous levels, may affect menstrual cycle length and decrease frequency of ovulation [71–73]. Thus, another mechanistic hypothesis for the exercise-related pathogenesis of ovarian cancer is that regular strenuous physical activity may reduce the risk of ovarian cancer through suppression of ovulation, although this mechanism only applies to premenopausal women. Further, physically active women are at lower risk of a number of common benign gynecologic conditions, including endometriosis [74–76]. Prior studies have identified endometriosis as a risk factor for ovarian cancer, with consistent findings of increased risks for endometrioid and clear cell ovarian cancer tumors [11, 77, 78].

Epidemiologic Evidence on Physical Activity and Ovarian Cancer Risk

Despite intriguing biological hypotheses indicating a plausible inverse association between physical activity and ovarian cancer, more than 20 population-based epidemiologic studies conducted over the last two decades have yielded mixed results. Early evidence regarding the association between physical activity and ovarian cancer risk was mostly from case-control studies. Most [79–86], but not all case-control studies [87–92], observed a statistically significant inverse association. Findings from a meta-analysis of nine case-control studies suggested 13% (95% CI: −5, −20) lower risk of ovarian cancer for moderate levels of non-occupational physical activity and 17% (95% CI: −9, −24) reduced risk for high levels, with no evidence of significant heterogeneity across studies (P-heterogeneity >0.17) [93]. A recent pooled analysis of nine population-based case-control studies from the Ovarian Cancer Association Consortium, including 8309 epithelial ovarian cancer cases, reported that chronic recreational physical inactivity was associated with 35% higher odds of ovarian cancer (95% CI: 1.14, 1.57) compared to women who were physically active at any level; the positive association between chronic physical inactivity and ovarian cancer risk was similar for different histologic subtypes [94].

However, these case-control studies were predominantly performed among white women residing in the North America or Europe. This limits the generalizability of the findings to other racial/ethnic populations or women living in other regions. For example, to our knowledge, there has been only one case-control study conducted in African American women, which reported mixed results [92]. While suggestively reduced ovarian cancer risk was observed for mild and strenuous physical activity, there was a significantly increased risk for moderate physical activity among African American women. Many studies utilized a sample of convenient controls, such as hospital controls, to represent the underlying study populations, which may further decrease the generalizability. Most importantly, as a result of the case-control design, physical activity was assessed in cases after diagnoses of ovarian cancer and in their matched controls. Self-reported physical activity may be biased due to differential recall, as women diagnosed with ovarian cancer may blame the disease for lack of regular physical activity and thus under-reported their usual physical activity levels. By contrast, control women, particularly healthy controls, may tend to over-report their physical activity levels [95, 96]. This could lead to a spurious inverse association between physical activity and ovarian cancer risk. Further, women were typically asked about participation in physical activity during the past 6 months or the past year. Preclinical disease symptoms for ovarian cancer during these time periods, such as pelvic pain, abdominal bloating and fatigue, may have compromised the ability to exercise and influenced the regular physical activity levels in cases. Therefore, inverse associations observed in case-control studies may be the consequence of reverse causation, and do not necessarily reflect the role of physical activity in ovarian carcinogenesis. In light of these limitations for case-control studies, our review will focus on studies of prospective design, which are less susceptible to such methodologic issues.

To date, a total of 14 studies [97–110], based on 11 independent cohorts, have been published to prospectively examine the association between physical activity and ovarian cancer risk (Table 13.1). While findings from case-control studies appear to support an inverse association between physical activity and ovarian cancer risk, prospective studies generally do not support a beneficial effect of physical activity on ovarian cancer. The first prospective study from well-established, large-scale cohorts is based on the Iowa Women's Health Study. Mink et al. examined the association between physical activity and ovarian cancer risk among 31,396 postmenopausal women aged 55–69 at baseline [97]. With 97 incident ovarian cancer cases during 7 years of follow-up, a significant positive trend was observed between a composite physical activity index (based on frequency and intensity) and ovarian cancer risk. Compared to a low physical activity index, the RRs (95% CIs) were 1.44 (0.86, 2.40) for moderate activity and 1.97 (1.22, 3.19) for high activity (p-trend = 0.006). The positive association was particularly strong among women participating in vigorous physical activity (RR comparing >4 times/week vs. rarely/ never: 2.52; 95% CI: 1.01, 6.28). A later investigation in this cohort with additional 8 years of follow-up and a total of 223 ovarian cancers reached essentially the same conclusion that high levels of physical activity, particularly vigorous physical activity, may increase ovarian cancer risk in postmenopausal women [99].

In the Nurses' Health Study, Bertone et al. followed 92,825 women from 1980 through 1996 and identified 377 ovarian cancer cases during follow-up [98]. Interestingly, a modest increase in ovarian cancer risk with higher physical activity was also noted in the study. This study used the metabolic equivalent task (MET) hours [111] as a composite measure to more accurately assess both duration and intensity of physical activity, which was calculated by assigning the MET scores to various types of physical activity to reflect their energy expenditure, multiplying each score with duration spent in the corresponding activity type, and summing the products over all activity types. Activities with a MET score ≥ 6 are usually considered to be vigorous; a physical activity level at 28 MET-hours/week is equivalent to an average of 1 h of brisk walking per day. Compared to inactive women (<2.5 MET-hours/week), those who had physical activity 20–30 MET-hours/week were at higher risk ovarian cancer (RR: 1.84; 95% CI: 1.12, 3.02). However, no significant risk increase was observed for ≥ 30 MET-hours/week, and overall there was no significant positive trend across categories of physical activity measured by MET-hours/week. Also, no association was observed when physical activity was measured only by frequency (e.g., times/week), suggesting that activity intensity, namely vigorous activity, may contribute to the observed increased risk.

Recently, we updated the investigation in the Nurses' Health Study and added the Nurses' Health Study II, an independent sister cohort, including a total of 815 incident ovarian cancer cases over 24 years of follow-up [109]. In addition to a similar but more modest elevation in ovarian cancer risk with high levels of physical activity as reported in the previous study [98], we also observed a slightly increased risk for very low levels of physical activity. Compared to 3–9 MET-hours/week, the RRs (95% CI) were 1.19 (0.94, 1.52) for <3 MET-hours/week and 1.26 (1.02, 1.55) for ≥ 27 MET-hours/week. Importantly, we leveraged the wide age distribution and long follow-up in the two cohorts to prospectively assess the impact of physical

Table 13.1 Selected characteristics of prospective studies on physical activity and ovarian cancer risk

First author, year, region,	Study population	Sample size (case/total)	Age (years)	Follow-up (years)	Physical activity assessment	Comparison and relative risks (95% CIs)	Direction of the association
Anderson et al., US [99]	Iowa Women's health study	223/41,835	55–69	15	Frequency (times/week) and intensity (moderate, vigorous)	For total activity,high vs. low level:1.42 (1.03, 1.97) for vigorous activity, >4 times/week vs. rarely/never:2.38 (1.29, 4.38)	Positive
Bertone et al., US [98]	Nurses' health study	377/92,825	30–55	16	Duration (hours/week) and type (running, jogging, tennis, etc.)	For total activity,20–30 vs. 0–2.5 MET-hours/week:1.84 (1.12, 3.02) >30 vs. 0–2.5 MET-hours/week:1.27 (0.75, 2.14)	Suggestively positive
Biesma et al., Netherland [102]	Netherlands cohort study on diet and cancer	252/62,573	55–69	11.3	Duration (hours/week) and type (biking/walking, gardening, etc.)	For total activity, >90 vs. <30 min/day:0.72 (0.48, 1.06)for biking/walking, >2 h/week vs. never:0.65 (0.41, 1.01)	Suggestively inverse

(continued)

Table 13.1 (continued)

First author, year, region	Study population	Sample size (case/total)	Age (years)	Follow-up (years)	Physical activity assessment	Comparison and relative risks (95% CIs)	Direction of the association
Chionh et al., Australia [112]	Melbourne collaborative cohort study	113/18,700	26–76	10.2	Frequency (times/week) and intensity (vigorous, less vigorous, walking)	For total activity,high vs. none:2.21 (1.16, 4.24)for less vigorous activity,≥3 times/week vs. none:1.62 (1.01, 2.61)for walking,≥3 times/week vs. none:1.62 (1.04, 2.52)	Positive
Hannan et al., US [100]	Breast cancer detectiondemonstration project follow-up cohort	121/27,365	61	8.3	Duration (hours/day) and intensity (sleep, light, moderate, vigorous)	For total activity in quintiles,Q2 vs. Q1: 0.73 (0.43, 1.25)Q3 vs. Q1: 0.84 (0.50, 1.41)Q4 vs. Q1: 0.56 (0.31, 1.01)Q5 vs. Q1: 0.71 (0.41, 1.22)	Suggestively inverse
Hildebrand et al., US [108]	Americancancer Society cancer prevention study II nutrition cohort	651/63,972	50–74	19	Duration (hours/week) and type (running, jogging, swimming, biking, etc.)	For total activity,≥17.5 MET-hours/week vs. none:0.95 (0.70, 1.29)for walking only,≥7 h/week vs. none:1.10 (0.72, 1.68)	Null

First author, year, region	Study population	Sample size (case/total)	Age (years)	Follow-up (years)	Physical activity assessment	Comparison and relative risks (95% CIs)	Direction of the association
Huang et al., US [109]	Nurses' health study and Nurses' health study II	601/85,462 and 214/112,679	30–55 and 25–42	24	Duration (hours/week) and type (running, jogging, tennis, etc.)	For total activity, <3 vs. 3–9 MET-hours/week (pooled):1.19 (0.94, 1.52)≥27 vs. 3–9 MET-hours/week (pooled):1.26 (1.02, 1.55) for premenopausal activity, <3 vs. 3–9 MET-hours/week (pooled):1.29 (0.95, 1.75)≥27 vs. 3–9 MET-hours/week (pooled):1.50 (1.13, 1.97)	Suggestively U-shaped
Lahmann et al., 10 European countries [110]	Europeanprospective investigation into cancer and nutrition	731/274,470	51.5	9.3	Duration and setting (recreational, household, and occupational)	For total activity,active vs. inactive:1.32 (0.93, 1.88) for recreational and household activity combined,>123 vs. <51 MET-hours/week:1.26 (0.99, 1.61)	Suggestively positive

(continued)

Table 13.1 (continued)

First author, year, region,	Study population	Sample size (case/ total)	Age (years)	Follow-up (years)	Physical activity assessment	Comparison and relative risks (95% CIs)	Direction of the association
Leitzmann et al. US [106]	NIH-AARP diet and health study	309/96,216	51–72	7	Duration and intensity (moderate, vigorous)	Moderate only vs. no activity:0.93 (0.66, 1.29) vigorous only vs. no activity:1.06 (0.74, 1.52) both vs. no activity:1.10 (0.82–1.48)	Null
Mink et al., US [97]	Iowa women's health study	97/31,396	55–69	7	Frequency (times/ week) and intensity (moderate, vigorous)	For total activity,moderate vs. low level:1.44 (0.86, 2.40)high vs. low level:1.97 (1.22, 3.19)	Positive
Patel et al., US [103]	Americancancer Society cancer prevention study II nutrition cohort	314/59,695	50–74	9	Duration (hours/ week) and type (running, jogging, swimming, biking, etc.)	For recreational activity, $\geq$ 31.5 MET-hours/week vs. none:0.73 (0.40, 1.34)for nonrecreational activity,$\geq$18.5 vs. 0–5 MET-hours/week:1.07 (0.79, 1.46)for recalled activity at age 40,$\geq$31.5 MET-hours/week vs. none:1.09 (0.68, 1.74)	Null

First author, year, region,	Study population	Sample size (case/total)	Age (years)	Follow-up (years)	Physical activity assessment	Comparison and relative risks (95% CIs)	Direction of the association
Schnohr et al., Denmark [101]	Copenhagen Centre for Prospective population studies	107/13,216	20–91	14	Cross-classification of duration and intensity in four categories	For recreational activity,moderate vs. low activity:0.72 (0.46, 1.13) vigorous vs. low activity:0.33 (0.16, 0.67)	Inverse
Weiderpass et al., Norway and Sweden [105]	Women's lifestyle and health study	264/96,541	30–49	11.1	A Likert scale of physical activity level at age 14, 30 and baseline	For activity at age 14,none vs. moderate:0.57 (0.21, 1.54)vigorous vs. moderate:0.99 (0.68, 1.42) for activity at age 30,none vs. moderate:0.76 (0.28, 2.07)high vs. none:1.10 (0.80, 1.50)for activity at baseline,none vs. moderate:0.96 (0.54, 1.71) vigorous vs. none:1.03 (0.64, 1.66)	Null

(continued)

Table 13.1 (continued)

First author, year, region,	Study population	Sample size (case/total)	Age (years)	Follow-up (years)	Physical activity assessment	Comparison and relative risks (95% CIs)	Direction of the association
Xiao et al., US [107]	NIH-AARP diet and health study	753/148,892	50–71	10	Frequency, duration and intensity of physical activity during different time periods	For baseline activity, 5+ vs. never/rarely: 1.04 (0.83, 1.30)for activity in the past 10 year, 7+ hours/week vs. never/rarely:0.84 (0.61, 1.14)for activity at age 35–39, 7+ hours/week vs. never/rarely:1.02 (0.71, 1.47)for activity at age 19–29, 7+ hours/week vs. never/rarely:0.95 (0.67, 1.35)for activity at age 15–18, 7+ hours/week vs. never/rarely:1.02 (0.76, 1.39)	Null

activity during different periods of life on ovarian cancer risk. We found that only physical activity during premenopausal years was associated with ovarian cancer risk; postmenopausal activity was not independently associated with the risk. Compared to premenopausal activity level at 3–9 MET-hours/week, the RRs (95% CI) were 1.29 (0.95, 1.75) for <3 MET-hours/week of premenopausal activity and 1.50 (1.13, 1.97) for ≥27 MET-hours/week of premenopausal activity. The corresponding risk estimates for postmenopausal activity were 1.05 (0.79, 1.40) and 1.03 (0.80, 1.33), respectively. Further analyses by histology suggested that high premenopausal activity was associated with increased risk of both serous and endometrioid tumors whereas low premenopausal activity was only strongly associated with endometrioid subtype. However, we observed no difference in the associations by intensity of physical activity, as observed in prior studies [97–99].

Neither moderate nor vigorous physical activity was associated with ovarian cancer in the NIH-AARP Diet and Health Study of 96,216 women aged 51–72 at baseline [106], although there was a suggestion of increased risk for serious subtype (RR comparing moderate/vigorous activity vs. neither: 1.42; 95% CI: 0.93, 2.17). Another study in this cohort examined physical activity during different periods of life in relation to ovarian cancer risk, and reported that recalled physical activity levels at age 15–18, age 19–29, age 35–39, or during the past 10 years were not associated with ovarian cancer risk [107]. Similarly, neither the original study [103] nor the updated study [108] in the American Cancer Society Cancer Prevention Study II Nutrition Cohort found compelling evidence for an association between physical activity and ovarian cancer.

Other population-based, prospective studies that have examined physical activity and ovarian cancer risk include the Netherlands Cohort Study on Diet and Cancer [102], Melbourne Collaborative Cohort Study [112], Breast Cancer Detection Demonstration Project follow-up cohort [100], European Prospective Investigation into Cancer and Nutrition [110], Copenhagen Centre for Prospective Population Studies [101] and Women's Lifestyle and Health Study [105]. Besides the Copenhagen Centre for Prospective Population Studies [101], which reported a strong inverse association between physical activity and ovarian cancer, findings from Netherlands Cohort Study on Diet and Cancer [102] and Breast Cancer Detection Demonstration Project follow-up cohort [100] also suggest a slightly reduced ovarian cancer risk for higher physical activity. Other studies, however, either reported no association or suggested a trend towards a positive association (Table 13.1).

In sharp contrast to case-control studies, prospective studies provide little support for the hypothetical benefits of physical activity on ovarian cancer. As expected, meta-analyses of nine of these prospective cohort studies result in a RR (95% CI) of 1.03 (0.87, 1.20) for any moderate-to-vigorous physical activity, 0.99 (0.86, 1.13) for moderate activity and 0.97 (0.74, 1.28) for vigorous activity, compared to low physical activity [93]. Significant between-study heterogeneity in the association was observed among these prospective cohorts (P-heterogeneity <0.05). There was even greater heterogeneity when estimates from case-control studies were considered simultaneously (P-heterogeneity <0.01). These statistics reflect the substantial inconsistency of the existing literature, a trend towards inverse associations in case-control studies but a trend towards positive or null associations in prospective studies.

The mechanisms underlying a potential positive association between physical activity and ovarian cancer remain unclear. This observation contradicts the prior biologic hypotheses described above. In the Nurses' Health Studies, we observed that increased ovarian cancer risk differed by menopausal status and was more strongly associated with premenopausal physical activity. We postulated that the increased risk may be explained by exercise-induced influence on reproductive function and ovulation that only occur during premenopausal period. Interestingly, a population-based case-control study in Canada reported a similar finding that physical activity in mid-teens and early 30s was positively associated with ovarian cancer risk but that physical activity during the last 2 years prior to diagnosis was inversely associated with ovarian cancer risk [91]. Another cohort study, however, did not find any association of physical activity in different periods of life with ovarian cancer risk [107]. The possibility that physical activity may interact with reproductive function to impact ovarian cancer risk is further enhanced by the fact that evidence linking other potential pathways (e.g., sex hormones, adiposity, IGF axis) with ovarian cancer development has been inconsistent, as reviewed above. By contrast, reproductive factors, particularly those related to frequency of ovulation (e.g., parity, oral contraceptive use), have been well established for ovarian cancer.

Indeed, the hypothesis that physical activity may reduce ovarian cancer risk through inhibition of ovulation is primarily based on studies among elite athletes or long-distance recreational runners, who had much more strenuous activity than the 'vigorous' activity in the general population [71–73, 113, 114]. Initiation of new exercise regimes, such as recreational running, did not appear to disturb menstrual cycle or ovulation in ordinary women [115, 116]. Further, it has been suggested that strenuous physical activity may induce reproductive dysfunction only if energy intake after exercise is limited (i.e., insufficient net influx of energy), as observed among agrarian female labors in the developing regions [117, 118]. Such interactions between physical activity and nutrition on ovarian function are also supported by experimental studies in monkeys [119, 120]. Given that energy surfeit is a worldwide phenomenon, particularly in the US and European countries, the very moderate activity level in the general population is unlikely to lead to suppression of ovulation. On the other hand, a prospective study in the Nurses' Health Study II has reported that higher level of vigorous physical activity was associated with lower risk of ovulatory disorder infertility, suggesting enhanced ovulation in the active women [121]. We have also shown that physical activity was positively associated with luteal progesterone level, an indicator for successful ovulation; the positive association between premenopausal activity and ovarian cancer risk was stronger in women who never used oral contraceptives, among whom the potential moderate ovulation-stimulating effects by physical activity may be more likely to be observed [109]. Collectively, the moderate positive association between physical activity and ovarian cancer risk observed in several large prospective studies may be mediated by more frequent ovulation facilitated by the physical activity levels typical in the general population. Additional studies are required to confirm these associations and elucidate the underlying biologic mechanisms.

Epidemiologic Evidence on Physical Activity and Ovarian Cancer Prognosis

While a large body of evidence suggests that both pre-diagnosis and post-diagnosis physical activity may improve survival among breast cancer and colorectal cancer patients [122–124], only two studies have evaluated the impact of pre-diagnosis physical activity on ovarian cancer survival [125, 126]. The study in the Ovarian Cancer Association Consortium, including 6806 invasive ovarian cancer cases, found that mortality was 34% (95% CI: 18, 52) higher in physically inactive women [125]. Similarly, participation in vigorous physical activity was associated with significantly lower risk of both cause-specific and all-cause mortality among 600 women diagnosed with ovarian cancer from the Women's Health Initiative [126]. Currently, an ongoing randomized controlled trial (Registration number: NCT00719303 at ClinicalTrials.gov) is being conducted to investigate whether a counseling program to change diet and physical activity vs. usual care may increase progression-free survival among women with previously treated stage II-IV ovarian cancer. Preliminary results from this trial suggest that ovarian cancer survivors were motivated to engage in physical activity at recommended levels, which improved health-related quality of life in a 6-month period [127]. Extended follow-up is needed to understand the longer-term prognostic outcomes associated with increased physical activity.

Sedentary Behavior and Ovarian Cancer Risk

As discussed above, higher systemic inflammation, such as increased circulating levels of CRP levels, have consistently been associated with increased risk of ovarian cancer [43–46]. Thus, modifying lifestyle exposures associated with higher levels of systemic inflammation markers may alter risk. While physical activity has been associated with lower inflammation, sedentary behavior, generally defined as time spent sitting (e.g., watching television), has been associated with increasing low grade inflammation [128–130], and those with both high physical activity and low sedentary behavior have the lowest CRP levels [130]. Despite this, the impact of sedentary behavior on ovarian cancer risk has received relatively little study, with reported data from three studies conducted within two prospective cohorts [103, 107, 108]. Non-occupational sitting time of ≥ 6 vs. <3 h per day was positively associated with 44% increased risk (95% CI: 12, 85) in the American Cancer Society Cancer Prevention Study II Nutrition Cohort, with over 650 ovarian cancer cases [108]. This association was stronger for serous cases (HR = 1.55), although there was not significant heterogeneity in the association. However, in the other cohort study, neither total sitting nor television watching at baseline were associated with risk [107]. In one case-control study, total sitting and hours watching television 5 years before diagnosis were associated with increased risk [131]. Among ovarian cancer patients, high sedentary behavior was associated with reduced quality of life in multiple domains, including physical, social, and sexual functioning [132]; however no studies have examined survival outcomes. Additional prospective studies in this area are warranted to evaluate the potential interactions between physical activity and sedentary behavior in ovarian carcinogenesis.

Limitations, Future Direction and Conclusion

Overall, the relationship between physical activity and sedentary behavior with ovarian cancer risk is not clear. Of particular note is that different study designs (i.e., case-control vs. prospective) have shown varying associations, suggesting that bias may be a challenge in interpreting the results. Given the reduced bias in prospective studies, increased weight should be given to these studies, especially those that carefully controlled for potential confounding factors such as adiposity. In general, these studies have observed either null or positive associations between physical activity and ovarian cancer risk, contrary to the putative biologic mechanisms that would suggest that activity should be associated with a lower risk as for other cancers. A key limitation for interpreting these studies is that each study asked about and characterized physical activity in a different manner, reducing ability to compare results across studies. Cross-cohort harmonization in the consortial setting is crucial to increasing sample size for assessment of activity relationships to cancer. A recent working group in the National Cancer Institute Cohort Consortium harmonized physical activity data from 12 prospective studies and evaluated associations with ovarian cancer (among others) with nearly 2300 cases. The overall association for ovarian cancer was null (HR, >90th vs. <10th percentile = 1.06, 95% CI: 0.93, 1.20), although there was a suggestive increased risk for never smokers (p-heterogeneity = 0.06) [133]. Future research should integrate more prospective studies to further increase sample size, allowing for in depth analysis by tumor histologic subtype and timing of activity (e.g., premenopausal vs. postmenopausal). Further, it will be crucial to better understand the relationship between physical activity and ovulation in premenopausal women who are not using oral contraceptives. Finally, additional work is needed to better evaluate the role of sedentary behavior, with an emphasis on the intersection with physical activity, on risk and the association of activity and sedentariness with survival among patients.

References

1. Lee IM, et al. Effect of physical inactivity on major non-communicable diseases worldwide: an analysis of burden of disease and life expectancy. Lancet. 2012;380(9838):219–29.
2. WHO (2016) Global strategy on diet, physical activity and health. http://www.who.int/dietphysicalactivity/factsheet_adults/en/.
3. Keum N, et al. Leisure-time physical activity and endometrial cancer risk: dose-response meta-analysis of epidemiological studies. Int J Cancer. 2014;135(3):682–94.
4. Schmid D, et al. A systematic review and meta-analysis of physical activity and endometrial cancer risk. Eur J Epidemiol. 2015;30(5):397–412.

5. National Cancer Institute (2009) Physical activity and cancer. https://www.cancer.gov/about-cancer/causes-prevention/risk/obesity/physical-activity-fact-sheet.
6. Torre LA, et al. Global cancer statistics, 2012. CA Cancer J Clin. 2015;65(2):87–108.
7. American Cancer Society. Cancer facts and figures 2013. Atlanta: American Cancer Society; 2013.
8. Buys SS, et al. Effect of screening on ovarian cancer mortality: the prostate, lung, colorectal and ovarian (PLCO) cancer screening randomized controlled trial. JAMA. 2011;305(22):2295–303.
9. Jacobs IJ, et al. Ovarian cancer screening and mortality in the UK collaborative trial of ovarian cancer screening (UKCTOCS): a randomised controlled trial. Lancet. 2016;387(10022):945–56.
10. Permuth-Wey J, Sellers TA. Epidemiology of ovarian cancer. Methods Mol Biol. 2009;472:413–37.
11. Wentzensen N, et al. Ovarian cancer risk factors by histologic subtype: an analysis from the ovarian cancer cohort Consortium. J Clin Oncol. 2016;34(24):2888–98.
12. Merritt MA, et al. Reproductive characteristics in relation to ovarian cancer risk by histologic pathways. Hum Reprod. 2013;28(5):1406–17.
13. Risch HA, et al. Differences in risk factors for epithelial ovarian cancer by histologic type. Results of a case-control study. Am J Epidemiol. 1996;144(4):363–72.
14. Lee IM, et al. Physical activity and weight gain prevention. JAMA. 2010;303(12):1173–9.
15. Mozaffarian D, et al. Changes in diet and lifestyle and long-term weight gain in women and men. N Engl J Med. 2011;364(25):2392–404.
16. Tian Y, et al. BMI, leisure-time physical activity, and physical fitness in adults in China: results from a series of national surveys, 2000-14. Lancet Diabetes Endocrinol. 2016;4(6):487–97.
17. Calle EE, Kaaks R. Overweight, obesity and cancer: epidemiological evidence and proposed mechanisms. Nat Rev Cancer. 2004;4(8):579–91.
18. Renehan AG, Zwahlen M, Egger M. Adiposity and cancer risk: new mechanistic insights from epidemiology. Nat Rev Cancer. 2015;15(8):484 98.
19. McTiernan A. Mechanisms linking physical activity with cancer. Nat Rev Cancer. 2008;8(3):205–11.
20. Nieman DC, Pedersen BK. Exercise and immune function. Recent developments. Sports Med. 1999;27(2):73–80.
21. Pedersen BK, Ullum H. NK cell response to physical activity: possible mechanisms of action. Med Sci Sports Exerc. 1994;26(2):140–6.
22. Shephard RJ, Shek PN. Effects of exercise and training on natural killer cell counts and cytolytic activity: a meta-analysis. Sports Med. 1999;28(3):177–95.
23. Jakobisiak M, Lasek W, Golab J. Natural mechanisms protecting against cancer. Immunol Lett. 2003;90(2–3):103–22.
24. Tworoger SS, Huang T. Obesity and ovarian cancer. Recent Results Cancer Res. 2016;208:155–76.
25. McTiernan A, et al. Relation of BMI and physical activity to sex hormones in postmenopausal women. Obesity (Silver Spring). 2006;14(9):1662–77.
26. McTiernan A, et al. Effect of exercise on serum estrogens in postmenopausal women: a 12-month randomized clinical trial. Cancer Res. 2004;64(8):2923–8.
27. Chan MF, et al. Usual physical activity and endogenous sex hormones in postmenopausal women: the European prospective investigation into cancer-norfolk population study. Cancer Epidemiol Biomark Prev. 2007;16(5):900–5.
28. Verkasalo PK, et al. Circulating levels of sex hormones and their relation to risk factors for breast cancer: a cross-sectional study in 1092 pre- and postmenopausal women (United Kingdom). Cancer Causes Control. 2001;12(1):47–59.
29. Ennour-Idrissi K, Maunsell E, Diorio C. Effect of physical activity on sex hormones in women: a systematic review and meta-analysis of randomized controlled trials. Breast Cancer Res. 2015;17(1):139.

30. Cunat S, Hoffmann P, Pujol P. Estrogens and epithelial ovarian cancer. Gynecol Oncol. 2004;94(1):25–32.
31. Lacey JV Jr, et al. Menopausal hormone replacement therapy and risk of ovarian cancer. JAMA. 2002;288(3):334–41.
32. Beral V, et al. Ovarian cancer and hormone replacement therapy in the Million Women study. Lancet. 2007;369(9574):1703–10.
33. Beral V, et al. Menopausal hormone use and ovarian cancer risk: individual participant meta-analysis of 52 epidemiological studies. Lancet. 2015;385(9980):1835–42.
34. Helzlsouer KJ, et al. Serum gonadotropins and steroid hormones and the development of ovarian cancer. JAMA. 1995;274(24):1926–30.
35. Schock H, et al. Early pregnancy sex steroids and maternal risk of epithelial ovarian cancer. Endocr Relat Cancer. 2014;21(6):831–44.
36. Lukanova A, et al. Circulating levels of sex steroid hormones and risk of ovarian cancer. Int J Cancer. 2003;104(5):636–42.
37. Hecht JL, et al. Relationship between epidemiologic risk factors and hormone receptor expression in ovarian cancer: results from the Nurses' Health study. Cancer Epidemiol Biomark Prev. 2009;18(5):1624–30.
38. Barry JA, Azizia MM, Hardiman PJ. Risk of endometrial, ovarian and breast cancer in women with polycystic ovary syndrome: a systematic review and meta-analysis. Hum Reprod Update. 2014;20(5):748–58.
39. Rinaldi S, et al. Endogenous androgens and risk of epithelial ovarian cancer: results from the European prospective investigation into cancer and nutrition (EPIC). Cancer Epidemiol Biomark Prev. 2007;16(1):23–9.
40. Tworoger SS, et al. Plasma androgen concentrations and risk of incident ovarian cancer. Am J Epidemiol. 2008;167(2):211–8.
41. Olsen CM, et al. Epithelial ovarian cancer: testing the 'androgens hypothesis'. Endocr Relat Cancer. 2008;15(4):1061–8.
42. Ose J, et al. Endogenous androgens and risk of epithelial invasive ovarian cancer by tumor characteristics in the European prospective investigation into cancer and nutrition. Int J Cancer. 2015;136(2):399–410.
43. McSorley MA, et al. C-reactive protein concentrations and subsequent ovarian cancer risk. Obstet Gynecol. 2007;109(4):933–41.
44. Ose J, et al. Inflammatory markers and risk of epithelial ovarian cancer by tumor subtypes: the EPIC cohort. Cancer Epidemiol Biomarkers Prev. 2015;24(6):951–61.
45. Poole EM, et al. A prospective study of circulating C-reactive protein, interleukin-6, and tumor necrosis factor alpha receptor 2 levels and risk of ovarian cancer. Am J Epidemiol. 2013;178(8):1256–64.
46. Zeng F, et al. Inflammatory markers of CRP, IL6, TNFalpha, and soluble TNFR2 and the risk of ovarian cancer: a meta-analysis of prospective studies. Cancer Epidemiol Biomark Prev. 2016;25(8):1231–9.
47. Maccio A, et al. High serum levels of soluble IL-2 receptor, cytokines, and C reactive protein correlate with impairment of T cell response in patients with advanced epithelial ovarian cancer. Gynecol Oncol. 1998;69(3):248–52.
48. Maccio A, Madeddu C. Inflammation and ovarian cancer. Cytokine. 2012;58(2):133–47.
49. Rzymski P, et al. Serum tumor necrosis factor alpha receptors p55/p75 ratio and ovarian cancer detection. Int J Gynaecol Obstet. 2005;88(3):292–8.
50. Lane D, et al. Prognostic significance of IL-6 and IL-8 ascites levels in ovarian cancer patients. BMC Cancer. 2011;11:210.
51. Lo CW, et al. IL-6 trans-signaling in formation and progression of malignant ascites in ovarian cancer. Cancer Res. 2011;71(2):424–34.
52. Mayer-Davis EJ, et al. Intensity and amount of physical activity in relation to insulin sensitivity: the insulin resistance atherosclerosis study. JAMA. 1998;279(9):669–74.

53. Assah FK, et al. The association of intensity and overall level of physical activity energy expenditure with a marker of insulin resistance. Diabetologia. 2008;51(8):1399–407.
54. Adler AI, et al. Is diabetes mellitus a risk factor for ovarian cancer? A case-control study in Utah and Washington (United States). Cancer Causes Control. 1996;7(4):475–8.
55. Inoue M, et al. Diabetes mellitus and the risk of cancer: results from a large-scale population-based cohort study in Japan. Arch Intern Med. 2006;166(17):1871–7.
56. Gapstur SM, et al. Type II diabetes mellitus and the incidence of epithelial ovarian cancer in the cancer prevention study-II nutrition cohort. Cancer Epidemiol Biomark Prev. 2012;21(11):2000–5.
57. Swerdlow AJ, et al. Cancer incidence and mortality in patients with insulin-treated diabetes: a UK cohort study. Br J Cancer. 2005;92(11):2070–5.
58. Resnicoff M, et al. Insulin-like growth factor-1 and its receptor mediate the autocrine proliferation of human ovarian carcinoma cell lines. Lab Investig. 1993;69(6):756–60.
59. Ji QS, et al. A novel, potent, and selective insulin-like growth factor-I receptor kinase inhibitor blocks insulin-like growth factor-I receptor signaling in vitro and inhibits insulin-like growth factor-I receptor dependent tumor growth in vivo. Mol Cancer Ther. 2007;6(8):2158–67.
60. Lukanova A, et al. Circulating levels of insulin-like growth factor-I and risk of ovarian cancer. Int J Cancer. 2002;101(6):549–54.
61. Peeters PH, et al. Serum IGF-I, its major binding protein (IGFBP-3) and epithelial ovarian cancer risk: the European prospective investigation into cancer and nutrition (EPIC). Endocr Relat Cancer. 2007;14(1):81–90.
62. Tworoger SS, et al. Insulin-like growth factors and ovarian cancer risk: a nested case-control study in three cohorts. Cancer Epidemiol Biomark Prev. 2007;16(8):1691–5.
63. Schock H, et al. Early pregnancy IGF-I and placental GH and risk of epithelial ovarian cancer: a nested case-control study. Int J Cancer. 2015;137(2):439–47.
64. Ose J, et al. Insulin-like growth factor I and risk of epithelial invasive ovarian cancer by tumour characteristics: results from the EPIC cohort. Br J Cancer. 2015;112(1):162–6.
65. Dal Maso L, et al. Association between components of the insulin-like growth factor system and epithelial ovarian cancer risk. Oncology. 2004;67(3–4):225–30.
66. Wang Q, et al. Association of circulating insulin-like growth factor 1 and insulin-like growth factor binding protein 3 with the risk of ovarian cancer: a systematic review and meta-analysis. Mol Clin Oncol. 2015;3(3):623–8.
67. Casagrande J, et al. "Incessant ovulation" and ovarian cancer. Lancet. 1979;314(8135):170–3.
68. Tung K-H, et al. Effect of anovulation factors on pre-and postmenopausal ovarian cancer risk: revisiting the incessant ovulation hypothesis. Am J Epidemiol. 2005;161(4):321–9.
69. Risch HA. Hormonal etiology of epithelial ovarian cancer, with a hypothesis concerning the role of androgens and progesterone. J Natl Cancer Inst. 1998;90(23):1774–86.
70. Ghahremani M, Foghi A, Dorrington JH. Etiology of ovarian cancer: a proposed mechanism. Med Hypotheses. 1999;52(1):23–6.
71. Bullen BA, et al. Induction of menstrual disorders by strenuous exercise in untrained women. N Engl J Med. 1985;312(21):1349–53.
72. Russell JB, et al. The relationship of exercise to anovulatory cycles in female athletes: hormonal and physical characteristics. Obstet Gynecol. 1984;63(4):452–6.
73. Shangold M, et al. The relationship between long-distance running, plasma progesterone, and luteal phase length. Fertil Steril. 1979;31(2):130–3.
74. Cramer DW, et al. The relation of endometriosis to menstrual characteristics, smoking, and exercise. JAMA. 1986;255(14):1904–8.
75. Dhillon PK, Holt VL. Recreational physical activity and endometrioma risk. Am J Epidemiol. 2003;158(2):156–64.
76. Vitonis AF, et al. Adult physical activity and endometriosis risk. Epidemiology. 2010;21(1):16–23.
77. Pearce CL, et al. Association between endometriosis and risk of histological subtypes of ovarian cancer: a pooled analysis of case-control studies. Lancet Oncol. 2012;13(4):385–94.

78. Mogensen JB, et al. Endometriosis and risks for ovarian, endometrial and breast cancers: a nationwide cohort study. Gynecol Oncol. 2016;143(1):87–92.
79. Cottreau CM, Ness RB, Kriska AM. Physical activity and reduced risk of ovarian cancer. Obstet Gynecol. 2000;96(4):609–14.
80. Freedman DM, Dosemeci M, McGlynn K. Sunlight and mortality from breast, ovarian, colon, prostate, and non-melanoma skin cancer: a composite death certificate based case-control study. Occup Environ Med. 2002;59(4):257–62.
81. Olsen CM, et al. Recreational physical activity and epithelial ovarian cancer: a case-control study, systematic review, and meta-analysis. Cancer Epidemiol Biomark Prev. 2007;16(11):2321–30.
82. Pan SY, Ugnat AM, Mao Y. Physical activity and the risk of ovarian cancer: a case-control study in Canada. Int J Cancer. 2005;117(2):300–7.
83. Riman T, et al. Some life-style factors and the risk of invasive epithelial ovarian cancer in Swedish women. Eur J Epidemiol. 2004;19(11):1011–9.
84. Tavani A, et al. Physical activity and risk of ovarian cancer: an Italian case-control study. Int J Cancer. 2001;91(3):407–11.
85. Zhang M, Lee AH, Binns CW. Physical activity and epithelial ovarian cancer risk: a case-control study in China. Int J Cancer. 2003;105(6):838–43.
86. Zheng W, et al. Occupational physical activity and the incidence of cancer of the breast, corpus uteri, and ovary in Shanghai. Cancer. 1993;71(11):3620–4.
87. Bertone ER, et al. Recreational physical activity and ovarian cancer in a population-based case-control study. Int J Cancer. 2002;99(3):431–6.
88. Chiaffarino F, et al. Risk factors for ovarian cancer histotypes. Eur J Cancer. 2007;43(7):1208–13.
89. Dosemeci M, et al. Occupational physical activity, socioeconomic status, and risks of 15 cancer sites in Turkey. Cancer Causes Control. 1993;4(4):313–21.
90. Moorman PG, et al. Recreational physical activity and ovarian cancer risk and survival. Ann Epidemiol. 2011;21(3):178–87.
91. Carnide N, Kreiger N, Cotterchio M. Association between frequency and intensity of recreational physical activity and epithelial ovarian cancer risk by age period. Eur J Cancer Prev. 2009;18(4):322–30.
92. Abbott SE, et al. Recreational physical activity and ovarian cancer risk in African American women. Cancer Med. 2016;5(6):1319–27.
93. Zhong S, et al. Nonoccupational physical activity and risk of ovarian cancer: a meta-analysis. Tumour Biol. 2014;35(11):11065–73.
94. Cannioto R, et al. Chronic recreational physical inactivity and epithelial ovarian cancer risk: evidence from the ovarian cancer Association Consortium. Cancer Epidemiol Biomark Prev. 2016;25(7):1114–24.
95. Adams SA, et al. The effect of social desirability and social approval on self-reports of physical activity. Am J Epidemiol. 2005;161(4):389–98.
96. Rzewnicki R, Vanden Auweele Y, De Bourdeaudhuij I. Addressing overreporting on the International Physical Activity Questionnaire (IPAQ) telephone survey with a population sample. Public Health Nutr. 2003;6(3):299–305.
97. Mink PJ, et al. Physical activity, waist-to-hip ratio, and other risk factors for ovarian cancer: a follow-up study of older women. Epidemiology. 1996;7(1):38–45.
98. Bertone ER, et al. Prospective study of recreational physical activity and ovarian cancer. J Natl Cancer Inst. 2001;93(12):942–8.
99. Anderson JP, Ross JA, Folsom AR. Anthropometric variables, physical activity, and incidence of ovarian cancer: the Iowa Women's Health study. Cancer. 2004;100(7):1515–21.
100. Hannan LM, et al. Physical activity and risk of ovarian cancer: a prospective cohort study in the United States. Cancer Epidemiol Biomark Prev. 2004;13(5):765–70.
101. Schnohr P, et al. Physical activity in leisure-time and risk of cancer: 14-year follow-up of 28,000 Danish men and women. Scand J Public Health. 2005;33(4):244–9.

102. Biesma RG, et al. Physical activity and risk of ovarian cancer: results from the Netherlands Cohort study (The Netherlands). Cancer Causes Control. 2006;17(1):109–15.
103. Patel AV, et al. Recreational physical activity and sedentary behavior in relation to ovarian cancer risk in a large cohort of US women. Am J Epidemiol. 2006;163(8):709–16.
104. Soll-Johanning H, Bach E. Occupational exposure to air pollution and cancer risk among Danish urban mail carriers. Int Arch Occup Environ Health. 2004;77(5):351–6.
105. Weiderpass E, et al. Prospective study of physical activity in different periods of life and the risk of ovarian cancer. Int J Cancer. 2006;118(12):3153–60.
106. Leitzmann MF, et al. Prospective study of physical activity and the risk of ovarian cancer. Cancer Causes Control. 2009;20(5):765–73.
107. Xiao Q, et al. Physical activity in different periods of life, sedentary behavior, and the risk of ovarian cancer in the NIH-AARP diet and health study. Cancer Epidemiol Biomark Prev. 2013;22(11):2000–8.
108. Hildebrand JS, et al. Moderate-to-vigorous physical activity and leisure-time sitting in relation to ovarian cancer risk in a large prospective US cohort. Cancer Causes Control. 2015;26(11):1691–7.
109. Huang T, et al. A prospective study of leisure-time physical activity and risk of incident epithelial ovarian cancer: impact by menopausal status. Int J Cancer. 2016;138(4):843–52.
110. Lahmann PH, et al. Physical activity and ovarian cancer risk: the European prospective investigation into cancer and nutrition. Cancer Epidemiol Biomark Prev. 2009;18(1):351–4.
111. Ainsworth BE, et al. Compendium of physical activities: classification of energy costs of human physical activities. Med Sci Sports Exerc. 1993;25(1):71–80.
112. Chionh F, et al. Physical activity, body size and composition, and risk of ovarian cancer. Cancer Causes Control. 2010;21(12):2183–94.
113. Carlberg K, et al. A survey of menstrual function in athletes. Eur J Appl Physiol Occup Physiol. 1983;51(2):211–22.
114. Frisch RE, et al. Delayed menarche and amenorrhea of college athletes in relation to age of onset of training. JAMA. 1981;246(14):1559–63.
115. Bonen A. Recreational exercise does not impair menstrual cycles: a prospective study. Int J Sports Med. 1992;13(2):110–20.
116. Rogol AD, et al. Durability of the reproductive axis in eumenorrheic women during 1 yr of endurance training. J Appl Physiol (1985). 1992;72(4):1571–80.
117. Ellison PT, Peacock NR, Lager C. Ecology and ovarian function among lese women of the Ituri Forest, Zaire. Am J Phys Anthropol. 1989;78(4):519–26.
118. Jasienska G, Ellison P. Heavy workload impairs ovarian function in Polish peasant women. Am J Phys Anthropol. 1993;16(Suppl):117–8.
119. Williams NI, et al. Evidence for a causal role of low energy availability in the induction of menstrual cycle disturbances during strenuous exercise training. J Clin Endocrinol Metab. 2001;86(11):5184–93.
120. Loucks AB. Energy availability, not body fatness, regulates reproductive function in women. Exerc Sport Sci Rev. 2003;31(3):144–8.
121. Rich-Edwards JW, et al. Physical activity, body mass index, and ovulatory disorder infertility. Epidemiology. 2002;13(2):184–90.
122. Holmes MD, et al. Physical activity and survival after breast cancer diagnosis. JAMA. 2005;293(20):2479–86.
123. Meyerhardt JA, et al. Physical activity and survival after colorectal cancer diagnosis. J Clin Oncol. 2006;24(22):3527–34.
124. Schmid D, Leitzmann MF. Association between physical activity and mortality among breast cancer and colorectal cancer survivors: a systematic review and meta-analysis. Ann Oncol. 2014;25(7):1293–311.
125. Cannioto RA, et al. Recreational physical inactivity and mortality in women with invasive epithelial ovarian cancer: evidence from the Ovarian Cancer Association Consortium. Br J Cancer. 2016;115(1):95–101.

126. Zhou Y, et al. Body mass index, physical activity, and mortality in women diagnosed with ovarian cancer: results from the Women's Health Initiative. Gynecol Oncol. 2014;133(1):4–10.
127. Zhou Y et al. (2015) Randomized trial of exercise on quality of life and fatigue in women diagnosed with ovarian cancer: the Women's Activity and Lifestyle Study in Connecticut (WALC). In: ASCO Annual Meeting Proceedings.
128. Zhou Y, Cartmel B, Gottlieb L, Ercolano EA, Li F, Harrigan M, McCorkle R, Ligibel JA, von Gruenigen VE, Gogoi R, Schwartz PE. Randomized trial of exercise on quality of life in women with ovarian cancer: women's activity and lifestyle study in connecticut (WALC). JNCI: J Natl Cancer Inst. 2017 Dec 1;109(12).
129. Hamer M, Smith L, Stamatakis E. Prospective association of TV viewing with acute phase reactants and coagulation markers: English Longitudinal study of ageing. Atherosclerosis. 2015;239(2):322–7.
130. Howard BJ, et al. Associations of overall sitting time and TV viewing time with fibrinogen and C reactive protein: the AusDiab study. Br J Sports Med. 2015;49(4):255–8.
131. Zhang M, et al. Sedentary behaviours and epithelial ovarian cancer risk. Cancer Causes Control. 2004;15(1):83–9.
132. Smits A, et al. Body mass index, physical activity and quality of life of ovarian cancer survivors: time to get moving? Gynecol Oncol. 2015;139(1):148–54.
133. Moore SC, et al. Association of leisure-time physical activity with risk of 26 types of cancer in 1.44 million adults. JAMA Intern Med. 2016;176(6):816–25.

Chapter 14
Impact of Obesity on Surgical Approaches to Gynecologic Malignancies

Amanika Kumar and William A. Cliby

Abstract As already described in previous chapters, the obesity epidemic in America is on the rise, with approximately 36% of Americans being obese, and more than 6% having Class III obesity (8% in women) defined as a BMI $\geq$40 kg/m². The rising obesity rate in women has profound effects on gynecologic malignancy occurrence and treatment. As surgery is a part of treating the majority of gynecologic malignancies, understanding the nuances of intra-operative and peri-operative management of the obese patient is an essential skill of the gynecologic oncologist. This chapter will briefly review the medical and anesthetic considerations for surgery in the obese woman with a gynecologic malignancy. It will focus on the impact of obesity in surgery in both endometrial cancer and in ovarian cancer as well as mention the impact on other gynecologic cancers. The chapter concludes with a mention of techniques that can be employed to facilitate surgery in obese women.

Keywords Perioperative management • Minimally invasive surgery endometrial cancer • Surgical staging endometrial cancer • Laparoscopic surgery endometrial cancer • LAP2 study • Robotic surgery endometrial cancer • Cytoreductive surgery ovarian cancer • Obesity paradox • Inguinal femoral lymph node dissection • Anesthesia in obese patients • Stomas • Surgical closures

Pre-Operative Assessment of the Obese Woman with a Gynecologic Malignancy

Pre-operative medical assessment of obese women is an important aspect of care for gynecologic cancer. Obesity-related diseases including obstructive sleep apnea and obesity hypoventilation syndrome, diabetes, cardiovascular disease, and hypertension all have impact on the intra-operative and post-operative management of patients [1, 2]. A proper medical history and medical assessment of the potential

A. Kumar, M.D. • W.A. Cliby, M.D. (✉)
Mayo Clinic, 200 First St SW, Rochester, MN 55905, USA
e-mail: Kumar.Amanika@mayo.edu; Cliby.william@mayo.edu

© Springer International Publishing AG 2018
N.A. Berger et al. (eds.), *Focus on Gynecologic Malignancies*, Energy Balance and Cancer 13, DOI 10.1007/978-3-319-63483-8_14

surgical patient may avoid potential complications in the post-operative period. It is well established that maintained glycemic control and continuation of peri-operative beta-blockers can help reduce risk of peri-operative morbidity, and these issues should be addressed pre-operatively. Plans for optimizing glycemic control during the post-operative course should be in place: utilizing an inpatient diabetes consult service can be quite effective if available. Cardiac risk should be assessed, knowing that patients with medically-complicated obesity will also have an increased risk of cardiac disease.

Proper management of the pre-operative medical issues in the morbidly obese gynecologic cancer patient is best done with a multidisciplinary team that is equipped and experienced in treating this population. These pre-existing conditions have significant impact on the ability for patients to quickly recover from surgery and move on to important adjuvant treatment. Avoidance of medical and surgical post-operative complications will allow for rapid recovery.

Endometrial Cancer

No gynecologic malignancy is more directly influenced by obesity than endometrial cancer. Both age and obesity are major risk factors for the development of endometrial cancer, and therefore, as our population continues to get older and more obese, gynecologic oncologists face the management of endometrial cancer in the obese patient on an almost daily basis. Here we will review the feasibility of surgery for endometrial cancer in the obese population, as well as discuss the role of minimally invasive surgery in these patients.

Endometrial cancer surgery ideally includes removal of the uterus, fallopian tubes and ovaries, and assessment of lymph nodes. Prior to the mid-2000s, the majority of endometrial cancer surgery was performed via a laparotomy. Studies have looked at the feasibility of surgical staging in the obese population via laparotomy and show that completeness of staging is possible in obese patients however is less frequently attempted. One retrospective study from Ohio examined 356 consecutive patients from 1997 to 2003. In this group, 22% had a BMI >40 kg/m^2; only 40% had a BMI <30 kg/m^2. Rates of staging did decrease with increasing BMI, with the rate of surgical staging in the BMI >40 kg/m^2 group dropping to 81%. The rate of para-aortic node assessment was significantly less in the BMI >40 kg/m^2 group, 48% vs. 74% in those patients with a BMI <30 kg/m^2. However, in the fully staged group, the number of lymph nodes removed did not differ by BMI, demonstrating the feasibility of surgical staging in the obese population when attempted. Regarding surgical risk, patients with a BMI >40 kg/m^2 had longer operative times and high blood loss, and a high incidence of wound infections (8%) and wound breakdowns (11%) [3].

Other studies confirm these findings. A retrospective study from 1990 to 2000 also examined 396 patients in three groups: BMI <30 kg/m^2 (41% of patients), BMI 30–40 kg/m^2 (32% of patients), and BMI >40 kg/m^2 (27% of patients). They also found longer operating room times and higher blood loss in patients with a

BMI > 40 kg/m^2. The study found differences in the rate of staging between BMI groups, 93.8% vs. 88.3% vs. 66.4% in BMI groups <30 kg/m^2, 30–40 kg/m^2, and >40 kg/m^2, respectively. The study confirms that equal numbers of lymph nodes were removed across each BMI group. Regarding complications and similar to the previously described study, this study found that patients with a BMI >40 kg/m^2 have a higher risk of wound complication, 8% vs. 1.9% in the BMI <30 kg/m^2 group [4]. These studies together demonstrate that in open surgery for endometrial cancer, morbidly obese patients are less likely to get staging and are more likely to have wound complications. If staging is performed, it is equal to staging in those patients who are not morbidly obese. Interestingly, both studies found that while extra-uterine disease was equally common across BMI groups, grade of disease was more commonly Grade 1 in the BMI >40 kg/m^2, leading some to consider hysterectomy alone for this group of patients. We will discuss this further after consideration of laparoscopic surgery.

The adoption of laparoscopic surgery and robotic-assisted laparoscopic surgery amongst gynecologic oncologists is high, and has had a profound influence on the management of endometrial cancer. Several retrospective trials have published on the feasibility and safety of laparoscopic surgical management of endometrial cancer. One early study reported on 42 obese women, mean BMI 35.8 kg/m^2 who underwent laparoscopic surgery for clinically stage I endometrial cancer. There was a low rate of conversion (7.5%) and patients had shorter hospital stay and lower pain scores than similar patients undergoing laparotomy. Surgery was longer in those patients undergoing laparoscopy. Patient's surgery, hysterectomy alone versus hysterectomy with lymphadenectomy, was not influenced by surgical approach and mean number of lymph nodes removed was higher in the laparoscopic group [5]. One retrospective matched cohort study compared patients with a planned laparoscopic lymphadenectomy to patients with a planned open lymphadenectomy. Overall success rate of the laparoscopic approach was 65%, however as BMI increased, successful laparoscopy without conversion decreased. Obesity was cited as the most common reason for conversion to laparotomy. As expected, laparoscopy was associated with shorter length of stay and fewer wound infections [6]. A large European retrospective study confirms the findings that laparoscopy is feasible and safer than laparotomy in obese patients with endometrial cancer. This study included four centers with 1266 patients, of whom 30.9% were obese: 18.8% had a BMI 30–35 kg/m^2, 7% had a BMI 35–40 kg/m^2, and 5.1% had a BMI >40 kg/m^2. Irrespective of obesity, patients in the laparotomy group had higher rates of complications than those in the laparoscopic group. Obese patients had a higher risk of venothromboembolism and wound complications than non-obese patients in both the laparotomy and laparoscopy groups. Increasing BMI was associated with high rates of conversion, with 8.6% of patients with a BMI >40 kg/m^2 experiencing a conversion vs. 1.1–2.2% in patients with a BMI <40 kg/m^2. As seen in other studies, as BMI increased, the rate of lymphadenectomy also decreased [7].

The randomized controlled data regarding laparoscopic surgery for endometrial cancer is a result of a cooperative group trial in the United states, LAP2 [8–10], and represents the strongest data on the feasibility and safety of minimally invasive surgery for endometrial cancer at this time. Patients in this trial were randomized to laparoscopy versus laparotomy for endometrial cancer. 1682 patients were enrolled in the laparoscopic arm with 920 patients enrolled in the laparotomy arm. Median BMI was the same in each group, however it is notable that the interquartile range of BMI in the groups was relatively low, 24–34 kg/m^2, likely reflective of surgeon bias toward enrolling thinner patients. In looking at the entire cohort, the laparoscopic arm had longer operative times, however patients who underwent laparoscopy had shorter hospital stays and fewer post-operative adverse events. Rates of pelvic lymphadenectomy did not differ between laparoscopy and laparotomy, 98% vs. 99%, while rates of para-aortic lymphadenectomy did, 94% vs. 97%. Overall survival, progression-free survival, and recurrence rates were similar between arms on the final analysis. Together, these results show that laparoscopy is both feasible and safe for endometrial cancer. There were however some important points raised by the study including a narrow range of BMI in patients included in the trial and the relatively high conversion rate, 42% of patients enrolled in LAP2 were obese: 21% BMI 30–35 kg/m^2, 11% BMI 30–40 kg/m^2, and 10% BMI >40 kg/m^2. BMI does play a role in conversion. The overall laparoscopic cohort had a conversion rate of 25.8%, however the risk of conversion increased with BMI, (OR = 1.11 for one unit increase in BMI, $p < 0.0001$). Conversion rate increased with increasing BMI regardless of age and metastatic disease. Regarding both the laparoscopic and laparotomy cohorts, similar to the retrospective data presented above, patients with a BMI >40 kg/m^2 had increased risk of hospitalization for >2 days, antibiotic use, wound infection (11.5%), and venothromboembolic event.

Interestingly, as BMI increased, the likelihood of low risk disease increased, adding to the evidence that obese patients may have lower risk disease and may not need surgical staging. These data combined with previously discussed retrospective data highlights the need to risk-stratify patients with endometrial cancer for those who need lymph node staging. One approach to surgical staging is the use of selective lymphadenectomy by uterine factors [11–14] and/or sentinel lymphadenectomy [15–19], thereby reducing the morbidity of lymphadenectomy in those patients who may not need lymph node assessment. In patients who do not need lymph node assessment, vaginal surgery may be a viable option for the treatment of endometrial cancer [20, 21]. The continued training in vaginal hysterectomy is an important part of gynecologic surgery training and a potential viable route of surgery to offer patients with low risk endometrial cancer.

An important consideration for lymphadenectomy is the extra-peritoneal laparoscopic approach to the para-aortic lymph nodes. This approach has been shown to be feasible for endometrial cancer, and feasible with obese patients. In our institution's experience, we found higher para-aortic lymph node retrieval in the obese group using the extra-peritoneal approach compared to laparotomy [22]. This approach should be considered for lymphadenectomy in obese patients.

While LAP2 demonstrated the efficacy and safety of the laparoscopic approach to endometrial cancer surgery, the adoption of minimally invasive approaches

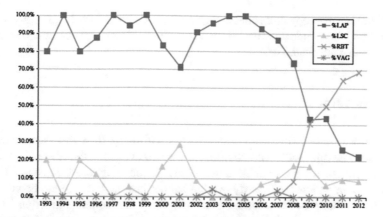

Fig. 14.1 Adopted from Leitao et al. [71]. Rates of laparotomy for endometrial cancer decrease sharply in the mid 2000s with the introduction and adoption of the robotic approach

increased exponentially with the FDA-approval of the Da Vinci® robotics system for gynecologic surgery in 2005 (Fig. 14.1). Many studies have compared a robotic approach versus an open approach and have demonstrated superiority of the robotic approach with regards to complications, particularly wound infections, blood loss, and hospital length of stay, particularly in the obese sub-population [23–25]. This is not surprising given the data on traditional laparoscopy versus laparotomy. One large study of 1000 robotic gynecologic surgeries in a single institution demonstrated an increase of mean BMI of patients over time, and despite the increasing BMI in the endometrial cancer cohort, there was no increase in cuff dehiscence, complication, conversion, and no decrease in lymph node acquisition [23].

The more important comparison is between types of minimally invasive surgery, robotics versus laparoscopy. One early study of obese and morbidly obese patients undergoing robotics versus laparoscopy for endometrial cancer showed a reduction in blood loss, shorter operative times and high lymph node retrieval (particularly in para-aortic lymph nodes) in the robotic cohort [26]. This study demonstrated no conversions in the robotics arm, but had a very low conversion risk in the laparoscopic arm (1/32 patients, 3.1%). These results were confirmed by a study of robotic surgery between 2006 and 2008 compared to a historical laparoscopic group in which they found the odds of conversion based on BMI to be 0.20 compared to the odds of conversion based on BMI in the laparoscopic group [27]. Large studies on robotic versus laparoscopic surgery in the obese population similarly demonstrate a lower blood loss, shorter operative time, and lower conversion rate with equal or better lymph node acquisition [28].

In conclusion, women with endometrial cancer and with a BMI >40 kg/m² have increased surgical risk. The mostly commonly cited risks include increase blood loss, lower likelihood of staging, and higher risks of wound complications [29, 30]. These risks can be reduced by using minimally invasive approaches. While both traditional laparoscopy and robotic surgery have benefits over laparotomy, robotic surgery may have benefits over laparoscopy, but this has not been confirmed by randomized control studies.

Ovarian Cancer

The surgical approach to ovarian cancer is quite different than that seen in endometrial cancer. As opposed to endometrial cancer where most patients are diagnosed in early stages, ovarian cancer is more likely to be diagnosed at Stage IIIC or IV. Surgery in patients with early ovarian cancer is aimed at staging, however surgery in advanced ovarian cancer is aimed at cytoreduction and often includes advanced procedures including upper abdominal surgery, bowel resection, and radical pelvic surgery. Few studies have specifically addresses the role of obesity in this surgery. The retrospective studies that have looked at all stages of ovarian cancer (Stage I–IV) have found no difference with regards to peri-operative outcomes in relation to BMI other than an increase in wound complications in those patients with higher BMI [31–34]. This is similar to results seen in a large group of general surgery patients ($n = 6336$) in which 9% had mild obesity and 4% have severe obesity. Overall there were no differences in post-operative complications other than wound complications [35].

Our group has examined the cohort of advanced ovarian cancer (Stage IIIc and IV) specifically, as these patients are the most frequent presenters of ovarian cancer and require high complexity surgery. In the largest published study of these patients, we found that patients with a BMI >40 kg/m^2 had an increased risk of severe complication (OR 2.93, $p < 0.01$) [36]. This group also had the highest rates of death within 90 days of surgery, 15.7% vs. 11.9 and 6.7% in normal and overweight/mildly obese patients, respectively. These data demonstrate the lowest complication and mortality risk in patients with a BMI 25.0–40.0 kg/m^2, which supports the concept of the "obesity paradox." (Fig. 14.2) The obesity paradox is a phenomenon demonstrated in other surgical populations in which the overweight/mildly obese patient population have the lowest complication risk. The underweight/normal weight and morbidly obese have the highest complications [37]. Certainly those patients who are morbidly obese are likely to have other co-morbidities, which can exacerbate complications and delay recovery from complications that do occur.

It is important to note that across all the studies in ovarian cancer, there was no difference in residual disease, and therefore ability to perform adequate surgery, across BMI groups, though the number of cases in the highest BMIs was limited. For example, in our cohort, there were only five patients with a BMI >50 kg/m^2 and only one with a BMI >60 kg/m^2. Undoubtedly there are limitations posed by higher BMI in terms of resectability, and in terms of the higher risk of complications. Surgeons should discuss with patients these limitations. Morbid obesity with BMI ≥40 kg/m^2 and certainly those with a BMI >50 kg/m^2 will present compromises in exposure and therefore safe resection when undertaking a high complexity surgical debulking. Fatty liver is a common

Fig. 14.2 Adopted from Kumar et al. [36]. This figures demonstrates the obesity paradox in which patients who are overweight or mildly obese have the lowest rates of mortality after ovarian cancer surgery

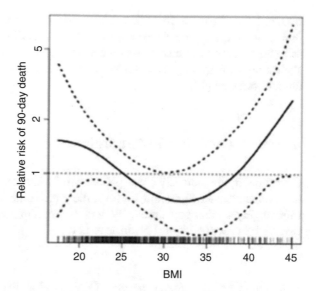

comorbidity in obese patients making liver mobilization and access to the diaphragm more problematic as well. While no hard and fast rules exist there is a BMI above which the benefits of resection will be limited by the technical feasibility and risks.

Other Gynecologic Malignancies

There is far less data available regarding the impact of obesity on surgery for cervical, vulvar, and vaginal cancers. Early cervical cancer treated with surgery is often approached with laparoscopic and robotic techniques. The data on feasibility of these approaches in the obese population derived from endometrial cancer studies likely applies to the obese cervical cancer population. The laparoscopic and robotic approaches likely have less morbidity and equal efficacy to laparotomy and should be considered when treatment planning for cervical cancer [38–40].

For difficult tumors in the deep pelvis (e.g., larger cervical cancers, pelvic recurrences for cervical/endometrial cancer) it is unavoidable the exposure and access will be compromised relative to thinner patients. Surgeons must take these limitations into account when considering operability and the ability to do an effective oncologic resection. Studies in both gynecologic and non-gynecologic pelvic tumors demonstrate the increased morbidity and less successful resection in obese patients, although data is sparse as most studies state morbid obesity as a contraindication to exenterative procedures [41–44].

Early vulvar cancers are often treated with local radical resection and lymph node assessment, which may include full inguinofemoral node dissection. The most frequent complications from this surgery include wound cellulitis, wound break-down, and lymphedema. Obesity is associated with all three of these outcomes [45, 46]. Techniques to reduce these outcomes include antibiotic use, drain use, and saphenous vein sparing, however none of these techniques have been tested in a randomized trial [47].

Anesthesia and Surgical Techniques

Operating on the morbidly obese patient can be challenging due to poor visualization and inadequate retraction, however there are some techniques that can assist in safe surgery in this population. We will review common issues relevant to open cases, MIS cases and issues germane to both.

Anesthesia Consideration and Patient Positioning

Anesthetic considerations include difficulty with obtaining and maintaining an airway. Obese patients often have shorter necks and excessively heavy chest walls that can make standard intubation difficulty. The use of fiber-optic intubation may be helpful in these patients. Ventilation becomes even more difficult with the addition of pneumoperitoneum used in laparoscopy and with steep Trendelenburg position used with robotic surgery. In obese patients, pulmonary compliance and functional residual capacity are reduced at baseline and peak airway pressures are high at baseline. Therefore, when adding in Trendelenburg and pneumoperitoneum, ventilation can be a challenge and peak and plateau airway pressures can rise by as much as 50% [48]. Ventilator interventions to decrease airway pressures to below 40 mmHg include reduction of intraabdominal pressure from our standard of 15–12 mmHg and changing from volume-controlled ventilation to pressure-controlled ventilation [48–50]. The potential hypercarbia that can ensue after prolonged robotic procedures can be corrected with hyperventilation. Intravenous and arterial access can also be a challenge in the morbidly obese, and sometimes may require the assistance of interventional radiology in order to secure intravenous access. Distribution of intravenous and inhalation anesthetic agents can be altered due to changes in total body water and increased adiposity [51].

Patient positioning is always important, especially for robotic cases or long oncologic cases. For robotic surgery requiring steep trendelenburg, we prefer Allen Yellow fin® stirrups. Patients are placed directly on a gel pad that sits on top of the surgical bed to prevent sliding when on the operating table. The use of a tight chest strap prevents further sliding, and we have found that shoulder pads or other barriers are not necessary even in our most obese patients. The chest strap does not impede proper ventilation when placed properly. One or both arms are left untucked but padded allowing access for anesthesia needs and for assessment during the case, as there have been rare cases of fluid infiltration and compartment syndrome in tucked arms. The arms are secured to arm boards in two locations to ensure they do not fall off arm boards, and are then draped in a sterile fashion so that the arm board can be moved as needed.

A similar set up is used for open gynecologic procedures in our institution, in part because the use of Trendelenburg can assist with pelvic visualization. Patients are placed on the operating room table with a Bair Hugger under the body to assist with maintenance of normothermia. They are either supine or in Allen yellow fin stirrups®, with a chest strap in place to ensure no slippage. These positioning techniques allow for safe Trendelenburg that is sometimes necessary for adequate visualization of the pelvis.

Other Surgical Techniques

The thoughtful use of retractors in open surgery can ensure adequate visualization. In our institution, we generally use a simple Balfour and a separate fixed upper abdominal retractor (Mayo-Brown, Omni). Others successfully employ the Bookwalter retractor, equipped with deep blades designed for the obese patient. The Alexis retractor is another options as they can assist in compressing the subcutaneous adipose tissue without introducing a mechanical obstacle to the surgical field. It has the added benefit of protecting the subcutaneous tissues, however is not routinely used in our division.

Proper placement of the abdominal incision can also help with surgical access— sometimes a supraumbilical incision will be superior access than an infraumbilical incision depending on the anatomy of a patient's pannus. Positioning the incision about the 'anaerobic zone' of the pannus may help reduce post-operative infections. Non-cosmetic panniculectomy with a long-transverse incision can be used to increased exposure by removing the large obstructing pannus transversely: the fascias is then opened vertically. Several papers describe the success of panniculectomy in obtaining pelvic access and demonstrate the safety of the procedure [52–57]. While the panniculectomy adds both time and blood loss to the procedure, these are minimal, and the ability to do lymphadenectomy in the obese patient increased from 45% in laparotomy alone to 70% with laparotomy including panniculectomy [55]. Rates of wound complications are 7.6–36%. Infectious complications can be reduced by the use of drains and extended post-operative antibiotics from 27.9 to 5.9%.

Stomas

Stoma creation is often necessary in the setting of malignant disease requiring bowel surgery. This is challenging with obese patients as the abdominal subcutaneous fat is thicker and the bowel mesentery can be redundant, leading to a more difficult mobilization of bowel through the abdominal wall. Stoma placement is important to consider pre-operatively. In general, the best location for a stoma is at the superior aspect of the inferior umbilical skin fold, however, in obese patients, stomas may need to be in the upper abdomen to ensure ability to visualize and care for the new stoma. In addition, the upper abdominal wall is usually less thick than the lower quadrants [58]. Stoma marking pre-operatively is ideal. Adequate bowel mobilization is the first step to creating a stoma, and as the thickness of the abdominal wall is greater in obese patients, more mobilization will be needed. The creation of a fascial incision for obese patients often needs to be larger in order to pull the thicker bowel through the abdominal wall. Some have advocated use of an Alexis retractor in this scenario [59]. These larger fascial defects can increase the risk of parastomal hernia, however in gynecologic patients, this is less commonly a concern due to the temporary nature or palliative nature of most ostomies. In likely permanent stomas, use of mesh at the site can decrease the risk of parastomal hernia, however this is not routine performed in oncologic patients. Ensuring adequate room at the level of the fascia is essential to proper blood supply to the new ostomy, particularly in obese patients where the stoma has a longer distance to travel in the abdominal wall. Delivery of the bowel through the abdominal wall takes patience and care, and reduction of appendices epiploicae and adequate fascial aperture can ensure a non-traumatic delivery. If mesentery is too thick or abdominal wall too thick, an end loop stoma can be created in lieu of split loop stoma, where the distal end is oversewn and left in the abdomen, but a proximal loop is brought out and matured as the stoma [58, 60].

Abdominal Closure

Effective fascial closure for abdominal surgery is particularly important in the obese population, as the rates of hernia and fascial dehiscence rises with rising obesity [61, 62]. Midline abdominal incisions should be closed with a continuous delayed absorbable or non-absorbable suture [63]. Some advocate closure of the fascia with smaller bites that are closer together as done in the STITCH trial however, the median BMI in this trial was quite low so it is yet to be determined whether this method of closure will improve outcomes in obese patients [64]. We do not recommend the use of prophylactic mesh for hernia prevention, particularly in the cancer patient.

Surgical site infection reduction bundles have been successful in gynecologic surgery in reducing the overall infection rates at institutions. Our experience with a bundle that includes patient education, chlorhexidine gluconate shower and surgical preparation, sterile closing tray and changing of surgical attire for closure, and dismissal with chlorhexidine wash has helped tremendously, reducing surgical site infection rate from 6.0 to 1.1% [65]. Other measures include maintenance of normothermia and administration of antibiotics pre-operatively [66, 67]. These measures should be routinely advocated in gynecologic surgery, particularly for those patients at highest risk.

Obese patients, especially those with diabetes or smokers, have increased rates in wound complications. The use of incisional wound vacuum assist devices has been advocated in high risk patients and has had some success in decreasing wound complications [68–70]. However this has not been studied in gynecologic surgery and warrants further investigation to identify the patients that will benefit from routine use of these devices. With these devices, the fascia, subcutaneous tissue, and skin are primarily closed in the usually fashion. A wound vacuum device is placed over the closed skin incision for 3–5 days.

Conclusions

The surgical management of obese gynecologic cancer patients is an ever more common task of the gynecologic oncologists. Proper pre-operative and peri-operative management of these patients is essential in their care, and collaboration with anesthesia, cardiology, and internal medicine departments can serve the patient well. More than any other gynecologic cancer, the impact of obesity in endometrial cancer has been profound, and the utilization of minimally invasive approach to staging endometrial cancer has resulted in equally oncologic outcomes with reduced post-operative morbidity. In ovarian cancer and other cancers, there is less data available about surgical management, however while surgery seems feasible, there are clearly limitations and possible some poorer outcomes in the morbidly obese patients. There are many surgical techniques including panniculectomy, proper retractor use, and incisional wound vacuum assist devices that may assist in proper surgery for the obese gynecologic patient.

References

1. Adams JP, Murphy PG. Obesity in anaesthesia and intensive care. Br J Anaesth. 2000;85(1):91–108.
2. Binks A. Anaesthesia in the obese patient. Endocrinology. 2008;9:299–302.
3. Pavelka JC, Ben-Shachar I, Fowler JM, Ramirez NC, Copeland LJ, Eaton LA, et al. Morbid obesity and endometrial cancer: surgical, clinical, and pathologic outcomes in surgically managed patients. Gynecol Oncol. 2004;95(3):588–92.
4. Everett E, Tamimi H, Greer B, Swisher E, Paley P, Mandel L, et al. The effect of body mass index on clinical/pathologic features, surgical morbidity, and outcome in patients with endometrial cancer. Gynecol Oncol. 2003;90(1):150–7.
5. Eltabbakh GH, Shamonki MI, Moody JM, Garafano LL. Hysterectomy for obese women with endometrial cancer: laparoscopy or laparotomy? Gynecol Oncol. 2000;78(3):329–35.
6. Scribner DR Jr, Walker JL, Johnson GA, McMeekin DS, Gold MA, Mannel RS. Laparoscopic pelvic and Paraaortic lymph node dissection in the obese. Gynecol Oncol. 2002;84(3):426–30.

7. Uccella S, Bonzini M, et al. Impact of obesity on surgical treatment for endometrial cancer: a multicenter study comparing laparoscopy vs open surgery, with propensity-matched analysis. J Minim Invasive Gynecol. 2016;23(1):53–61.
8. Walker JL, Piedmonte MR, Spirtos NM, Eisenkop SM, Schlaerth JB, Mannel RS, et al. Laparoscopy compared with laparotomy for comprehensive surgical staging of uterine cancer: gynecologic oncology group study LAP2. J Clin Oncol. 2009;27(32):5331–6.
9. Walker JL, Piedmonte MR, Spirtos NM, Eisenkop SM, Schlaerth JB, Mannel RS, et al. Recurrence and survival after random assignment to laparoscopy versus laparotomy for comprehensive surgical staging of uterine cancer: gynecologic oncology group LAP2 study. J Clin Oncol. 2012;30(7):695–700.
10. Gunderson CC, Java J, Moore KN, Walker JL. The impact of obesity on surgical staging, complications, and survival in uterine cancer: a gynecologic oncology group LAP2 ancillary study. Gynecol Oncol. 2014;133(1):23–7.
11. Mariani A, Keeney GL, Aletti G, Webb MJ, Haddock MG, Podratz KC. Endometrial carcinoma: paraaortic dissemination. Gynecol Oncol. 2004;92(3):833–8.
12. Mariani A, Webb MJ, Keeney GL, Aletti G, Podratz KC. Predictors of lymphatic failure in endometrial cancer. Gynecol Oncol. 2002;84(3):437–42.
13. Mariani A, Dowdy SC, Cliby WA, Gostout BS, Jones MB, Wilson TO, et al. Prospective assessment of lymphatic dissemination in endometrial cancer: a paradigm shift in surgical staging. Gynecol Oncol. 2008;109(1):11–8.
14. Dowdy SC, Borah BJ, Bakkum-Gamez JN, Weaver AL, McGree ME, Haas LR, et al. A prospective assessment of survival, morbidity, and cost associated with lymphadenectomy in low-risk endometrial cancer. Gynecol Oncol. 2012;127(1):5–10.
15. Niikura H, Okamura C, Utsunomiya H, Yoshinaga K, Akahira J, Ito K, et al. Sentinel lymph node detection in patients with endometrial cancer. Gynecol Oncol. 2004;92(2):669–74.
16. Lopes L, Nicolau S, et al. Sentinel lymph node in endometrial cancer. Int J Gynecol Cancer. 2007;17(5):1113–7.
17. Abu-Rustum NR, Khoury-Collado F, Gemignani ML. Techniques of sentinel lymph node identification for early-stage cervical and uterine cancer. Gynecol Oncol. 2008;111(S):S44–50.
18. Khoury-Collado F, Murray MP, Hensley ML, Sonoda Y, Alektiar KM, Levine DA, et al. Sentinel lymph node mapping for endometrial cancer improves the detection of metastatic disease to regional lymph nodes gynecologic oncology. Gynecol Oncol. 2011;122(2):251–4.
19. Levenback CF, Ali S, Coleman RL, Gold MA, Fowler JM, Judson PL, et al. Lymphatic mapping and sentinel lymph node biopsy in women with squamous cell carcinoma of the vulva: a gynecologic oncology group study. J Clin Oncol. 2012;30(31):3786–91.
20. Beck T, Morse C, Gray H, et al. Route of hysterectomy and surgical outcomes from a statewide gynecologic oncology population: is there are role for vaginal hysterectomy? Am J Obstet Gynecol. 2016;214(3):348.e1–9.
21. Bakkum J. Refining the definition of low-risk endometrial cancer: improving value. Gynecol Oncol. 2016;141(2):189–90.
22. Dowdy SC, Aletti G, Cliby WA, Podratz KC, Mariani A. Extra-peritoneal laparoscopic paraaortic lymphadenectomy. Gynecol Oncol. 2008;111(3):418–24.
23. Paley PJ, Veljovich DS, Shah CA, Everett EN, Bondurant AE, Drescher CW, et al. Surgical outcomes in gynecologic oncology in the era of robotics: analysis of first 1000 cases. Am J Obstet Gynecol. 2011;204(6):551.e1–9.
24. Bernardini MQ, Gien LT, Tipping H, Murphy J, Rosen BP. Surgical outcome of robotic surgery in morbidly obese patient with endometrial cancer compared to laparotomy. Int J Gynecol Cancer. 2012;22(1):76–81.
25. Hinshaw SJ, Gunderson S, Eastwood D, Bradley WH. Endometrial carcinoma: the perioperative and long-term outcomes of robotic surgery in the morbidly obese. J Surg Oncol. 2016;114(7):884–7.

26. Gehrig PA, Cantrell LA, Shafer A, Abaid LN, Mendivil A, Boggess JF. What is the optimal minimally invasive surgical procedure for endometrial cancer staging in the obese and morbidly obese woman? Gynecol Oncol. 2008;111(1):41–5.
27. Seamon LG, Cohn DE, Henretta MS, Kim KH, Carlson MJ, Phillips GS, et al. Minimally invasive comprehensive surgical staging for endometrial cancer: robotics or laparoscopy. Gynecol Oncol. 2009;113(1):36–41.
28. Freeman AH, Barrie A, Lyon L, Garcia C, Littell RD, Powell CB. Should we recommend robotic surgery rather than traditional laparoscopy for obese women? A comprehensive comparison of surgical outcomes for endometrial cancer. Gynecol Oncol. 2015;139(1):192–3.
29. Bouwman F, Smits A, Lopes A, Das N, Pollard A, Massuger L, et al. Impact of BMI on surgical complications and outcome: an institutional study and systematic review of the literature. Gynecol Oncol. 2015;139(2):369–76.
30. Martinek IE, Haldar K, Tozzi R. Laparoscopic surgery for gynaecological cancers in obese women. Maturitas. 2010;65(4):320–4.
31. Matthews KS, Straughn JM Jr, Kemper MK, Hoskins KE, Wang W, Rocconi RP. The effect of obesity on survival in patients with ovarian cancer. Gynecol Oncol. 2009;112(2):389–93.
32. Suh DH, Kim HS, Chung HH, Kim JW, Park NH, Song YS, et al. Body mass index and survival in patients with epithelial ovarian cancer. J Obstet Gynaecol Res. 2011;38(1):70–6.
33. Fotopoulou C, Richter R, Braicu E-I, Kuhberg M, Feldheiser A, Schefold JC, et al. Impact of obesity on operative morbidity and clinical outcome in primary epithelial ovarian cancer after optimal primary tumor Debulking. Ann Surg Oncol. 2011;18(9):2629–37.
34. Smits A, Smits E, Lopes A, Das N, Hughes G, Talaat A, et al. Body mass index, physical activity and quality of life of ovarian cancer survivors: time to get moving? Gynecol Oncol. 2015;139(1):148–54.
35. Dindo D, Muller MK, Weber M, Clavien P-A. Obesity in general elective surgery. Lancet. 2005;361:2032–5.
36. Kumar A, Bakkum-Gamez JN, Weaver AL, McGree ME, Cliby WA. Impact of obesity on surgical and oncologic outcomes in ovarian cancer. Gynecol Oncol. 2014;135(1):19–24.
37. Mullen JT, Davenport DL, Hutter MM, Hosokawa PW, Henderson WG, Khuri SF, et al. Impact of body mass index on perioperative outcomes in patients undergoing major intra-abdominal cancer surgery. Ann Surg Oncol. 2008;15(8):2164–72.
38. Spirtos NM, Eisenkop SM, Schlaerth JB, Ballon SC. Laparoscopic radical hysterectomy (type III) with aortic and pelvic lymphadenectomy in patients with stage I cervical cancer: surgical morbidity and intermediate follow-up. Am J Obstet Gynecol. 2002;187(2):340–8.
39. Malzoni M, Tinelli R, Cosentino F, Perone C, Iuzzolino D, Rasile M, et al. Laparoscopic radical hysterectomy with lymphadenectomy in patients with early cervical cancer: our instruments and technique. Surg Oncol. 2009;18(4):289–97.
40. Pomel C. Laparoscopic radical hysterectomy for invasive cervical cancer: 8-year experience of a pilot study. Gynecol Oncol. 2003;91(3):534–9.
41. Fleisch MC, Pantke P, Beckmann MW, Schnuerch HG, Ackermann R, Grimm MO, et al. Predictors for long-term survival after interdisciplinary salvage surgery for advanced or recurrent gynecologic cancers. J Surg Oncol. 2007;95(6):476–84.
42. Domes T. Total pelvic exenteration for rectal cancer: outcomes and prognostic factors. Can J Surg. 2011;54(6):387–93.
43. Berek JS, Howe C, Lagasse LD, Hacker NF. Pelvic exenteration for recurrent gynecologic malignancy: survival and morbidity analysis of the 45-year experience at UCLA. Gynecol Oncol. 2005;99(1):153–9.
44. Benn T, Brooks RA, Zhang Q, Powell MA, Thaker PH, Mutch DG, et al. Pelvic exenteration in gynecologic oncology: a single institution study over 20 years. Gynecol Oncol. 2011;122(1):14–8.
45. Rouzier R, Haddad B, Dubernard G, Dubois P, Paniel B-J. Inguinofemoral dissection for carcinoma of the vulva: effect of modifications of extent and technique on morbidity and survival. J Am Coll Surg. 2003;196(3):442–50.

46. Wills A, Obermair A. A review of complications associated with the surgical treatment of vulvar cancer. Gynecol Oncol. 2013;131(2):467–79.
47. Dardarian TS, Gray HJ, Morgan MA, Rubin SC, Randall TC. Saphenous vein sparing during inguinal lymphadenectomy to reduce morbidity in patients with vulvar carcinoma. Gynecol Oncol. 2006;101(1):140–2.
48. Danic MJ, Chow M, Alexander G, Bhandari A, Menon M, Brown M. Anesthesia considerations for robotic-assisted laparoscopic prostatectomy: a review of 1,500 cases. J Robotic Surg. 2007;1(2):119–23.
49. Ogurlu M, Kucuk M, et al. Pressure-controlled vs volume-controlled ventilation during laparoscopic gynecologic surgery. J Minim Invasive Gynecol. 2010;17(3):295–300.
50. Badawy M, Beique F, et al. Anesthetic considerations for robotic surgery in gynecologic oncology. J Robot Surg. 2011;5(4):235–9.
51. Casati A, Putzu M. Anesthesia in the obese patient: pharmacokinetic considerations. J Clin Anesth. 2005;17(2):134–45.
52. Hopkins MP, Shriner AM, Parker MG, Scott L. Panniculectomy at the time of gynecologic surgery in morbidly obese patients. Am J Obstet Gynecol. 2000;182(6):1502–5.
53. Tillmanns TD, Kamelle SA, Abudayyeh I, McMeekin SD, Gold MA, Korkos TG, et al. Panniculectomy with simultaneous gynecologic oncology surgery. Gynecol Oncol. 2001;83(3):518–22.
54. Wright JD, Rosenbush EJ, Powell MA, Rader JS, Mutch DG, Gao F, et al. Long-term outcome of women who undergo panniculectomy at the time of gynecologic surgery. Gynecol Oncol. 2006;102(1):86–91.
55. Eisenhauer EL, Wypych KA, Mehrara BJ, Lawson C, Chi DS, Barakat RR, et al. Comparing surgical outcomes in obese women undergoing laparotomy, laparoscopy, or laparotomy with Panniculectomy for the staging of uterine malignancy. Ann Surg Oncol. 2007;14(8):2384–91.
56. Hardy JE, Salgado CJ, Matthews MS, Chamoun G, Fahey AL. The safety of pelvic surgery in the morbidly obese with and without combined Panniculectomy. Ann Plast Surg. 2008;60(1):10–3.
57. Matory WE, O'Sullivan J, Fudem G. Abdominal surgery in patients with severe morbid obesity. Plast Reconstr Surg. 1994;94(7):976–87.
58. Brand M, Dujovny N. Preoperative considerations and creation of normal Ostomies. Clin Colon Rectal Surg. 2008;21(1):5–16.
59. Meagher AP, Owen G, Gett R. An improved technique for end stoma creation in obese patients. Dis Colon Rectum. 2009;52(3):531–3.
60. Colwell JC, Fichera A. Care of the obese patient with an ostomy. J Wound Ostomy Continence Nurs. 2005;32(6):378–83.
61. Makela J, Kiviniemi H, Juvonen T. Factors influencing wound dehiscence after midline laparotomy. Am J Surg. 1995;170:387–90.
62. Webster C, Neumayer L. Prognostic models of abdominal wound dehiscence after laparotomy. J Surg Res. 2003;109:130–7.
63. Riet MV, Steyerberg EW, Bonjer HJ, Jeekel J. Meta-analysis of techniques for closure of midline abdominal incisions. Br J Surg. 2002;89:1350–6.
64. Deerenberg E, Harlaar J, et al. Small bites versus large bites for closure of abdominal midline incisions (STITCH): a double-blind, multicentre, randomised controlled trial. Lancet. 2015;386(10000):1254–60.
65. Johnson MP, Kim SJ, Langstraat CL, Jain S, Habermann EB, Wentink JE, et al. Using bundled interventions to reduce surgical site infection after major gynecologic cancer surgery. Obstet Gynecol. 2016;127(6):1135–44.
66. Cima R, Dankbar E, Lovely J, et al. Colorectal surgery surgical site infection reduction program: a National Surgical Quality Improvement programe driven multidisciplinary single-institution experience. J Am Coll Surg. 2013;216(1):23–33.
67. Bratzler DW. The surgical infection prevention and surgical care improvement projects: national initiatives to improve outcomes for patients having surgery. Clin Infect Dis. 2006;43:322–30.

68. Gomoll A, Lin A, Harris MB. Incisional vacuum-assisted closure therapy. J Orthop Trauma. 2006;20(10):705–9.
69. Condé-Green A, Chung TL, Holton LH III, Hui-Chou HG, Zhu Y, Wang H, et al. Incisional negative-pressure wound therapy versus conventional dressings following abdominal wall reconstruction. Ann Plast Surg. 2013;71(4):394–7.
70. Stannard JP, Atkins BZ, O'Malley D, Singh H. Use of negative pressure therapy on closed surgical incisions: a case series. Ostomy Wound Manage. 2009;55(8):58–66.
71. Leitao MM Jr, Narain WR, Boccamazzo D. Impact of robotic platforms on surgical approach and costs in the management of morbidly obese patients with newly diagnosed uterine cancer. Ann Surg Oncol. 2016;23(7):2192–8.

Chapter 15
Obesity, Fertility Preservation and Gynecologic Cancers

Terri L. Woodard and Jessica Rubin

Abstract A small but significant number of gynecologic cancers are diagnosed in women less than 40 years old. Many of these women will have not started or fulfilled their plans to have children and will desire to preserve their fertility, in spite of their cancer diagnosis. The field of Oncofertility utilizes multidisciplinary collaboration between reproductive medicine specialists and oncology providers to inform patients of the potential for cancer-related infertility and present options for fertility preservation (FP) while balancing disease treatment and fertility goals.

While FP offers hope for future parenthood in reproductive age women with cancer, it is important to recognize that obesity also presents unique challenges in terms of treatment and reproductive outcomes. Currently, there are limited data on FP outcomes in this population. Here we review the impact of obesity and cancer treatment on fertility, options for fertility preservation, and special considerations in the reproductive management of obese women with gynecologic malignancies.

Keywords Ovulatory dysfunction • Assisted reproductive technology • Gonadotoxic therapy • Ovarian reserve • Cryopreservation—embryo • Oocyte • Ovarian tissue • Gonadal shielding • In vitro fertilization

T.L. Woodard, M.D. (✉)
The University of Texas MD Anderson Cancer Center,
1155 Pressler St., Unit Number 1362, Room Number CPB6.3546, Houston, TX 77030, USA

Division of Reproductive Endocrinology and Infertility, Baylor College of Medicine,
One Baylor Plaza MS:BCM610, Houston, TX 77030, USA
e-mail: tlwoodard@mdanderson.org

J. Rubin, M.D.
Division of Reproductive Endocrinology and Infertility, Baylor College of Medicine,
One Baylor Plaza MS:BCM610, Houston, TX 77030, USA
e-mail: jessica.rubin@bcm.edu

© Springer International Publishing AG 2018
N.A. Berger et al. (eds.), *Focus on Gynecologic Malignancies*, Energy Balance and Cancer 13, DOI 10.1007/978-3-319-63483-8_15

Introduction

Obesity and Impaired Fertility

The prevalence of obesity has increased over the past few decades. Among reproductive age females, approximately half of women in the United States and one third of women worldwide are overweight or obese [1, 2]. Obese women have an increased risk of medical comorbidities including hypertension, cardiovascular disease, respiratory problems, gynecologic malignancies, and impaired fertility. Additionally, obese women who conceive have a higher incidence of antenatal, intrapartum, and perinatal complications.

Obesity can impair reproductive success. Women who are overweight or obese have decreased pregnancy rates compared to women with a normal BMI, even in the presence of regular menstrual cycles. Gaskins and colleagues reported that the time to pregnancy increases proportionally with BMI. After adjustment for age, race, smoking and marital status, every 5 kg of weight gain after age 18 increases the time to conception by 1.8 months [3]. A reduction in fecundity has also been reported following significant weight gain during adolescence. Women with a BMI above 24 at age 23 or younger have an increased risk of anovulatory infertility during their reproductive years. This finding remains significant regardless of subsequent weight loss and pre-pregnancy BMI [4].

Obese women exhibit decreased fecundity for several reasons. An elevated BMI is associated with menstrual and ovulatory dysfunction. Women with a BMI above 27 have a relative risk of anovulatory infertility of 3.1 compared to lean women [5]. Data also suggests that obese women with an increased abdominal fat distribution experience higher rates of anovulation compared to BMI matched controls [6]. Potential mechanisms to explain ovulatory dysfunction in obese women include polycystic ovarian syndrome, increased conversion of androgens to estrogen by adipose aromatase, and insulin-induced suppression of sex hormone-binding globulin [2]. Obese women also have a diminished ovarian response to ovarian stimulation and require higher doses of fertility medications, likely due to leptin-induced impairment of follicle stimulating hormone (FSH) and insulin-like growth factor 1 activity in granulosa cell steroidogenesis [7, 8]. Furthermore, data suggests obesity may impair oocyte morphology and quality, leading to decreased fertilization and pregnancy rates [9].

Obesity and Gynecologic Malignancies

The rise in obesity may be partially responsible for the increase in reproductive age women diagnosed with cancer. Obesity increases the risk of several malignancies, including breast, colorectal and esophageal cancers. With regard to gynecologic malignancies, the connection between obesity and endometrial cancer has been long appreciated. The link between obesity and cervical or ovarian cancers is inconsistent, though there may be some association in certain subcategories of disease, such as cervical adenocarcinomas and premenopausal low grade serous and non-serous ovarian cancers. [10].

Obesity causes environmental alterations that may promote carcinogenesis, most notably a change in hormonal milieu. Overweight women have elevated estrogen levels derived from adrenal and ovarian androgen secretion, increased aromatase activity in adipose tissue, decreased sex hormone binding globulin production resulting in elevated free hormone levels, and lower progesterone levels from anovulation [10]. Elevated estrogen levels can promote proliferation of hormonally sensitive malignancies. In addition to unopposed estrogen exposure, other factors including adipocytokines and inflammatory mediators produced by adipose tissue may contribute to carcinogenesis and tumor proliferation in obese women [11, 12].

Effects of Cancer Treatment on Fertility

Cancer treatment often involves chemotherapy radiation, and/or surgery, all of which can have deleterious effects on reproductive capacity. Women with obesity-related infertility may experience a more exaggerated decline in fecundity following cancer therapy.

Ovarian hormones regulate the hypothalamic-pituitary-gonadal axis to promote follicular growth, ovulation, and endometrial thickening for pregnancy implantation. Ovarian function is crucial for reproductive success with autologous gametes. One challenge for assisted reproductive technology (ART) centers on the finite quantity of female gametes. In females, the number of primordial oocytes naturally declines with age. Women have approximately two million oocytes at birth, which decreases to 200,000–500,000 at menarche and 400 around the onset of menopause [13]. Exposure to gonadotoxic agents accelerates the decline of primordial follicles (see Fig. 15.1).

Chemotherapeutic agents decrease the number of primordial follicles and damage granulosa cells, diminishing steroid hormone production [14]. The degree of gonadal damage is dependent on numerous factors, which include age at diagnosis, baseline ovarian reserve, type of agent, total dosage, and treatment duration. Data on the gonadotoxic effects of chemotherapy is not comprehensive, but medications have been stratified into the following risk categories: high, intermediate risk, and low risk [15] (see Table 15.1). However, many cancer patients are treated with multi-agent regimens, and it is challenging to accurately estimate the risk of ovarian insufficiency or failure following cancer therapy.

Women who have received gonadotoxic therapy have an increased risk of premature ovarian failure and infertility. The risk of amenorrhea following chemotherapy has been reported to range from 10% to 90% and is partially dependent on a woman's age and oocyte quantity. Per Bines, the resumption of menses in women less than 40 years of age compared to women over 40 is 39–55% and 0–11%, respectively [13].

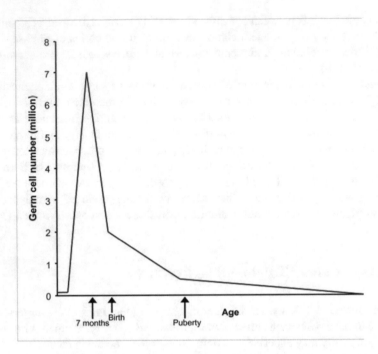

Changes in human oocyte number during prenatal and postnatal development.

Fig. 15.1 Risk of gonadal damage by chemotherapy type (from source [12])

Table 15.1 The degree of gonadal damage by chemotherapy (from source [12])

High risk	Intermediate risk	Low risk
Cyclophosphamide	Cisplatin	Methotrexate
Chlorambucil	Adriamycin	5-Fluorouracil
Melphalan		Vincristine
Busulfan		Bleomycin
Nitrogen mustard		Actinomycin D
Procarbazine		

Clin Exp Reprod Med. 2012 Jun; 39(2): 46–51
Published online 2012 Jun 30. doi:10.5653/cerm.2012.39.2.46

It is important to emphasize that resumption of menses is not indicative of "normal" fertility or ovarian function. Survivors who resume menstrual cycles still remain at increased risk for premature ovarian failure. The average age of menopause for the general population is 52 years, compared to 38–46 years in women previously treated with chemotherapy [13]. Therefore, women in remission who have received medical clearance for pregnancy should be encouraged to pursue pregnancy as soon as reasonably possible [16].

Radiation therapy is another significant risk factor for ovarian failure and infertility. The patient's age, dose, and fractionation schedule influence the degree of gonadal damage. Irradiation of 1–2 Gy in adolescents and 3–4 Gy in adults has been associated with significant depletion of primordial follicles. The location of irradiation also impacts the risk of gonadal toxicity. Total body irradiation, a previously common treatment for children and young adolescents with malignancies, requires an average dose of 20–30 Gy and is associated with a 90–97% risk of ovarian failure [17]. Wallace and colleagues developed a mathematical model to predict the age of ovarian failure following a known dosage of pelvic radiotherapy. The effective sterilizing dose, defined as premature ovarian failure in 97.5% of patients, was reported to be 20.3, 18.4, 16.5, and 14.3 Gy following pelvic irradiation at birth, 10, 20, and 30 years of age respectively [18]. Radiation to the pelvis also causes deleterious effects on the uterus with irreversible damage to the uterine musculature and vasculature. Pelvic and whole body irradiation have been associated with an increased prevalence of miscarriage, mid-trimester pregnancy loss, preterm delivery and intrauterine growth restriction [19]. While not directly gonadotoxic, irradiation of cranial tissue above 5 Gy is associated with hypogonadotropic hypogonadism and ovarian dysfunction, which also results in impaired fertility [20].

Surgery that necessitates the removal of reproductive organs can also cause infertility. Surgery requiring the resection of ovarian tissue will decrease ovarian reserve. In situations where there is a high suspicion for ovarian tumor recurrence or reoperation, such as ovarian borderline tumors, fertility preservation should be considered. Other scenarios where FP can be offered include women with cervical or endometrial cancers who proceed with a hysterectomy but elect to leave the ovaries in situ. Following completion of therapy, these patients can utilize in vitro fertilization (IVF) to obtain embryos that can be transplanted into a gestational carrier.

Integrating Fertility Preservation Counseling into Cancer Care

The current survival rate for reproductive age women and men with cancer is 87% [21]. In 2010, one in every 715 adults was estimated to be childhood cancer survivor [22]. The number of cancer survivors will continue to grow as screening modalities and treatments improve. Necessarily, treatment planning is evolving to consider disease survival as well as quality of life, which includes concerns about future fertility and family building. The desire for genetic offspring among cancer survivors is significant; for cancer patients younger than 45 years of age, 33–78% desire biological offspring [23–26]. When presented with the risks of impaired fertility following cancer treatment, women will consider both standard and experimental fertility preservation techniques to preserve future childbearing. Among female teenagers diagnosed with malignancy, 80% of patients and 90% of their parents would consider experimental fertility preservation procedures [27]. Despite the desire for biological children, cancer survivors are less likely to parent a child using autologous gametes [28, 29].

Although cancer survivors often express a desire for future childbearing, they often have a limited understanding of the gonadotoxic effects of cancer therapy and available fertility preservation options [23]. In 2006, the American Society of Clinical Oncology (ASCO) developed practice guidelines on fertility preservation for individuals with cancer. Current ASCO guidelines recommend that all health care providers counsel patients on the potential gonadotoxic effects of treatment and that discussions about fertility preservation be initiated as early as possible during treatment planning to help expand the number of options that are available. Patients should also be referred to reproductive specialists, if desired [30, 31].

The decision to pursue fertility preservation prior to cancer treatment is dependent on many factors, including the patient's desire for future fertility, estimated risk of infertility, cancer prognosis, and availability of financial resources. Time constraints are another important consideration, with many providers and patients feeling urgency to initiate cancer treatment as soon as possible. However, Lohrisch reported in a retrospective study of over 2500 women with stage 1–2 breast cancer that intervals of less than 12 weeks between definitive surgery and the initiation of chemotherapy have no impact on survival, whereas prolongation longer than 12 weeks between surgery and chemotherapy can have adverse effects [32]. Thus, the decision to postpone cancer treatment to allow time for fertility preservation should be considered in medically appropriate scenarios.

Discussions on fertility preservation allow patients to play an active role in treatment decisions and to provide hope for quality survival [33]. Regardless of whether the gametes were later used for reproduction, cancer survivors recall banking gametes prior to therapy as a positive experience [34].

Determination of Ovarian Reserve

Ovarian reserve refers to reproductive potential as a function of the number and quality of remaining oocytes a woman has [35]. Oocyte quantity declines with age, but the rate of decline is variable between individuals. Ovarian reserve testing can help establish a baseline while also helping to identify individuals who are at risk for diminished ovarian reserve (DOR). There is no consensus on the definition of DOR, but women with diminished reserve may experience a limited response to ovarian stimulation or decreased fecundity rates.

Ovarian reserve is assessed using ultrasound measurements and hormonal testing. On transvaginal ultrasound, antral follicles can be visualized within the ovary as circular, anechoic masses measuring 2–10 mm. The presence of 10–12 antral follicles between both ovaries represents a normal antral follicle count. Traditionally, FSH and estradiol levels have been collected on day 3 of the menstrual cycle. As the quantity of oocytes diminishes, there are fewer follicles to secrete inhibin-B and provide negative feedback on the pituitary release of FSH. Women with DOR may exhibit elevated FSH and/or estradiol values. A newer assay to test ovarian reserve measures anti-mullerian hormone (AMH). AMH is produced by primary follicles and has a positive correlation with ovarian reserve [36]. It is thought to be a more sensitive marker of ovarian reserve and has the added benefit of being able to be assessed during any time of a woman's menstrual cycle. For women who are newly diagnosed with cancer and need fertility preservation urgently, an antral follicle count and AMH should be assessed to estimate her baseline ovarian reserve, risk of cancer-related infertility, and anticipated response to ovarian stimulation. As a woman becomes older, the genetic quality of her oocytes diminishes and pregnancy in older women increases the risk for offspring with genetic abnormalities, such as trisomy 21. All women with cancer who desire future fertility should receive ovarian reserve testing and review their results with a reproductive health specialist, so that individualized estimates of risk and outcomes can be discussed.

Obesity has been negatively associated with ovarian reserve. Data has shown an inverse relationship between obesity and AMH values [37, 38]. Proposed mechanisms for oocyte depletion in this population have not been elucidated. Overweight and obese women pursuing IVF require higher doses of medications for ovarian stimulation, and we can infer that obese women have a lower ovarian reserve and/or a decreased response to gonadotropin stimulation [39, 40].

Fertility Preservation Options

The most established and successful methods of preserving fertility in women utilize ART (i.e., embryo and oocyte cryopreservation), however, there are experimental options that may be available if ART is not an option. Even if FP is not desired, all women should still be familiar with protective measures that can minimize the risk of infertility when applicable [41].

Embryo and Oocyte Cryopreservation

Embryo and oocyte cryopreservation are the only standard of care methods of fertility preservation recognized by the American Society for Reproductive Medicine and the European Society of Human Reproduction and Embryology. In humans, the first IVF pregnancy was reported in 1973 by Carl Wood and John Leeton, and the first child born following IVF occurred in 1978 [42]. Embryo and oocyte cryopreservation technology has progressed significantly over the last few decades as knowledge in the field continues to advance.

The goal of assisted reproduction is to increase follicular recruitment and maturation. During IVF, gonadotropins are administered to recruit the development of multiple follicles, termed controlled ovarian hyperstimulation (COH). Serial transvaginal ultrasounds and hormonal labs are performed to monitor follicular development and gonadotropin doses are adjusted in accordance with follicular growth. On average, COH protocols involve 10–12 days of gonadotropin administration. When the largest follicles grow to approximately 18–20 mm, human chorionic gonadotropin or leuprolide are administered to trigger ovulation and the oocyte retrieval is scheduled for 36 h later.

Oocytes are retrieved from the ovary via transvaginal oocyte aspiration, which is generally performed under intravenous sedation. A transvaginal ultrasound probe with an attached needle is placed into the vagina. Under ultrasound guidance, the needle is advanced through the vaginal wall to puncture the ovarian follicles and aspirate follicular fluid. The oocyte-cumulus complex is aspirated in the follicular fluid and then passed to the embryologists, who identify the oocytes and place the gametes in culture media. The transvaginal oocyte retrieval lasts approximately 15–20 min.

If a woman does not have a partner, has ethical or legal concerns about cryopreserving embryos, or desires complete reproductive autonomy, she can elect to cryopreserve unfertilized oocytes. Oocytes can be cryopreserved and stored and then warmed or thawed to be inseminated at a later date. Otherwise, oocytes can be fertilized in vitro with sperm using conventional insemination or intracytoplasmic sperm injection to form embryos. Embryos may be cryopreserved at the pronuclear state or cultured in vitro until they reach the blastocyst stage and then cryopreserved, depending on patient and provider preferences. Embryos that are cryopreserved can be stored for decades, if not longer. Vitrification is currently the preferred method for gamete cryopreservation due to increased tissue survival, pregnancy implantation, and live birth rates compared to the traditional slow freeze technique [43].

All patients who pursue ART should be advised regarding the possibility of a poor response to ovarian stimulation and the chance of an unsuccessful pregnancy outcome, as well as the risks inherent in the IVF process. The most common side effect from IVF stimulation is abdominal bloating. Other risks include allergic reactions to stimulation medications, discomfort or infection at the injection site, and the risks associated with the oocyte aspiration procedure such as bleeding, infection, and injury to pelvic organs. The most serious complication from COH is ovarian hyperstimulation syndrome (OHSS), which is characterized by increased vessel permeability and extravascular fluid accumulation. OHSS patients can present with shortness of breath, significant edema, pleural effusions, ascites, and venous thrombosis. Cancer patients pursuing ART should be counseled regarding the following risk factors for venous thrombosis: OHSS, malignancy, and elevated estrogen levels during hormonal stimulation [41]. They should be also counseled that development of severe OHSS can potentially delay initiation of cancer treatment.

Obese women pursuing ART may have additional complications. Overweight and obese women require higher doses of gonadotropins during IVF stimulation and data suggests the total FSH dose is positively correlated with BMI [44]. As medication dosage increases, patients are subject to more potential side effects. Research on the potential difference in oocyte quality, fertilization, and embryo development between obese women compared and lean controls in conflicting [39, 40]. Both rodent and human oocyte models suggest obesity may be associated with increased metabolic abnormalities, oxidative stress, embryonic lipid deposition, and abnormal embryo development [45, 46]. Furthermore, gynecologic surgical procedures on obese patients have been associated with increased blood loss and operative time; however, there is limited data on the prevalence of surgical complications in obese women following transvaginal oocyte aspiration for ART [47].

Special Considerations for Patients with Cancer Pursuing Egg and/or Embryo Cryopreservation

- Concerns about ovarian reserve: The success of ovarian stimulation is primarily dependent on the woman's age and ovarian reserve. It is debated whether females with a genetic predisposition or diagnosis of malignancy have impaired success rates with ovarian stimulation. Women with BRCA-1 mutations and malignancy prior to treatment have been reported to produce decreased oocyte yields following assisted reproduction [48, 49]. However, other studies report that cancer patients do not have impaired success with ART. Robertson and colleagues concluded that cancer patients prior to gonadotoxic therapy had no change in gonadotropin dose requirement, oocyte yield, or number of embryos cryopreserved compared to women without malignancy [50]. More research investigating ART success in cancer patients is needed to determine if ovarian stimulation and oocyte yield is influenced by the specific cancer diagnosis [51].
- Timing of stimulation: Providers and patients should be informed that oocyte and embryo cryopreservation can be completed within 2–3 weeks. Although ovarian stimulation is typically initiated during the early follicular phase of the menstrual cycle, women who need to initiate cancer treatment more urgently can initiate fertility preservation immediately. With "random start" IVF protocols, gonadotropin stimulation is started on any day of the woman's menstrual cycle. Since multiple cohorts of ovarian follicles develop each month, the phase of the menstrual cycle in which ovarian stimulation is initiated does not affect the number of mature oocytes recovered [52, 53]. There is limited data on the long-term outcomes of oocyte quality and live birth rates from 'random start' protocols since many of these patients are just beginning to return for embryo transfer [41]. If a woman has several weeks prior to the initiation of gonadotoxic therapy, she may be able to pursue two consecutive COH cycles to increase gamete yield. Data on consecutive ART cycles has shown good ovarian response and increased oocyte yield during the second stimulation cycle [54].
- Stimulation in women with hormone sensitive malignancies: In women with estrogen sensitive malignancies, there is concern that elevated estrogen levels might contribute to cancer progression. A normal, unstimulated ovulatory cycle produces an estradiol level of approximately 300 pg/mL, whereas COH can produce estradiol concentrations that exceed 3000 pg/mL. There is a theoretical

concern that the elevated steroid hormones in COH cycles can stimulate the growth of hormone dependent breast and endometrial malignancies. Current data have not shown an increased risk of breast cancer recurrence or death following IVF over an average of 50–63 months [55]. However, given the theoretical risk of cancer progression with ART, novel ovarian stimulation protocols have been designed to stimulate multiple follicles without achieving supra-physiologic estradiol levels.

- In women with hormonally sensitive malignancies, reproductive endocrinologists should consider adding letrozole to IVF ovarian stimulation regimens. Letrozole is an aromatase inhibitor and prevents the conversion of androgen precursors to estrogen in numerous tissues, including granulosa cells of the ovary. By decreasing estrone and estradiol levels, aromatase inhibitors decrease negative feedback on FSH secretion and the rise in FSH promotes follicular growth. Oktay initially reported on the addition of letrozole to gonadotropin IVF cycles to minimize serum estradiol levels. The addition of letrozole to gonadotropin IVF cycles results in a significant reduction in estrogen exposure while maintaining a similar gonadotropin dose, oocyte yield, oocyte fertilization rate, and number of cryopreserved embryos compared to traditional COH protocols. Tamoxifen has also been used to decrease estradiol levels during COH, however, compared to letrozole, the addition of tamoxifen to gonadotropin IVF cycles produces increased peak estradiol levels [56]. Thus, the supplementation of letrozole is preferred over tamoxifen. Another option is to pursue a natural IVF cycle without the administration of exogenous gonadotropins; however, the oocyte yield is very low and not cost-effective.

- Availability of preimplantation genetic diagnosis (PGD) : Women with a hereditary cancer syndrome may have a decreased interest in fertility due to concerns about transmitting their mutation to their offspring. Premenopausal breast cancer is often associated with hereditary mutations in BRCA1 and BRCA2 genes, which also increase the risk of ovarian cancer. Women with BRCA mutations have been reported to express a decreased interest in future childbearing and struggle with the decision regarding fertility preservation [57, 58]. Genetic testing of embryos using PGD involves biopsying embryos to test for a specific mutation. This technology has broadened reproductive options for women, since they can elect to only transfer embryos that do not harbor the mutation. PGD is a valid option for women at high risk of having a child with a monogenetic disease, however data is lacking regarding the efficacy of different molecular techniques used. The optimal method of PGD for BRCA carriers is controversial, and some data suggests PCR remains superior to whole genome application, however further research is needed [59].

Ovarian Tissue Cryopreservation

Ovarian tissue cryopreservation (OTC) is an experimental FP technique. This procedure is the only option for pre-pubertal girls who desire fertility preservation, since they cannot be hormonally stimulated for gamete preservation. OTC is also an option for women with inadequate time to complete oocyte stimulation prior to cancer therapy [60]. The American Society of Reproductive Medicine and the European Society of Human Reproduction and Embryology consider OTC investigational, but this technique has advanced significantly over the last few decades. The first successful live birth following fresh ovarian tissue cortical graft placement occurred in monozygotic twins discordant for premature ovarian failure [61]. Around the same time, the first cryopreserved ovarian transplant was performed for fertility preservation following cancer treatment [62]. To date, worldwide there have been over 70 live births following ovarian tissue transplantation, and many of these pregnancies occurred spontaneously after tissue transplant without requiring ovarian stimulation [63].

Ideally, ovarian tissue is removed prior to gonadotoxic treatment, with the exception of leukemia [64]. In leukemia patients, the ideal time for ovarian tissue excision and cryopreservation is after remission in order to decrease the likelihood of residual malignancy in the tissue [65]. Ovarian tissue is usually removed laparoscopically. Oocytes are located within the follicles of the ovarian cortex, and both cortical strip and whole ovary transplantation have resulted in successful live births. Advantages of removing the entire ovary and vascular pedicle include an immediate blood supply for the graft and a larger volume of oocytes at the time of transplantation; however, whole ovary transplantation is also associated with increased operative time, possible vascular pedicle ischemia, and increased technical challenges during cryopreservation. Given these potential disadvantages, many providers have investigated partitioning the ovary into 0.3–2 mm sections to cryopreserve ovarian cortical strips [60].

Ovarian tissue can be cryopreserved with slow freeze or vitrification protocols. Both techniques have similar outcomes on the morphologic integrity of ovarian specimens, but vitrification is associated with less laboratory processing time and financial burden [66]. When the patient has completed gonadotoxic therapy and desires fertility, cryopreserved ovarian tissue can be warmed and transplanted into an orthotopic or heterotopic location. Orthotopic transplantation can occur in the remaining medullary portion of the ovary or the ovarian fossa peritoneum. Heterotopic transplantation of ovarian tissue has been reported in the abdominal wall, chest, and forearm. Resumption of hormonal function and normal menses with ovulation can occur within 4–9 months of transplant. The duration of ovarian function is variable, and transplanted ovarian tissue has been found to retain hormonal function for at least 6 years in both sheep and human studies [64, 67]. Successful pregnancy outcomes have been reported following the transplantation of fresh and cryopreserved cortical tissue, as well as fresh whole ovaries. To date there have been no reported cases of pregnancy following transplant of a cryopreserved whole ovary, but data is scarce given the recent development and implementation of this technology.

Cryopreservation of ovarian tissue should be considered for fertility preservation, especially in prepubertal adolescents following a careful assessment of the potential benefits and risks. Risks of OTC include the reintroduction of malignant cells following graft placement, surgical complications during graft transplant, and failure to obtain successful pregnancy outcomes. Furthermore, a significant limitation to OTC centers on the limited patient access to this service. OTC is not currently offered at most hospitals in the United States. New research suggests that the reproductive potential of primordial follicles can be maintained for at least 20 h prior to cryopreservation if the tissue is stored at 4 °C following oophorectomy [68]. Therefore, even if a patient receives treatment at a facility that does not provide OTC services but the surgeons are trained to perform an oophorectomy, there is a possibility that these specimens could be transported to designated facilities for gonadal cryopreservation.

Another emerging aspect of ART involves the process of in vitro maturation of oocytes. Current research focuses on activating dormant primordial follicles via biochemical and mechanical signal pathways. Data on in vitro maturation of oocytes remains controversial and limited pregnancies have been reported. If maturation of female gametes can be achieved, this would shift the paradigm of fertility care for many patients [69].

Ovarian Suppression

Hormonal agents can be used to suppress the ovaries during cancer treatment, potentially diminishing the gonadotoxic effects of chemotherapy; however, reports of the efficacy of these agents is mixed and their use remains controversial. The mechanism by which gonadotropin releasing hormone (GnRH) agonists could minimize the gonadotoxic effects of chemotherapy are not understood. One theory is that GnRH agonists suppress pituitary FSH release to prevent follicle recruitment. However, less than 10% of follicles are estimated to be growing and destined for ovulation or atresia, so this may not explain the complete protective mechanism. Other proposed mechanisms include an increase in the production of apoptotic molecules such as sphingosine-1-phosphate, a direct protective influence on ovarian cells, or a decrease in ovarian perfusion and chemotherapy exposure [70]. In rodents, Kitajima showed that GnRH agonist therapy decreases ovarian vascular permeability and blood flow [71]. However, the effect of GnRH agonists on ovarian vasculature in humans remains controversial [72].

Long-term data on the effect of GnRH agonist therapy on ovarian function in women who have received chemotherapy remains inadequate for many reasons. Cancer patients are often on multi-drug regimens, confounding gonadotoxic effects and preventing appropriate comparisons. In addition, a woman's age, pubertal status and ovarian reserve play a fundamental role in her fertility and there is variability between women on the same treatment regimen. Current clinical trials are assessing the role of GnRH agonist therapy for ovarian protection.

Ovarian Transposition

Ovarian transposition, or oophoropexy, is method that can be used to minimize gonadal damage from pelvic and/or abdominal radiation. Using a laparoscopic or open technique, the fallopian tube and ovary are mobilized by transecting the utero-ovarian ligament and mesovarium with bipolar energy or sharp dissection. Historically, the ovary was positioned behind the posterior aspect of the uterus. Conventional practice is to mobilize the ovary and distal fallopian tube outside of the pelvis to the pelvic brim, ideally 3–5 cm superior to the radiation field. Surgeons should maintain the proximity of the ovary and distal tube to allow for natural ovum pickup [73]. Transposed ovaries can retain ovarian hormonal function following radiotherapy. In a sample size of 18 women, Husseinzadeh reported continued ovarian function and normal gonadotropin levels in 88% of women less than 40 years of age who elected for ovarian transposition prior to pelvic irradiaton [74]. Barahmeh similarly reported in a study of 14 women with ovarian transposition prior to pelvic radiation, 93% maintained ovarian function during the mean 42 month follow up period [75]. However, the presence of ovarian hormone production should not be considered to be indicative of fertility. Limited knowledge exists regarding long-term ovarian function or pregnancy rates following ovarian transposition. Reports have shown women to have earlier menopause onset after transposition compared to the general population, but it is unclear if this association is secondary to surgical technique or potential vascular compromise. Furthermore, there have been reported cases of ovarian torsion following laparoscopic ovarian transposition and patients should be counseled regarding potential risks [76, 77].

Gonadal Shielding

Gonadal shielding is recommended for women exposed to abdominal or pelvic irradiation [15]. Careful attention should be paid to ensure the shield is positioned and sized correctly. The ovaries are located in the lateral pelvic sidewall, referred to as the ovarian fossa. The ovary is anchored by three structures: the uteroovarian ligament to the uterus, the mesovarium to the posterior broad ligament, and the suspensory ligament to the pelvic sidewall. Anatomical presentation of the ovary is variable between individuals, and when permissible, abdominal shielding should protect both the midline and the lateral aspects of the pelvis [78].

Fertility-Sparing Management of Gynecologic Cancers

Fertility sparing interventions should be considered in the management of women with early gynecologic cancers, when appropriate per oncology treatment guidelines. Women with early cervical cancer who desire future fertility may avoid a hysterectomy and instead opt for a trachelectomy. Multiple studies have confirmed that trachelectomy done abdominally, laparoscopically and robotically have oncologic outcomes similar to radical hysterectomy. Lanowska and colleagues reported patients with early stage cervical cancer treated with radical vaginal trachelectomy and laparoscopic lymphadenectomy have a 5-year survival rate above 90% and a 5-year recurrence rate of 3–6% [79]. Patients considering trachelectomy should be counseled that the procedure is associated with a twofold increase in preterm delivery [80]. They should also be aware of a 10–12% risk of incompletion, with the possibility of conversion to chemoradiation. In those instances, meeting with a reproductive endocrinologist can help with treatment planning. Other complications include isthmic stenosis and amenorrhea.

Women with early ovarian cancers that are limited to one ovary, such as in non-epithelial origin, may be candidates for unilateral oophorectomy. Data on outcomes is somewhat limited, but Maltaris et al. reported that out of a total of 282 patients with early epithelial ovarian cancer who were treated conservatively, 113 became pregnant with 87 subsequent term deliveries. There were 33 relapses and 16 disease-related deaths in this sample of patients [81]. In the case of borderline ovarian tumors, cystectomy or unilateral salpingoophorectomy can be considered. While fertility-sparing surgery has a higher rate of recurrence, there is no difference in survival rates. Approximately 50% spontaneously conceived [82, 83].

Obese women are at increased risk of endometrial cancer due to infertility and body habitus. Women diagnosed with endometrial cancer often have concurrent medical comorbidities, such as obesity, polycystic ovarian syndrome, metabolic syndrome, and chronic anovulation. Treatment options may include lifestyle modification, metformin, and fertility sparing therapies. Fertility sparing options for reproductive age women with early endometrial cancer are treatment with a levonorgestrel intrauterine device (IUD) or oral progestins. The IUD is preferable, as oral progestins are associated with significant weight gain. Surgical resection has also been proposed; however, reproductive age women with early disease typically receive non-surgical treatment with biopsies every 3 months until absence of disease. The desired number of biopsies without evidence of malignancy varies by clinician. Once cleared with normal endometrial biopsies, the patient is encouraged to become pregnant as soon as possible. Regression rates for endometrial cancer are approximately 76.3%, however there is a relapse rate of approximately 40%. Live birth rates following endometrial cancer are approximately 30% [84]. Fertility preservation treatment strategies should be discussed when indicated, but persistent disease often warrants a hysterectomy. IVF can be performed prior to or after hysterectomy and pregnancy can later be achieved with use of a gestational carrier.

Fertility and Family Building After Cancer

Patients present with varying levels of ovarian function after cancer treatment, however, remain at risk for diminished ovarian reserve and premature ovarian failure. Some women will be able to conceive spontaneously, while others may need assistance. Reassessment of ovarian reserve at least 1 year after completion of treatment may be helpful in identifying women with DOR and empowering them to consider seeking fertility assistance.

Women are generally advised to wait at least 2 years following treatment before attempting pregnancy, when the likelihood of recurrence has decreased, but this timing is variable based on age and diagnosis. Data thus far does not show that pregnancy in women with a history of cancer affects recurrence or disease survival rates [16]. However, patients should seek consultation with their oncology provider and obstetrician prior to conception to ensure that health status is optimized. For patients who may be at a higher-risk for obstetrical complications, a preconception consultation with a maternal-fetal medicine specialist is warranted.

In the event a woman experiences ovarian failure, it is important to inform her that she still has options for family building available to her. If she chose to cryopreserve oocytes or embryos, she can utilize them and transfer them back to her uterus, even if she is menopausal, or can use a gestational carrier. If not, other options include the use of donor egg, donor embryo, and adoption.

Conclusion

The potential to have children in the future is a priority for many cancer patients. Cancer treatment can impair fertility, limiting the reproductive options of cancer survivors. All patients at risk of cancer-related infertility should be informed of their risk and availability of options for fertility preservation prior to the initiation of gonadotoxic treatment.

Providing FP counseling and services to women is an important component of comprehensive cancer care. Viable options for FP exist; however, obesity can present challenges that affect reproductive outcomes. More data is needed to improve the care of this patient population. Collaboration between reproductive specialists and oncology providers creates an opportunity to maximize oncologic and reproductive outcomes.

References

1. Vahratian A. Prevalence of overweight and obesity among women of childbearing age: results from the 2002 National Survey of Family Growth. Matern Child Health J. 2009;13(2):268–73.
2. Practice Committee of the American Society for Reproductive Medicine. Obesity and reproduction: a committee opinion. Fertil Steril. 2015;104(5):1116–26.
3. Gaskins AJ, et al. Association of fecundity with changes in adult female weight. Obstet Gynecol. 2015;126(4):850–8.
4. Lake JK, Power C, Cole TJ. Women's reproductive health: the role of body mass index in early and adult life. Int J Obes Relat Metab Disord. 1997;21(6):432–8.
5. Grodstein F, Goldman MB, Cramer DW. Body mass index and ovulatory infertility. Epidemiology. 1994;5(2):247–50.
6. Kuchenbecker WK, et al. The subcutaneous abdominal fat and not the intraabdominal fat compartment is associated with anovulation in women with obesity and infertility. J Clin Endocrinol Metab. 2010;95(5):2107–12.
7. Greisen S, et al. Effects of leptin on basal and FSH stimulated steroidogenesis in human granulosa luteal cells. Acta Obstet Gynecol Scand. 2000;79(11):931–5.
8. Mulders AG, et al. Patient predictors for outcome of gonadotrophin ovulation induction in women with normogonadotrophic anovulatory infertility: a meta-analysis. Hum Reprod Update. 2003;9(5):429–49.
9. Leary C, Leese HJ, Sturmey RG. Human embryos from overweight and obese women display phenotypic and metabolic abnormalities. Hum Reprod. 2015;30(1):122–32.
10. Modesitt SC, van Nagell JR Jr. The impact of obesity on the incidence and treatment of gynecologic cancers: a review. Obstet Gynecol Surv. 2005;60(10):683–92.
11. Lee H, Lee IS, Choue R. Obesity, inflammation and diet. Pediatr Gastroenterol Hepatol Nutr. 2013;16(3):143–52.

12. Tao W, Lagergren J. Clinical management of obese patients with cancer. Nat Rev Clin Oncol. 2013;10(9):519–33.
13. Bines J, Oleske DM, Cobleigh MA. Ovarian function in premenopausal women treated with adjuvant chemotherapy for breast cancer. J Clin Oncol. 1996;14(5):1718–29.
14. Familiari G, et al. Ultrastructure of human ovarian primordial follicles after combination chemotherapy for Hodgkin's disease. Hum Reprod. 1993;8(12):2080–7.
15. Lee S, et al. Fertility preservation in women with cancer. Clin Exp Reprod Med. 2012;39(2):46–51.
16. Lee MC, et al. Fertility and reproductive considerations in premenopausal patients with breast cancer. Cancer Control. 2010;17(3):162–72.
17. Sanders JE, et al. Late effects on gonadal function of cyclophosphamide, total-body irradiation, and marrow transplantation. Transplantation. 1983;36(3):252–5.
18. Wallace WH, et al. Predicting age of ovarian failure after radiation to a field that includes the ovaries. Int J Radiat Oncol Biol Phys. 2005;62(3):738–44.
19. Critchley HO, Wallace WH. Impact of cancer treatment on uterine function. J Natl Cancer Inst Monogr. 2005;34:64–8.
20. Gonfloni S, et al. Inhibition of the c-Abl-TAp63 pathway protects mouse oocytes from chemotherapy-induced death. Nat Med. 2009;15(10):1179–85.
21. Wallace WH, Kelsey TW, Anderson RA. Fertility preservation in pre-pubertal girls with cancer: the role of ovarian tissue cryopreservation. Fertil Steril. 2016;105(1):6–12.
22. Wallace WH, Anderson RA, Irvine DS. Fertility preservation for young patients with cancer: who is at risk and what can be offered? Lancet Oncol. 2005;6(4):209–18.
23. Peate M, et al. It's now or never: fertility-related knowledge, decision-making preferences, and treatment intentions in young women with breast cancer—an Australian fertility decision aid collaborative group study. J Clin Oncol. 2011;29(13):1670–7.
24. Schover LR, et al. Having children after cancer. A pilot survey of survivors' attitudes and experiences. Cancer. 1999;86(4):697–709.
25. Mancini J, et al. Barriers to procreational intentions among cancer survivors 2 years after diagnosis: a French national cross-sectional survey. Psychooncology. 2011;20(1):12–8.
26. Quinn GP, et al. Discussion of fertility preservation with newly diagnosed patients: oncologists' views. J Cancer Surviv. 2007;1(2):146–55.
27. Burns KC, Boudreau C, Panepinto JA. Attitudes regarding fertility preservation in female adolescent cancer patients. J Pediatr Hematol Oncol. 2006;28(6):350–4.
28. Madanat LM, et al. Probability of parenthood after early onset cancer: a population-based study. Int J Cancer. 2008;123(12):2891–8.
29. Syse A, Kravdal O, Tretli S. Parenthood after cancer – a population-based study. Psychooncology. 2007;16(10):920–7.
30. Loren AW, et al. Fertility preservation for patients with cancer: American Society of Clinical Oncology clinical practice guideline update. J Clin Oncol. 2013;31(19):2500–10.
31. Lee SJ, et al. American Society of Clinical Oncology recommendations on fertility preservation in cancer patients. J Clin Oncol. 2006;24(18):2917–31.
32. Lohrisch C, et al. Impact on survival of time from definitive surgery to initiation of adjuvant chemotherapy for early-stage breast cancer. J Clin Oncol. 2006;24(30):4888–94.
33. Quinn GP, et al. Physician referral for fertility preservation in oncology patients: a national study of practice behaviors. J Clin Oncol. 2009;27(35):5952–7.
34. Bahadur G. Fertility issues for cancer patients. Mol Cell Endocrinol. 2000;169(1–2):117–22.
35. Practice Committee of the American Society for Reproductive Medicine. Testing and interpreting measures of ovarian reserve: a committee opinion. Fertil Steril. 2015;103(3):e9–e17.
36. Committee on Gynecologic Practice. Committee opinion no. 618: ovarian reserve testing. Obstet Gynecol. 2015;125(1):268–73.
37. Durmanova AK, et al. Ovarian reserve and adipokine levels in reproductive-aged obese women. Ter Arkh. 2016;88(10):46–50.
38. Moy V, et al. Obesity adversely affects serum anti-mullerian hormone (AMH) levels in Caucasian women. J Assist Reprod Genet. 2015;32(9):1305–11.

39. Depalo R, et al. Oocyte morphological abnormalities in overweight women undergoing in vitro fertilization cycles. Gynecol Endocrinol. 2011;27(11):880–4.
40. Zhang D, et al. Overweight and obesity negatively affect the outcomes of ovarian stimulation and in vitro fertilisation: a cohort study of 2628 Chinese women. Gynecol Endocrinol. 2010;26(5):325–32.
41. Benard J, et al. Freezing oocytes or embryos after controlled ovarian hyperstimulation in cancer patients: the state of the art. Future Oncol. 2016;12(14):1731–41.
42. Kamel RM. Assisted reproductive technology after the birth of louise brown. J Reprod Infertil. 2013;14(3):96–109.
43. Rezazadeh Valojerdi M, et al. Vitrification versus slow freezing gives excellent survival, post warming embryo morphology and pregnancy outcomes for human cleaved embryos. J Assist Reprod Genet. 2009;26(6):347–54.
44. Christensen MW, et al. Effect of female body mass index on oocyte quantity in fertility treatments (IVF): treatment cycle number is a possible effect modifier. A register-based cohort study. PLoS ONE. 2016;11(9):e0163393.
45. Luzzo KM, et al. High fat diet induced developmental defects in the mouse: oocyte meiotic aneuploidy and fetal growth retardation/brain defects. PLoS One. 2012;7(11):e49217.
46. Wu LL, et al. High-fat diet causes lipotoxicity responses in cumulus-oocyte complexes and decreased fertilization rates. Endocrinology. 2010;151(11):5438–45.
47. Bohlin KS, et al. Influence of the modifiable life-style factors body mass index and smoking on the outcome of hysterectomy. Acta Obstet Gynecol Scand. 2016;95(1):65–73.
48. Domingo J, et al. Ovarian response to controlled ovarian hyperstimulation in cancer patients is diminished even before oncological treatment. Fertil Steril. 2012;97(4):930–4.
49. Friedler S, et al. Ovarian response to stimulation for fertility preservation in women with malignant disease: a systematic review and meta-analysis. Fertil Steril. 2012;97(1):125–33.
50. Robertson AD, Missmer SA, Ginsburg ES. Embryo yield after in vitro fertilization in women undergoing embryo banking for fertility preservation before chemotherapy. Fertil Steril. 2011;95(2):588–91.
51. Alvarez RM, Ramanathan P. Fertility preservation in female oncology patients: the influence of the type of cancer on ovarian stimulation response. Hum Reprod. 2016;pii:dew158.
52. Bedoschi GM, et al. Ovarian stimulation during the luteal phase for fertility preservation of cancer patients: case reports and review of the literature. J Assist Reprod Genet. 2010;27(8):491–4.
53. von Wolff M, et al. Timing of ovarian stimulation in patients prior to gonadotoxic therapy: an analysis of 684 stimulations. Eur J Obstet Gynecol Reprod Biol. 2016;199:146–9.
54. Turan V, et al. Safety and feasibility of performing two consecutive ovarian stimulation cycles with the use of letrozole-gonadotropin protocol for fertility preservation in breast cancer patients. Fertil Steril. 2013;100(6):1681–5 e1.
55. Goldrat O, et al. Pregnancy following breast cancer using assisted reproduction and its effect on long-term outcome. Eur J Cancer. 2015;51(12):1490–6.
56. Oktay K, et al. Fertility preservation in breast cancer patients: a prospective controlled comparison of ovarian stimulation with tamoxifen and letrozole for embryo cryopreservation. J Clin Oncol. 2005;23(19):4347–53.
57. Woodson AH, et al. Breast cancer, BRCA mutations, and attitudes regarding pregnancy and preimplantation genetic diagnosis. Oncologist. 2014;19(8):797–804.
58. Staton AD, et al. Cancer risk reduction and reproductive concerns in female BRCA1/2 mutation carriers. Familial Cancer. 2008;7(2):179–86.
59. Michalska D, et al. Comparison of whole genome amplification and nested-PCR methods for preimplantation genetic diagnosis for BRCA1 gene mutation on unfertilized oocytes-a pilot study. Hered Cancer Clin Pract. 2013;11(1):10.
60. Practice Committee of American Society for Reproductive Medicine. Ovarian tissue cryopreservation: a committee opinion. Fertil Steril. 2014;101(5):1237–43.
61. Silber SJ, et al. Ovarian transplantation between monozygotic twins discordant for premature ovarian failure. N Engl J Med. 2005;353(1):58–63.

62. Donnez J, et al. Livebirth after orthotopic transplantation of cryopreserved ovarian tissue. Lancet. 2004;364(9443):1405–10.
63. Silber S. Ovarian tissue cryopreservation and transplantation: scientific implications. J Assist Reprod Genet. 2016;33(12):1595–603.
64. Silber SJ. Ovary cryopreservation and transplantation for fertility preservation. Mol Hum Reprod. 2012;18(2):59–67.
65. Greve T, et al. Cryopreserved ovarian cortex from patients with leukemia in complete remission contains no apparent viable malignant cells. Blood. 2012;120(22):4311–6.
66. Campos AL, et al. Comparison between slow freezing and vitrification in terms of ovarian tissue viability in a bovine model. Rev Bras Ginecol Obstet. 2016;38(7):333–9.
67. Arav A, et al. Ovarian function 6 years after cryopreservation and transplantation of whole sheep ovaries. Reprod Biomed Online. 2010;20(1):48–52.
68. Duncan FE, et al. Ovarian tissue transport for fertility preservation: from animals to human. Reproduction. 2016;152(6):R201–10.
69. Yin O, Cayton K, Segars JH. In vitro activation: a dip into the primordial follicle pool? J Clin Endocrinol Metab. 2016;101(10):3568–70.
70. Garrido-Oyarzun MF, Castelo-Branco C. Controversies over the use of GnRH agonists for reduction of chemotherapy-induced gonadotoxicity. Climacteric. 2016;19:522–5.
71. Kitajima Y, et al. Hyperstimulation and a gonadotropin-releasing hormone agonist modulate ovarian vascular permeability by altering expression of the tight junction protein claudin-5. Endocrinology. 2006;147(2):694–9.
72. Yu Ng EH, et al. Effect of pituitary downregulation on antral follicle count, ovarian volume and stromal blood flow measured by three-dimensional ultrasound with power Doppler prior to ovarian stimulation. Hum Reprod. 2004;19(12):2811–5.
73. Martin JR, et al. Ovarian cryopreservation with transposition of a contralateral ovary: a combined approach for fertility preservation in women receiving pelvic radiation. Fertil Steril. 2007;87(1):189 e5–7.
74. Husseinzadeh N, et al. The preservation of ovarian function in young women undergoing pelvic radiation therapy. Gynecol Oncol. 1984;18(3):373–9.
75. Barahmeh S, et al. Ovarian transposition before pelvic irradiation: indications and functional outcome. J Obstet Gynaecol Res. 2013;39(11):1533–7.
76. Delotte J, Bongain A. Ovarian torsion after transposition in patients with gynecologic cancer. J Minim Invasive Gynecol. 2016;23(1):139.
77. Gomez-Hidalgo NR, et al. Ovarian torsion after laparoscopic ovarian transposition in patients with gynecologic cancer: a report of two cases. J Minim Invasive Gynecol. 2015;22(4):687–90.
78. Tsai YS, et al. Shielding during x-ray examination of pediatric female patients with developmental dysplasia of the hip. J Radiol Prot. 2014;34(4):801–9.
79. Lanowska M, et al. Radical vaginal trachelectomy (RVT) combined with laparoscopic lymphadenectomy: prospective study of 225 patients with early-stage cervical cancer. Int J Gynecol Cancer. 2011;21(8):1458–64.
80. Denschlag D, Reed NS, Rodolakis A. Fertility-sparing approaches in gynecologic cancers: a review of ESGO task force activities. Curr Oncol Rep. 2012;14(6):535–8.
81. Maltaris T, et al. Reproduction beyond cancer: a message of hope for young women. Gynecol Oncol. 2006;103(3):1109–21.
82. Morice P. Borderline tumours of the ovary and fertility. Eur J Cancer. 2006;42(2):149–58.
83. Seong SJ, et al. Controversies in borderline ovarian tumors. J Gynecol Oncol. 2015;26(4):343–9.
84. Gallos ID, et al. Regression, relapse, and live birth rates with fertility-sparing therapy for endometrial cancer and atypical complex endometrial hyperplasia: a systematic review and metaanalysis. Am J Obstet Gynecol. 2012;207(4):266 e1–12.

Chapter 16
Metformin as Adjuvant Therapy in Ovarian and Endometrial Cancers

Leslie H. Clark and Victoria L. Bae-Jump

Abstract Obesity has been linked with increased risk for and worse outcomes from cancer, including gynecologic cancers. Metformin (1,1-dimethylbiguanide) is a biguanide anti-hyperglycemic widely used for the treatment of type 2 diabetes. Epidemiologic studies suggest metformin both lowers cancer risk and improves cancer outcomes in diabetic patients when compared to those treated with other anti-diabetic medications. This epidemiologic evidence prompted pre-clinical investigation of the effects of metformin in cancer. In vitro and in vivo data find that metformin possesses anti-cancer effects through both indirect and direct effects on tumor growth. Indirect effects are likely due to inhibition of hepatic gluconcogenesis, resulting in reduced circulating glucose and insulin levels, which may decrease growth factor-stimulated tumor growth. Metformin may directly affect tumor growth through inhibition of mitochondrial complex 1 and activation of adenosine monophosphate-activated protein kinase (AMPK), resulting in the regulation of multiple downstream signaling pathways that control cell proliferation and metabolism, including inhibition of the mammalian target of rapamycin (mTOR) pathway as well as decreased fatty acid and lipid sythesis.

Keywords Biguanides • Metformin—anti cancer effects • Polycystic ovary syndrome • LKBI • AMPK • Hyperinsulinemia • Organic cation transporters • Preoperative metformin

Introduction

This chapter will review the underlying biologic mechanisms of metformin's anti-tumorigenic effects as a possible adjuvant treatment for ovarian and endometrial cancer. We will assess the epidemiologic and pre-clinical data that supports the use

L.H. Clark, M.D. • V.L. Bae-Jump, M.D., Ph.D. (✉)
University of North Carolina School of Medicine,
101 Manning Drive, First Floor, Chapel Hill, NC 27514, USA
e-mail: Leslie.Clark@unchealth.unc.edu; vbae@unch.unc.edu

© Springer International Publishing AG 2018   279
N.A. Berger et al. (eds.), *Focus on Gynecologic Malignancies*, Energy Balance
and Cancer 13, DOI 10.1007/978-3-319-63483-8_16

of metformin in patients with endometrial and ovarian cancer and explore its potential for the prevention and treatment of both of these cancers. Finally, we will review current and future clinical trials that incorporate metformin as a prevention or treatment strategy for gynecological cancers.

Overview of Metformin

Metformin is a member of the biguanide class of drugs. It is widely used as the first line treatment of type 2 diabetes [1]. Metformin was approved in the United States in 1994 and is known to be effective, well-tolerated and inexpensive [2]. Additional clinical uses of metformin in women include the treatment of menstrual dysfunction and infertility due to polycystic ovarian syndrome (PCOS). Furthermore, metformin has been used to prevent the development of diabetes in patients with obesity and the metabolic syndrome [3, 4]. Mounting epidemiological evidence finds that metformin reduces cancer incidence and death in diabetic patients [5–9]. This data led to an interest in the use of metformin for both cancer treatment and prevention. Metformin is currently undergoing investigation for the treatment and prevention of several cancers, including breast, colon and prostate cancer, as well as being explored in gynecologic cancers [10–16].

Metformin's Anti-tumorigenic Effects

Metformin is believed to have both indirect and direct effects on tumor growth. It is controversial which of these effects are the most important for metformin's anti-tumorigenic activity (Fig. 16.1) [9]. One proposed indirect mechanism is that through suppression of hepatic gluconeogenesis, metformin increases insulin sensitivity and reduces circulating glucose and insulin levels resulting in decreased growth factor stimulation of tumor cells [17]. Additionally, metformin enhances peripheral glucose uptake and decreases absorption of glucose from the gastrointestinal tract [18]. Furthermore, metformin may antagonize the action of glucagon, resulting in decreased fasting glucose levels [19]. It is also hypothesized that increases in peripheral utilization of glucose may be secondary to improved insulin binding to insulin receptors seen with metformin treatment [20]. Metformin has also been shown to modulate the gut microbiota, by increasing the mucin-degrading bacterium Akkermansia, in obese mice [21].

On the cellular or direct level, metformin enters cells through cation-selective transporters, inhibits mitochondrial respiratory complex 1, leading to suppression of tricarboxylic acid (TCA) cycle flux, interrupted oxidative phosphorylation and decreased mitochondrial ATP production [9, 22–24]. Tumors engineered to express a surrogate for complex 1 that is refractory to metformin were found to be resistant to metformin in vivo [24], supporting that metformin's effects on mitochondrial

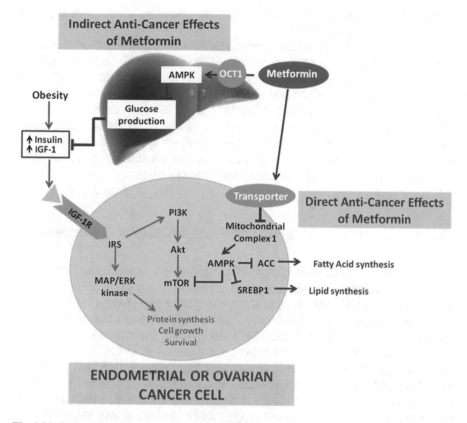

Fig. 16.1 Indirect and direct anti-cancer effects of metformin

metabolism are critical to direct inhibition of tumor growth. The resulting cellular energetic stress from inhibition of complex 1 raises the AMP/ATP ratio, resulting in increased AMPK signaling via phsophorylation by LKB1 as well as stimulated glycolysis and fatty acid oxidation. AMPK is a central regulator of multiple signaling pathways that control cellular proliferation and metabolism, including inhibition of the mTOR pathway (i.e. specifically mTORC1 inhibition) [9]. In addition, metformin has been found to inhibit the mTOR pathway via AMPK-independent mechanisms, potentially through its effects on the Ragulator complex and REDD1 upregulation or *via* enhanced PRAS40 binding to RAPTOR [9, 25–28].

Hyperinsulinemia, IGF-1 and IGF-1R levels are important in both endometrial and ovarian cancer development and progression. Signaling through the IGF-1R pathway leads to activation of the PI3K/Akt/mTOR pathway [29–34]. Activation of the PI3K/Akt/mTOR pathway, through PIK3CA amplifications, PIK3CA/PIK3R1/PIK3R2 mutations and phosphatase and tensin homolog (PTEN) mutations/loss of function, is common in endometrial cancer and has been linked to more aggressive tumor behavior [35–38]. Similar to endometrial cancer, components of the mTOR pathway, including Akt, PI3K and PTEN, are often mutated, amplified or aberrantly expressed in ovarian cancers [39–44].

Taken together, obesity is a high-energy, pro-inflammatory condition that culminates in increased growth factor signaling via the insulin/IGF-1 axis, as well as a nutrient-saturated environment via increased glucose (and other nutrients), ultimately resulting in excessive stimulation of the PI3K/Akt/mTOR pathway [45–48]. In experimental animal models, diet-induced obesity leads to activation of Akt and mTOR in epithelial tissues [49, 50]. Conversely, calorie restriction represses signaling through this pathway [49, 50]. Therefore, obesity may create a unique environment that can be exploited by a therapeutic approach, such as metformin, resulting in improved outcomes for both endometrial and ovarian cancer.

Cation-Selective Transporters Mediate Efficacy of Metformin

Metformin is one of the most hydrophilic drugs known, necessitating transporters to facilitate cell uptake. Metformin uptake is mediated by organic cation transporters (OCT)1–3 and the plasma membrane monoamine transporter (PMAT), and its extrusion is dependent on the human multidrug and toxin extrusion (MATE) transporters 1 and 2 [51–57]. MATE1/2 have been typically implicated in the extrusion of compounds from cells; however, there is evidence that MATE1/2 may be bidirectional transporters and facilitate uptake of compounds into cells [58]. The expression patterns of these transporters differs significantly between normal and tumor tissues, but all have been found in both ovarian and endometrial cancers [59, 60]. Recent studies in breast cancer suggest that metformin transporter expression may play a critical role in tumor responsiveness to metformin [61]. Metformin uptake into human breast cancer cell lines has been shown to be dictated by the expression levels of these cation-selective transporters [61]. Furthermore, in xenograft mouse models of breast cancer, metformin was more effective in shrinking tumors developed from an OCT3-overexpressing breast cancer cell line versus tumors developed from wild-type cells [61]. These results suggest that variation in expression of transporters may contribute to differential susceptibility of cancers to metformin's anti-tumorigenic effects and may even serve as a biomarker predictive of response to this agent, given that metformin can only have activity if it is able to enter tumor cells.

It is also reasonable to postulate that genetic diversity in cation-selective transporters could affect outcomes of metformin treatment in cancer, as genetic variations in transporters have been shown to influence metformin's pharmacokinetics and glucose-lowering effects in humans [59, 62–65]. Single nucleotide polymorphisms (SNPs) are the most common genetic variations in the human genome; therefore, SNPs in transporters can cause variability in response to drug treatment. The effect of genetic variations in transporters is currently being explored in some of the ongoing clinical trials of metformin for cancer treatment.

Alternative Biguanides to Metformin

Phenformin is another biguanide with anti-diabetic as well as anti-tumorigenic activity. Phenformin is almost 50 times as potent as metformin for the treatment of diabetes, but it was withdrawn from the market in the United States in 1977 due to a small increased risk of lactic acidosis (64 cases per 100,000 patient-years), higher than that seen with metformin (3 per 100,000 years) [66]. Lactic acid is formed because biguanides impair mitochondrial respiration via inhibition of complex I, which can result in a compensatory acceleration of glycolysis to counteract the reduced ATP production via oxidative phosphorylation [67]. Metformin is a less powerful inhibitor of the mitochondrial respiratory chain, which may decrease its risk for lactic acidosis [22]. The increased incidence of lactic acidosis with phenformin may also occur through its inhibition of lactate oxidation [68, 69] and stimulation of lactate release from muscle. In contrast, metformin increases lactate oxidation and does not alter the release of lactate from muscle [70]. Nonetheless, given that phenformin is safer and has fewer side effects than many of the typical cytotoxic and targeted agents used for cancer treatment, this potential increased risk may be tolerated if phenformin has greater anti-neoplastic properties than metformin.

As previously mentioned, metformin is highly hydrophilic with a net positive charge at all physiologic pH values; and therefore, requires cation-selective transporter proteins that mediate its entry into cells [71]. Phenformin is more lipophilic and is not reliant on these transporter proteins, allowing for higher concentrations of this biguanide over metformin to accumulate intracellularly. It has been theorized that phenformin may have heightened anti-tumorigenic efficacy as compared to metformin, due to increased uptake of this drug by tumor cells. In vitro and in vivo studies in a variety of cancer types demonstrate that phenformin is more potent for inhibiting cell proliferation and tumor growth than metformin [72–79]. Although the risk/benefit ratio clearly favors metformin over phenformin for the treatment of diabetes, this may not hold true for the treatment of cancer if phenformin was found to have superior efficacy. Metformin and phenformin have not been compared head-to-head in cell lines and mouse models for either ovarian or endometrial cancer.

Efforts are also underway to pharmacologically improve on metformin for both the treatment of diabetes and cancer. The understanding of metformin's complex pharmacology drives the design of novel biguanides with improved potency and transporter selectivity. The ability of metformin to lower blood glucose is dependent on OCT1 [22, 59]. OCT2 is predominantly expressed in the kidney and is responsible for metformin clearance in the urine [22, 59, 80]. OCT3 is thought to be particularly important in the uptake of metformin in muscle [22, 59]. OCT1 and OCT3 are highly expressed in epithelial ovarian cancer and ovarian germ cell tumors, respectively [81, 82]. Thus, novel biguanides with increased affinity for OCT1 and 3 and lower affinity for OCT2 may provide more potent and ovarian cancer selective AMPK activators, with a longer plasma half-life than metformin. This profile is also anticipated to have a profound effect on metabolic parameters; since OCT1 is expressed at high levels in the liver [83] where an AMPK activator is likely to reduce glucose levels and insulin secretion.

NovaTarg Therapeutics has designed, synthesized and screened ~140 biguanides to identify compounds that have high affinity for OCT1 and 3 with reduced activity at OCT2, in order to find compounds that would be effective in treating diabetes and cancer. Of these compounds, NT1014 has displayed particularly promising activity in ovarian cancer. NovaTarg has demonstrated the anti-diabetic effects of these agents in animal models. In all experiments, NT1014 was more effective than the gold standard of metformin at 1/5th of the dose [84]. The anti-tumorigenic effects of NT1014 have also been examined in human ovarian cancer cell lines and a genetically engineered mouse model of high grade serous ovarian cancer [84]. NT1014 significantly inhibited cell proliferation in the ovarian cancer cell lines, at doses that where 2–5 times lower than that for metformin in these cell lines [84]. In addition, NT1014 activated AMPK, inhibited downstream targets of the mTOR pathway, induced G1 cell cycle arrest/apoptosis/cellular stress, altered glycolysis and reduced invasion/adhesion in both ovarian cancer cell lines [84]. Similar to its anti-proliferative effects in vitro, NT1014 decreased tumor growth in a ovarian cancer mouse model and showed more significant inhibition compared to metformin at the same dose, as evidenced by a decrease in tumor weight of approximately 70% in the NT1014 group and 46% in the metformin group [84]. Thus, novel biguanides, such as NT1014, may have increased efficacy over metformin, but their efficacy even more so than metformin may be critically dependent on transporter expression in the tumors themselves.

Lastly, another approach to increasing the potency and efficacy of metformin would be to use supratherapeutic dosing. All clinical trials to date of metformin for the treatment of cancer, including the ongoing trials in ovarian and endometrial cancer, have used typical diabetic dosing of the drug. Higher doses of metformin should be associated with increased penetration of drug to tumor, which may align with improved efficacy as compared to traditional diabetic dosing of metformin. As ongoing clinical trials unfold and if metformin has proven anti-cancer efficacy, the question of adequate dosing should be further addressed.

Pre-clinical Studies of Metformin and Endometrial and Ovarian Cancer

Metformin has been studied in multiple cancer types, including endometrial and ovarian cancer, in the pre-clinical setting. This biguanide has been consistently found to decrease tumor growth both in vitro and in xenograft and genetically engineered mouse models [9]. Metformin-mediated AMPK activation has been found to decrease endometrial cancer cell growth via inhibition of mTOR signaling [85–87]. Some studies have noted differential AMPK activation dependent on mutational status, with K-Ras mutated tumors being more responsive to metformin treatment [86]. In a mouse model of endometrial hyperplasia, metformin induced anti-proliferative effects on the endometrium that coincided with inhibition of downstream targets of the mTOR pathway [88]. In vitro, treatment of endometrial cancer cells with metformin via serum from PCOS patients after 6 months of treatment with metformin (850 mg twice daily) significantly reduced invasion compared to matched controls [89]. Furthermore, metformin appears to hinder estrogen-mediated endometrial proliferation in obese rats compared to untreated controls [90].

Additionally, pre-clinical data findss that metformin in combination with paclitaxel or cisplatin has synergistic, anti-proliferative effects in endometrial cancer cell lines [91, 92]. Metformin has also been shown to reverse progestin resistance in endometrial cancer cell lines, suggesting that metformin and progestins used in combination may be a promising therapeutic strategy in endometrial cancer [93–95].

In ovarian cancer, metformin has been found to inhibit cell proliferation, migration, angiogenesis, invasion and adhesion in human ovarian cancer cell lines and mouse models [96–103]. Metformin has been shown to have anti-proliferative effects in both platinum-sensitive and platinum-resistant ovarian cancer cell lines [104]. Furthermore, metformin has been found to behave synergistically when used in combination with platinum (i.e. carboplatin or cisplatin) in ovarian cancer cell lines in both primary isolates from ovarian cancer patients and ovarian cancer mouse models [100, 105–107]. Metformin has also been shown to inhibit ovarian cancer stem cells both in vitro and in vivo [106].

Recently metformin has been combined with the poly-ADP ribose polymerase (PARP) inhibitor, olaparib, in ovarian cancer with promising results. PARP inhibitors are a novel class of therapeutics being evaluated in ovarian cancer with particular affinity for BRCA mutated tumors. The addition of metformin to olaparib therapy resulted in greater effects on inhibition of cell and tumor growth in BRCA mutated ovarian cancer cell lines and mouse models, respectively [108]. The combination of meformin and olabarib also led to a potentiation of cisplatin sensitivity in vitro and in vivo as well as increased activation of AMPK [108].

Some preclinical data in animal models suggests that the anti-tumorigenic efficacy of metformin is dependent on the metabolic composition of its host. Metformin has been found to be more effective in inhibiting tumor growth in obese and insulin resistant animals compared to their lean counterparts in a variety of tumor types, including breast, lung, and ovarian cancer [109–111]. In particular for ovarian cancer, diet induced-obesity promoted more aggressive tumor growth in a genetically engineered mouse model of high grade serous ovarian cancer [112], coincident with mitochondrial dysfunction and energy supplied by fatty acid oxidation rather than glycolysis in tumors from obese versus lean mice [113]. Furthermore, metformin was found to be more efficacious in the inhibition of OC tumor growth in obese versus lean mice, which corresponded with inhibition of mitochondrial complex I, halting of fatty acid oxidation and reversion back to glycolysis in *only* tumors from obese mice [113]. In a randomized, placebo-controlled pre-operative window study in breast cancer patients, women with higher BMIs and HOMA indexes had a greater response to metformin as evidenced by a decrease in Ki-67 staining [10]. These findings suggest that the anti-tumorigenic effects of metformin may be heightened in the setting of obesity and insulin resistance, due to its ability to improve the metabolic milieu of patients either indirectly or directly.

However, in striking contrast, metformin treatment has been found to elicit greater reductions in tumor growth in normoglycemic versus hyperglycemic conditions in a syngeneic ovarian cancer mouse model [114], suggesting the opposite effect in that metformin may have greater anti-tumorigenic efficacy in non-diabetic as opposed to diabetic patients. Alternatively, it could be argued that hyperglycemia and obesity may not be interchangeable in their impact on modifying metformin response for cancer treatment. Nonetheless, this data underscores the importance of evaluating the metabolic milieu of a patient as a potential biomarker of metformin response in cancer therapeutic trials using evolving technologies such as metabolomic profiling, discussed later in this chapter. Tissue specific biomarkers capable of predicting response to metformin treatment are still needed. There is some preclinical data to suggest that changes in expression of cell growth regulator with ring finger domain 1 (CGRRF1), a tumor suppressor gene thought to reflect the insulin-sensitivity of tissues in response to metformin treatment, may have utility in predicting response to metformin treatment in obese individuals [115]. However, further exploration of this hypothesis is needed.

Epidemiology of Metformin and Endometrial Cancer

Endometrial cancer is the most common cancer of the female genital tract and the fourth most common cancer in women in the United States [116]. The incidence of endometrial cancer in the United States has been increasing, secondary to an aging female population and changes in dietary and hormonal factors. Particularly, the ongoing obesity epidemic in the United States and across developed countries is a major culprit. In 2016, approximately 60,050 new cases of endometrial cancer will be diagnosed with 10,470 deaths [117]. Obesity, diabetes and insulin resistance are risk factors known to drive the development of endometrial cancer [118–121]. For each increase in BMI of 5 kg/m^2, there is a significantly increased risk of developing endometrial cancer [122]. Obesity is not only a risk factor for developing endometrial cancer, but may be associated with an increased risk of death [121, 123–126]. Women with endometrial cancer who have a BMI over 40 kg/m^2 have a sixfold increased risk of death compared to their non-obese counterparts [124], although it is controversial if this is related to all-cause versus cancer-specific mortality.

Overall, up to 25% of those patients diagnosed with local disease and 50% of those with advanced disease will die of their endometrial cancer despite currently available therapies [127]. Thus, novel therapeutic strategies are greatly needed in endometrial cancer, particularly for advanced and recurrent disease. Given the high incidence of obesity in endometrial cancer, therapeutics like metformin that target obesity and insulin-resistance are particularly relevant for this disease.

Endometrial cancer has been subdivided into two main categories, type I (85%) and type II (15%) disease, based on clinical and pathologic variation [128]. Type I endometrial cancers are composed of tumors with endometrioid histology and typically arise due to excess estrogen from chronic anovulation and obesity. Type I tumors occur more frequently in younger, Caucasian women than type II tumors. In addition, type I tumors are often diagnosed at an early stage and are associated with a good prognosis. In contrast, type II endometrial cancers, or those of non-endometrioid histology, are predominantly serous and tend to occur in the older postmenopausal population. These tumors affect a greater percent of African American women. By definition, type II tumors are poorly differentiated and often diagnosed at advanced stages. Type II tumors carry a poor prognosis compared to type I tumors. Increasing evidence suggests that obesity and diabetes are strong risk factors for both type I and II endometrial cancers despite traditional teaching that obesity is solely associated with type I tumors [118, 120].

Several epidemiologic studies evaluating the impact of metformin on endometrial cancer outcomes are listed in Table 16.1. Currie et al. found that diabetic women who were taking metformin at the time of ovarian or endometrial cancer diagnosis had half the risk of death compared to non-metformin users (HR: 0.48, 95% CI: 0.28–0.81) [129]. However, limitations to this study included a lack of information on pathology, treatment and stage, all of which can significantly alter cancer outcomes. A retrospective study of type II endometrial cancers also showed improved survival in diabetics who were taking metformin compared to non-metformin users and non-diabetics [130]. Ko et al. conducted a multi-institutional retrospective cohort study of endometrial cancer patients with diabetes and compared outcomes between metformin and non-metformin users [131]. Nearly all patient in both groups were obese, and the majority had hypertension. Metformin users were found to have improved recurrence free survival and overall survival, even after adjusting for age, stage, grade, histology and adjuvant treatment [131]. However, metformin use was not associated with improvements in time-to-recurrence (TTR) [131]. This epidemiologic data suggests that metformin may offer a survival benefit from all-cause mortality, but its potential impact on cancer specific outcomes remains less certain.

The relationship between metformin use and risk of developing endometrial cancer has also been explored. In a study of the General Practice Research Database, "any prior use of metformin" was compared to "no prior use" and was not associated with an altered risk of endometrial cancer in either the main analysis (adjusted OR 0.86, 95% CI 0.63–1.18) or the analysis restricted to diabetic cases and controls (adjusted OR 0.87, 95% CI 0.63–1.21) [132]. The authors note several limitations to this study including lack of histological data and the inability to adjust for common variables associated with the risk of endometrial cancer such as physical activity, parity, race and genetic predisposition [132]. Similar findings were seen in a population cohort analysis using the Truven Health Analytics MarketScan® database [133]. The findings of these studies is disappointing given than metformin would seem to be a logical agent for endometrial cancer prevention. Given the discrepancies between the promising pre-clinical studies and these epidemiological findings, further research will be needed to determine the role of metformin in the prevention of endometrial cancer.

Table 16.1 Epidemiologic data on metformin and gynecologic cancer

Investigator [reference]	Subjects enrolled	Study type	Primary site	Database (years collected)	Findings
Bodmer et al. [142]	1611	Retrospective case-control	Ovarian	General Practice Research Database (1995–2009)	Metformin use associated with decreased risk of cancer (OR: 0.61, 95% CI 0.30–1.25)
Romero et al. [143]	341	Retrospective cohort	Ovarian	Single institution database (1992–2010)	Improved PFS and OS in type 2 diabetics on metformin (PFS = 51%, OS = 63%) vs. non-diabetics (PFS = 23%, OS = 37%) and diabetics not on metformin (PFS = 8%, OS = 23%), $p = 0.03$ and $p = 0.03$, respectively
Kumar et al. [144]	239	Retrospective case-control	Ovarian	Single institution database (1995–2010)	Metformin use associated with improved survival (67% vs. 47%), $p = 0.007$
Currie et al. [129]	112,408	Retrospective cohort	Ovarian and endometrial	More than 350 primary care centers in the U.K. (1990–2009)	Diabetics taking metformin at the time of diagnosis, had half the risk of dying when compared to non-metformin users (HR: 0.48, 95% CI: 0.28–0.81)
Becker et al. [132]	2554	Retrospective case-control	Endometrial	General Practice Research Database (1995–2012)	Metformin use did not impact risk of developing endometrial cancer (adjusted OR 0.86, 95% CI 0.63–1.18)
Nevadunsky et al. [130]	985	Retrospective cohort	Endometrial (non-endometrioid histologies only)	Single institution database (1999–2009)	Improved OS in diabetics on metformin (HR: 0.54, 95% CI: 0.30–0.97)
Ko et al. [133]	1561	Retrospective cohort	Endometrial	Multi-institutional database (2005–2010)	Non-metformin users had 1.8 times worse RFS (95% CI: 1.1–2.9, $p = 0.02$) and 2.3 times worse OS (95% CI: 1.3–4.2, $p = 0.005$)

OR odds ratio, *HR* hazard ratio, *CI* confidence interval, *PFS* progression free survival, *RFS* recurrence free survival, *OS* overall survival.

Epidemiology of Metformin and Ovarian Cancer

Epithelial ovarian cancer is the second most common cancer of the female genital tract, with an estimated 22,280 cases in 2016 [117]. Ovarian cancer is often diagnosed at a late stage making it one of the most deadly cancers with an overall 5-year survival of only 30–40%, including 14,240 deaths in 2016 alone [117, 134, 135].

There are several important prognostic indicators for ovarian cancer, which include stage, age, histology, success of debulking surgery and performance status [136]. Additionally, increasing evidence suggests that obesity is a significant risk factor for ovarian cancer development and is associated with worse disease outcomes, including an up to 1.6-fold increased risk of death [124]. Three meta-analyses looking at the effect of obesity on ovarian cancer survival have demonstrated increased risks associated with obesity [137–139]. Timing of obesity exposure may also be particularly important. Adolescence and early adulthood may represent a particularly vulnerable time for exposure to obesity. One study found that individuals who were overweight or obese at ages 18–29 had the highest risk of ovarian cancer mortality [138]. While other studies have shown that adolescent exposure to obesity bears the greatest risk for future ovarian cancer development [139–141].

In addition to the previously mentioned analysis by Curric et al. [129], three studies have found metformin use to be associated with decreased risk and improved outcomes in diabetic ovarian cancer patients. These studies are listed in Table 16.1. The first study is a case control design using the United Kingdom General Practice Research Database [142]. Diabetic metformin users had a decreased risk of ovarian cancer compared to non-metformin users. Another study showed that diabetic ovarian cancer patients on metformin had improved progression-free survival compared to non-diabetics and diabetics not on metformin [143]. A final retrospective case-control study of ovarian cancer patients found that metformin users had improved overall survival compared to non-metformin users (67% vs. 47%), even after controlling for stage, grade, histology, chemotherapy, BMI and degree of surgical cytoreduction [144].

Pre-operative Window Studies of Metformin in Endometrial Cancer

Pre-operative window studies, or phase 0 studies, take advantage of a natural gap in cancer care such as the time from diagnosis until surgery to test a potential therapeutic agent. These studies use biomarker endpoints as surrogates to determine the potential efficacy of a drug [145]. By comparing pre- and post-treatment samples, such studies can give a glimpse into the potential therapeutic effects of a drug of interest. To be successful, there must be a testable biomarker in the pre- and post-treatment tissue [145]. Window studies have been utilized in numerous disease sites including breast, colon, prostate and gynecologic cancers [10, 146–150]. Antigen Ki-67 is a human nuclear protein that is associated with and may be necessary for cellular proliferation, making it a popular marker to demonstrate the effects of a given drug in pre-operative window studies [151]. Other potential biomarkers for window studies of metformin are AMPK, phosphorylated-S6 and other downstream markers of the AMPK/mTOR pathway. Pre-operative window studies in breast and prostate cancer have found metformin to reduce Ki-67 staining, signifying decreases in cellular proliferation with metformin treatment [10, 150, 152].

To date, there have been five reported preoperative window studies of metformin in gynecologic cancers, and all have been conducted in endometrial cancer patients [153–158]. There are also two ongoing window trials of metformin in endometrial cancer being conducted with one at the University of Arkansas with ongoing recruitment and one trial combining metformin with doxycycline in uterine or breast cancer at Thomas Jefferson University. These seven window of opportunity trials evaluating metformin are summarized in Table 16.2.

Regarding the five completed window trials, the first was reported by Mitsuhashi et al., and this study evaluated 31 endometrial cancer patients with grade 1 or 2 endometrioid adenocarcinoma treated with 750 mg of metformin increased weekly to a maximum dose of 1500–2250 mg daily for 4–6 weeks preoperatively [158]. When comparing pre-metformin treatment curettage specimen to post-treatment hysterectomy specimen, the authors noted a 44.2% reduction in Ki-67 expression ($p < 0.001$). Overall, 28 patients (90%) responded to treatment. Ten control specimens were retrospectively obtained and showed no change in Ki-67 expression from diagnostic biopsy to hysterectomy specimen. The median age on this trial was 51 years (range 27–72 years) with a mean BMI of 28 kg/m^2 (range 18–42 kg/m^2). Serum insulin, glucose, IGF-1 and leptin levels also decreased with metformin treatment.

Laskov et al. evaluated 11 non-diabetic patients with endometrial cancer (eight with endometrioid histology and three with non-endometrioid histology) who underwent treatment with metformin 500 mg three times daily from diagnosis until surgery for a mean of 36.6 days [158]. They found a reduction in serum insulin, IGF-1 and IGF binding protein levels following metformin treatment. When comparing pre-treatment endometrial biopsies to post-treatment hysterectomy specimens, there was a 9.7% reduction in Ki-67 staining ($p = 0.02$) and a 31% reduction in phosphorylated-S6 ($p = 0.03$). Furthermore, this study evaluated 10 control patients and noted no change in Ki-67 or phosphorylated-S6 from diagnostic biopsy to hysterectomy specimen, indicating that observed changes in the treatment arm were due to metformin treatment and not related to simply comparing an endometrial biopsy to a hysterectomy specimen [153].

In a study by Schuler et al., 20 obese women who were to undergo surgical staging for endometrial cancer received short-term metformin treatment (850 mg once a day) until the day before their surgery [154]. Diabetic women on insulin or metformin therapy were excluded from this trial. The mean age was 58.8 years, and the mean BMI was 39.6 kg/m^2 (range 30.8–52.2 kg/m^2). Patients received metformin for a mean duration of 14.6 days (range of 7–28 days). When comparing pre-treatment endometrial biopsies to post-treatment hysterectomy specimens, metformin significantly reduced Ki-67 staining by 11.8% ($p = 0.008$). Overall, 65% of patients (13/20) responded to metformin treatment, with a mean decrease in Ki-67 staining of 21.9%

Table 16.2 Window of opportunity trials evaluating metformin in endometrial cancer.

Investigator	Subjects enrolled	Dose	Duration	Status	Results	Biomarkers	Clinical trial identifier [reference]
Schuler et al.	20	850 mg daily	Mean of 14.6 days (range 7–28)	Published	11.8% reduction in Ki-67	Metabolomics with alterations in lipid, amino acid and microbiome metabolism greater in responders	NCT01911247 [154]
Soliman et al.	20	850 mg daily	Median of 9.5 days (range 7–24)	Published	No change in Ki-67	Reductions in glucose, IGF-1, omentin, insulin, c-peptide, leptin and adiponectin	NCT01205672
Mitsuhashi et al.	31	1500–2250 mg daily	Range 4–6 weeks	Published	44.2% reduction in Ki-67	Reductions in glucose, insulin, IGF-1, HOMA-R, leptin and adiponectin	[158]
Laskov et al.	11	500 mg three times daily	Mean of 36.6 days	Published	9.7% reduction in Ki-67	Reductions in insulin, IGF-1, IGFBP-1	[153]
Sivalingam et al.	40 (28 treated)	850 mg twice daily	Median of 20 days (range 7–28)	Published	12.9% reduction in Ki-67	Evaluated insulin, glucose, HOMA-R and leptin but no statistical difference	[155] [156]
Burnett et al.	Goal = 40	500 mg twice daily	14–21 days	Recruiting	N/A	N/A	NCT01877564
Johnson et al.	Goal = 74	Not provided (combined with doxycycline)	7–14 days	Recruiting[a]	N/A	N/A	NCT02874430

IGF-1 insulin-like growth factor 1, *HOMA-R* homeostasis model assessment of insulin resistance, *IGFBP-1* insulin-like growth factor binding protein 1
[a]Includes breast and uterine cancer

among responders to metformin. Responders to metformin treatment were defined as those patients with an absolute decrease in percent of Ki-67 staining (observed range: 7–50%). Non-responders were defined as those who had no decrease in percent of Ki-67 staining. Glucose levels decreased in both responders and non-responders, but were only statistically significant in responders. Pre-treatment Ki-67 indices were significantly higher in responders than non-responders (47.3% vs. 24.9%, $p = 0.004$), suggesting highly proliferative tumors may be more sensitive to metformin's anti-tumorigenic effects. Metformin also decreased expression of downstream targets of the insulin/IGF-1 and mTOR pathway in the endometrial tumors, including phosphorylated-IGF1R, phosphorylated-S6 and phosphorylated-4E-BP-1, as demonstrated by immunohistochemistry [154, 159]. Expression of the metformin transporter, MATE2, decreased with metformin treatment, and approached significance in predicting response to metformin ($p = 0.0625$) [159].

For the endometrial cancer patients enrolled on this phase 0 clinical trial, metabolomic profiling was performed on serum pre- and post-metformin treatment. By Random Forest (RF) analysis, responders and non-responders to metformin treatment were predicted with 100% and 66.6% accuracy, respectively and an overall accuracy of 88% (OOB error rate of 11.76%). When comparing pre- and post-treatment serum, metformin significantly altered the concentration of 173 metabolites (37 up and 136 down) in the obese endometrial cancer patients [154]. Comparison of global biochemical serum profiles revealed several key metabolic differences between metformin responders and non-responders. Metformin-driven metabolic alterations in the responders were primarily related to elevated lipolysis, more efficient amino acid metabolism and altered gut microbiome-associated metabolites. The metabolic changes in the serum of responders as compared to non-responders to metformin treatment were co-incident with metabolic changes in their corresponding endometrial tumors [154]. In addition, responders had higher pre-metformin treatment serum levels of amino acids, dipeptides, glycolytic intermediates, arachidonic acid, monohydroxy fatty acids and lysolipids when compared to non-responders [159]. Higher pre-treatment serum levels of several fatty acids and glycolipids could be indicative of increased insulin resistance underlying increased benefit to metformin therapy. These metabolites could serve as potential biomarkers predictive of response to metformin treatment.

A similar pre-operative window study of metformin in 20 patients with endometrial cancer treated with metformin 850 mg daily by Soliman et al. found a decrease in expression of phosphorylated-Akt, phosphorylated-S6rp, and Ras-Mitogen activated protein kinase (Ras-MAPK), all of which are downstream targets of the metformin signaling cascades [157, 160]. Median treatment duration was 9.5 days (range 7–24), and the median BMI was 34.5 (range, 21.9–50.0). Insulin, IGF-1, omentin, C-peptide and leptin levels in serum were reduced with metformin treatment. In this study, the investigators did not find a difference in Ki-67 staining [160].

Finally, Sivalingam et al. published their window trial of 28 endometrial cancer patients treated with 850 mg of metformin twice daily for a 1–4 weeks preoperatively with a median treatment duration of 20 days (range 7–34 days) [155]. This study included 12 contemporaneous control patients recruited and compared for a total of 40 samples. The median age was 64 years with 60% of patients being obese and 55% with undiagnosed diabetes or insulin resistance based on enrollment serum testing. These authors found a 12.9% decrease in Ki-67 staining in the metformin treated group ($p = 0.008$), but did not see a decrease in phosphorylation of AKT or markers of insulin resistance [155]. Of note, these authors express concern regarding the use of hysterectomy specimens for evaluation of phosphorylation events due to concerns regarding devascularization of the uterus prior to preservation. While they noted no difference in Ki-67 expression using the technique of comparing endometrial biopsies to devascularized hysterectomy specimens, changes in both the control and treatment groups in protein phosphyorylation of PI3K-AKT-mTOR proteins raises concerns for evaluating these pathway changes using endometrial biopsies compared to hysterectomy specimens [156].

Overall, four of the five reported window trials of metformin in endometrial cancer show a reduction in cell proliferation as measured by Ki-67 staining of the endometrium following short term treatment with metformin prior to surgical staging. These trials demonstrate that metformin has promise as an anti-tumorigenic agent in endometrial cancer warranting its further evaluation. Furthermore, the only trial not to note a reduction in Ki-67 staining had the shortest duration of exposure (9.5 days), which may be the cause of discrepant results in this outlier trial. There are currently no window trials in ovarian cancer: however, given the recent uptake in neoadjuvant chemotherapy in patients with medical comorbidities or in cases in which complete tumor debulking is deemed unlikely, this represents an area for potential evaluation.

Completed Clinical Trials of Metformin and Cancer

Given the emerging pre-clinical and epidemiological data supporting the use of metformin in cancer treatment and prevention, multiple clinical trials are ongoing evaluating the effect of metformin in a variety of cancers. In fact, there are more than 200 clinical trials listed on www.clinicaltrials.gov for metformin in regards to cancer, including translational and pre-operative window studies, chemotherapeutic trials, prevention trials and survivorship studies.

Some of the key advantages for using metformin in cancer treatment include its low cost, oral route of administration and relatively low toxicity profile. In fact, the main side effect of metformin is gastrointestinal distress, which generally manifests as transient nausea and diarrhea. The level of gastrointestinal distress observed with metformin rarely requires discontinuation of the drug. Regarding cost, metformin is approximately one dollar per day depending on dosing which is a significant bargain relative to other emerging targeted cancer therapies.

While there are many ongoing trials for metformin for cancer treatment and prevention, there are fewer clinical trials that have been completed and reported in the literature. Of the reported trials in other cancer types, it has been demonstrated that one month of metformin treatment resulted in decreased proliferation in the size and number of colorectal aberrant crypt foci, an endoscopic surrogate marker of colorectal cancer [12]. Two similar phase I studies of temsirolimus and metformin in advanced solid tumors have been completed and demonstrate acceptable toxicity and promising response rates in heavily pre-treated patients, including a eight patients with a gynecologic malignancy (endometrial = 4, uterine carcinosarcoma = 2, ovarian = 2) [13, 161]. The aromatase inhibitor, exemastane, has been combined with metformin and rosiglitazone in obese post-menopausal women with hormone-receptor positive metastatic breast cancer and found to be well-tolerated [11]. A phase II trial of metformin and paclitaxel in advanced pancreatic cancer showed no benefit, but moderate benefit was seen when metformin was combined with 5-FU in advanced colorectal cancer [162, 163]. Metformin has also been shown to improve weight, circulating insulin levels, glucose, leptin and CRP following 6 months of treatment in non-diabetic patients who had completed surgery and neoadjuvant or adjuvant therapy for breast cancer [164].

Aside from the window studies of metformin in endometrial cancer reviewed above, there is only one resulted clinical trial of metformin in gynecologic malignancies. Mitsuhashi et al. evaluated the therapeutic benefit of combining medroxyprogesterone acetate (MPA) and metformin for fertility-preserving treatment of endometrial hyperplasia with atypia and grade 1 endometrial cancer [165]. This phase II trial enrolled 17 women with hyperplasia and 19 with endometrial cancer. Patients were treated with MPA 400 mg daily and metformin 750–2250 mg daily for 24–36 weeks. After 36 weeks of treatment, 81% of patients achieved a complete response and 14% achieved a partial response. Two patients showed progression at 12 weeks and were removed from the study. There was a 10% relapse rate during follow up for a median of 38 months [165]. There were no severe toxicities observed; however, three patients developed asymptomatic liver dysfunction attributed to fatty liver with one patient stopping metformin treatment at 23 months due to grade 2 liver dysfunction. Grade 2 gastrointestinal toxicity was seen in six patients with diarrhea and/or nausea at a dose of 2250 mg daily. Symptoms resolved in four women with dose reduction to 1500 mg daily and did not require cessation of therapy. There were no treatment related deaths or lactic acidosis; and thus, metformin treatment was overall well tolerated. Furthermore, the authors noted improvement in all translational endpoints including reduction in BMI ($31.4–29.2$ kg/m^2, $p < 0.001$), insulin ($18.4–10$ U/mL, $p < 0.001$), glucose ($107–92$ g/dL, $p < 0.001$) and homeostasis model of insulin resistance score ($5.2–2.3$, $p < 0.001$).

Ongoing Clinical Trials of Metformin and Gynecologic Cancers

There are a number of ongoing clinical trials in ovarian cancer and endometrial hyperplasia and cancer. These trials are summarized in Table 16.3. Five of these trials are focused on metformin and ovarian cancer. The University of Michigan is conducting a phase II, open label evaluation of metformin in combination with

Table 16.3 Ongoing clinical trials of metformin in ovarian and uterine cancer

Disease site	Phase	Status	Site	Regimen	Clinical trial identifier
Ovary/fallopian/peritoneal, stage III-IV	Phase II	Recruiting	University of Chicago	Metformin and combination chemotherapy	NCT02122185
Advanced ovarian	Phase IB	Recruiting	University Medical Center Gronigen	Metformin in Combination With Carboplatin and Paclitaxel	NCT02312661
Stage II–IV ovary/fallopian/peritoneal	Phase II	Recruiting	Gynecologic Oncology Associates	Metformin in Combination With Carboplatin and Paclitaxel	NCT02437812
Recurrent platinum sensitive ovarian cancer	Phase I	Withdrawn	Fox Chase Cancer Center	Metformin in Combination With Carboplatin and Paclitaxel	NCT02050009
Advanced ovarian and fallopian tube	Phase II	Active, not recruiting	University of Michigan	Metformin in Combination With Carboplatin and Paclitaxel	NCT 01579812
Endometrial hyperplasia	Phase II	Not recruiting	University of North Carolina	Metformin	NCT01685762
Endometrial hyperplasia with atypia and early endometrial cancer	Phase II	Recruiting	China	Megestrol acetate ± metformin	NCT01968317
Early endometrial cancer	Phase II	Recruiting	University of Queenslanc̄	Mirena® ± metformin ± weight loss intervention	NCT01686126
Early endometrial cancer	Phase II	Recruiting	University of North Carolina	Levonorgesterol IUD with metformin	NCT02035787
Advanced or recurrent endometrial cancer	Phase II	Active, not recruiting	MD Anderson	Everolimus, letrozole, and metformin	NCT01797523
Advanced or recurrent endometrial cancer	Phase II/III	Suspended, not recruiting	Muti-institution, GOG study	Paclitaxel/carboplatin ± metformin	NCT02065687
Advanced or recurrent endometrial cancer	Phase I/II	Not yet recruiting	France	Cyclophosphamide, metformin, and olaparib	NCT 02755844

adjuvant or neoadjuvant chemotherapy for the treatment of advanced ovarian/ fallopian tube and primary peritoneal cancer (NCT01579812). The University of Chicago is conducting a phase II, randomized-controlled trial of metformin in combination with standard chemotherapy in advanced ovarian/fallopian tube and primary peritoneal cancer (NCT02122185). The Fox Chase Cancer Center has proposed a phase II, open label trial of metformin, paclitaxel and carboplatin in recurrent, platinum sensitive ovarian cancer patients (NCT02050009). The Gynecologic Oncology Associates in conjunction with the University of North Carolina are conducting a phase II, open label, non-randomized pilot study of metformin in combination with paclitaxel/carboplatin therapy for stage II–IV ovarian/ fallopian tube/peritoneal cancer (NCT02437812). Finally, the University Medical Center Gronigen in the Netherlands has a phase Ib study of metformin combined with platinum/taxane therapy in advanced ovarian cancer (NCT02312661).

There are eight trials that are being conducted for endometrial hyperplasia and cancer including a clinical trial of single agent metformin for the treatment of endometrial hyperplasia (NCT01685762), a chemoprevention study in obese women (NCT01697566), and three trials evaluating metformin in combination with progesterone therapy (either using the levonorgestrel-releasing intrauterine device or megestrol acetate) in non-surgical patients with endometrial cancer or complex endometrial hyperplasia with atypia (NCT02035787, NCT01686126, NCT01968317). There are also three trials evaluating metformin in combination with cytotoxic chemotherapy.

The first of the three cytotoxic combination trials is being conducted by MD Anderson Cancer Center. It is a phase II trial of metformin, letrozole and everolimus in advanced and recurrent endometrial cancer patients (NCT01797523). The primary endpoint was evaluation of clinical benefit rate determined by combining the complete response rate, partial response rate and stable disease rate. Response was evaluated by repeat imaging (CT or MRI) using RECIST 1.1 at the completion of the second cycle. Preliminary results show a 67% clinical benefit rate and suggest a role for this triplet combination in advanced and recurrent endometrial cancer [166].

The Gynecologic Oncology Group (GOG) has an ongoing two arm, randomized, placebo-controlled phase II/III trial designed to assess the efficacy and safety of metformin in combination with paclitaxel and carboplatin versus paclitaxel and carboplatin alone in women with advanced and recurrent endometrial cancer (GOG 286B) (NCT02065687). The primary endpoints of the phase II and III trials are progression-free survival and overall survival, respectively. The key secondary endpoint of this trial is to estimate the differences in recurrence rate, progression-free survival, overall survival and toxicity rates for the treatment regimens by the patients' level of obesity in order to determine if obesity and insulin resistance predict responsiveness to metformin treatment, as some of the pre-clinical studies and animal models suggest. In addition to obesity, other metabolic characteristics will be followed throughout this trial, including hip-to-waist ratio and fasting insulin and glucose levels. Translational components of this trial include investigating potential biomarkers of response to treatment with metformin, including downstream targets of the metformin/mTOR signaling pathway and expression of the metformin transporter proteins (OCT1–3, PMAT, and MATE1–2. The phase 2 portion of this trial has completed and will be moving to phase 3 in December of 2016.

Finally, a phase I/II trial is planned to open in France evaluating the safety and efficacy of cyclophosphamide, metformin and olaparib in recurrent or advanced endometrial cancer (NCT02755844).

Results from these large-scale clinical trials evaluating metformin's therapeutic effect in endometrial and ovarian cancer are eagerly awaited. The repurposing of metformin as a novel therapeutic agent appears to have great potential for both of these cancers, and these ongoing clinical trials should hopefully shed light on its efficacy and most critically, related modifiers of response which could include both metabolic (i.e. obesity, insulin resistance, hyperglycemia) and molecular factors (i.e. transporters, IGF-1 and mTOR pathway activation).

Conclusions

The pre-clinical, epidemiologic and clinical data supporting the use of metformin in the prevention and treatment of cancers is building. There is a particularly large growing body of evidence in endometrial and ovarian cancer. The association between obesity, insulin resistance and increased risk of endometrial and ovarian cancer makes metformin an attractive agent for the prevention and treatment of these diseases. Furthermore, the potential therapeutic benefit seen in pre-clinical and clinical trials, as well as the low cost and favorable toxicity profile makes this agent a particularly appealing choice. However, there remain many unanswered questions for metformin and cancer. It remains to be seen if metformin will be universally effective in cancer treatment and prevention, or rather if this agent will be more efficacious in the obese and/or insulin resistant population. It is also unclear as to the key mechanisms of metformin's anti-tumorigenic activity as both indirect and direct effects have been noted. Lastly, the optimal dose of metformin for cancer treatment is unknown. Most clinical trials are using conventional anti-diabetic doses, but perhaps higher doses would improve the efficacy of metformin for cancer treatment with a tolerable side effect profile. Alternatively, phenformin or other novel biguanides may pharmacologically improve on the anti-tumorigenic benefits of metformin. With multiple clinical trials in progress, the hope is that many of these remaining questions will be answered in the not too distant future and valuable information gained on the potential benefits of metformin in the management of gynecologic cancer patients.

References

1. Inzucchi SE, et al. Management of hyperglycaemia in type 2 diabetes: a patient-centered approach. Position statement of the American Diabetes Association (ADA) and the European Association for the Study of Diabetes (EASD). Diabetologia. 2012;55(6):1577–96.
2. Quinn BJ, et al. Repositioning metformin for cancer prevention and treatment. Trends Endocrinol Metab. 2013;24(9):469–80.

3. Knowler WC, et al. Reduction in the incidence of type 2 diabetes with lifestyle intervention or metformin. N Engl J Med. 2002;346(6):393–403.
4. Dronavalli S, Ehrmann DA. Pharmacologic therapy of polycystic ovary syndrome. Clin Obstet Gynecol. 2007;50(1):244–54.
5. Decensi A, et al. Metformin and cancer risk in diabetic patients: a systematic review and meta-analysis. Cancer Prev Res (Phila). 2010;3(11):1451–61.
6. Evans JM, et al. Metformin and reduced risk of cancer in diabetic patients. BMJ. 2005;330(7503):1304–5.
7. Bowker SL, et al. Increased cancer-related mortality for patients with type 2 diabetes who use sulfonylureas or insulin. Diabetes Care. 2006;29(2):254–8.
8. Libby G, et al. New users of metformin are at low risk of incident cancer: a cohort study among people with type 2 diabetes. Diabetes Care. 2009;32(9):1620–5.
9. Pollak MN. Investigating metformin for cancer prevention and treatment: the end of the beginning. Cancer Discov. 2012;2(9):778–90.
10. Bonanni B, et al. Dual effect of metformin on breast cancer proliferation in a randomized presurgical trial. J Clin Oncol. 2012;30(21):2593–600.
11. Esteva FJ, et al. Phase I trial of exemestane in combination with metformin and rosiglitazone in nondiabetic obese postmenopausal women with hormone receptor-positive metastatic breast cancer. Cancer Chemother Pharmacol. 2013;71(1):63–72.
12. Hosono K, et al. Metformin suppresses colorectal aberrant crypt foci in a short-term clinical trial. Cancer Prev Res (Phila). 2010;3(9):1077–83.
13. MacKenzie MJ, et al. A phase I study of temsirolimus and metformin in advanced solid tumours. Investig New Drugs. 2012;30(2):647–52.
14. Nobes JP, et al. A prospective, randomized pilot study evaluating the effects of metformin and lifestyle intervention on patients with prostate cancer receiving androgen deprivation therapy. BJU Int. 2012;109(10):1495–502.
15. He X, et al. Metformin and thiazolidinediones are associated with improved breast cancer-specific survival of diabetic women with HER2+ breast cancer. Ann Oncol. 2012;23(7):1771–80.
16. He XX, et al. Thiazolidinediones and metformin associated with improved survival of diabetic prostate cancer patients. Ann Oncol. 2011;22(12):2640–5.
17. Kirpichnikov D, McFarlane SI, Sowers JR. Metformin: an update. Ann Intern Med. 2002;137(1):25–33.
18. Collier CA, et al. Metformin counters the insulin-induced suppression of fatty acid oxidation and stimulation of triacylglycerol storage in rodent skeletal muscle. Am J Physiol Endocrinol Metab. 2006;291(1):E182–9.
19. Miller RA, et al. Biguanides suppress hepatic glucagon signalling by decreasing production of cyclic AMP. Nature. 2013;494(7436):256–60.
20. Bailey CJ, Turner RC. Metformin. N Engl J Med. 1996;334(9):574–9.
21. Shin NR, et al. An increase in the Akkermansia spp. population induced by metformin treatment improves glucose homeostasis in diet-induced obese mice. Gut. 2014;63(5):727–35.
22. Pernicova I, Korbonits M. Metformin—mode of action and clinical implications for diabetes and cancer. Nat Rev Endocrinol. 2014;10(3):143–56.
23. Morales DR, Morris AD. Metformin in cancer treatment and prevention. Annu Rev Med. 2015;66:17–29.
24. Wheaton WW, et al. Metformin inhibits mitochondrial complex I of cancer cells to reduce tumorigenesis. elife. 2014;3:e02242.
25. Liu X, et al. Discrete mechanisms of mTOR and cell cycle regulation by AMPK agonists independent of AMPK. Proc Natl Acad Sci U S A. 2014;111(4):E435–44.
26. Pierotti MA, et al. Targeting metabolism for cancer treatment and prevention: metformin, an old drug with multi-faceted effects. Oncogene. 2013;32(12):1475–87.
27. Ben Sahra I, et al. Metformin, independent of AMPK, induces mTOR inhibition and cell-cycle arrest through REDD1. Cancer Res. 2011;71(13):4366–72.
28. Gou S, et al. Low concentrations of metformin selectively inhibit CD133(+) cell proliferation in pancreatic cancer and have anticancer action. PLoS One. 2013;8(5):e63969.

29. Gunter MJ, et al. A prospective evaluation of insulin and insulin-like growth factor-i as risk factors for endometrial cancer. Cancer Epidemiol Biomark Prev. 2008;17(4):921–9.
30. Berns EM, et al. Receptors for hormones and growth factors and (onco)-gene amplification in human ovarian cancer. Int J Cancer. 1992;52(2):218–24.
31. van Dam PA, et al. Expression of c-erbB-2, c-myc, and c-ras oncoproteins, insulin-like growth factor receptor I, and epidermal growth factor receptor in ovarian carcinoma. J Clin Pathol. 1994;47(10):914–9.
32. Brokaw J, et al. IGF-I in epithelial ovarian cancer and its role in disease progression. Growth Factors. 2007;25(5):346–54.
33. Spentzos D, et al. IGF axis gene expression patterns are prognostic of survival in epithelial ovarian cancer. Endocr Relat Cancer. 2007;14(3):781–90.
34. McCampbell AS, et al. Overexpression of the insulin-like growth factor I receptor and activation of the AKT pathway in hyperplastic endometrium. Clin Cancer Res. 2006;12(21):6373–8.
35. Dedes KJ, et al. Emerging therapeutic targets in endometrial cancer. Nat Rev Clin Oncol. 2011;8(5):261–71.
36. Salvesen HB, et al. Integrated genomic profiling of endometrial carcinoma associates aggressive tumors with indicators of PI3 kinase activation. Proc Natl Acad Sci U S A. 2009;106(12):4834–9.
37. Cheung LW, et al. High frequency of PIK3R1 and PIK3R2 mutations in endometrial cancer elucidates a novel mechanism for regulation of PTEN protein stability. Cancer Discov. 2011;1(2):170–85.
38. Kandoth C, et al. Integrated genomic characterization of endometrial carcinoma. Nature. 2013;497(7447):67–73.
39. Sun M, et al. AKT1/PKBalpha kinase is frequently elevated in human cancers and its constitutive activation is required for oncogenic transformation in NIH3T3 cells. Am J Pathol. 2001,159(2).431–7.
40. Bellacosa A, et al. Molecular alterations of the AKT2 oncogene in ovarian and breast carcinomas. Int J Cancer. 1995;64(4):280–5.
41. Shayesteh L, et al. PIK3CA is implicated as an oncogene in ovarian cancer. Nat Genet. 1999;21(1):99–102.
42. Levine DA, et al. Frequent mutation of the PIK3CA gene in ovarian and breast cancers. Clin Cancer Res. 2005;11(8):2875–8.
43. Philp AJ, et al. The phosphatidylinositol 3′-kinase p85alpha gene is an oncogene in human ovarian and colon tumors. Cancer Res. 2001;61(20):7426–9.
44. Saito M, et al. Allelic imbalance and mutations of the PTEN gene in ovarian cancer. Int J Cancer. 2000;85(2):160–5.
45. Hursting SD, et al. Reducing the weight of cancer: mechanistic targets for breaking the obesity-carcinogenesis link. Best Pract Res Clin Endocrinol Metab. 2008;22(4):659–69.
46. Dann SG, Selvaraj A, Thomas G. mTOR Complex1-S6K1 signaling: at the crossroads of obesity, diabetes and cancer. Trends Mol Med. 2007;13(6):252–9.
47. Wysocki PJ, Wierusz-Wysocka B. Obesity, hyperinsulinemia and breast cancer: novel targets and a novel role for metformin. Expert Rev Mol Diagn. 2010;10(4):509–19.
48. Gonzalez-Angulo AM, Meric-Bernstam F. Metformin: a therapeutic opportunity in breast cancer. Clin Cancer Res. 2010;16(6):1695–700.
49. Jiang W, Zhu Z, Thompson HJ. Dietary energy restriction modulates the activity of AMP-activated protein kinase, Akt, and mammalian target of rapamycin in mammary carcinomas, mammary gland, and liver. Cancer Res. 2008;68(13):5492–9.
50. Moore T, et al. Dietary energy balance modulates signaling through the Akt/mammalian target of rapamycin pathways in multiple epithelial tissues. Cancer Prev Res (Phila). 2008;1(1):65–76.
51. Wang DS, et al. Involvement of organic cation transporter 1 in hepatic and intestinal distribution of metformin. J Pharmacol Exp Ther. 2002;302(2):510–5.
52. Kimura N, et al. Metformin is a superior substrate for renal organic cation transporter OCT2 rather than hepatic OCT1. Drug Metab Pharmacokinet. 2005;20(5):379–86.

53. Kimura N, Okuda M, Inui K. Metformin transport by renal basolateral organic cation transporter hOCT2. Pharm Res. 2005;22(2):255–9.
54. Terada T, et al. Molecular cloning, functional characterization and tissue distribution of rat H+/organic cation antiporter MATE1. Pharm Res. 2006;23(8):1696–701.
55. Masuda S, et al. Identification and functional characterization of a new human kidney-specific H+/organic cation antiporter, kidney-specific multidrug and toxin extrusion 2. J Am Soc Nephrol. 2006;17(8):2127–35.
56. Zhou M, Xia L, Wang J. Metformin transport by a newly cloned proton-stimulated organic cation transporter (plasma membrane monoamine transporter) expressed in human intestine. Drug Metab Dispos. 2007;35(10):1956–62.
57. Han, T., Proctor W, Costales C, Everett R, Thakker D. The role of the organic cation transporter 1 (OCT1) and plasma membrane monoamine transporter (PMAT) in metformin apical uptake in Caco-2 cells. Proceedings of the annual meeting of the American association of pharmaceutical scientists, 2011.
58. Winter TN, Elmquist WF, Fairbanks CA. OCT2 and MATE1 provide bidirectional agmatine transport. Mol Pharm. 2011;8(1):133–42.
59. Emami Riedmaier A, et al. Metformin and cancer: from the old medicine cabinet to pharmacological pitfalls and prospects. Trends Pharmacol Sci. 2013;34(2):126–35.
60. Schaeffeler E, et al. DNA methylation is associated with downregulation of the organic cation transporter OCT1 (SLC22A1) in human hepatocellular carcinoma. Genome Med. 2011;3(12):82.
61. Cai H, et al. Cation-selective transporters are critical to the AMPK-mediated antiproliferative effects of metformin in human breast cancer cells. Int J Cancer. 2016;138(9):2281–92.
62. Shu Y, et al. Effect of genetic variation in the organic cation transporter 1, OCT1, on metformin pharmacokinetics. Clin Pharmacol Ther. 2008;83(2):273–80.
63. Shu Y, et al. Effect of genetic variation in the organic cation transporter 1 (OCT1) on metformin action. J Clin Invest. 2007;117(5):1422–31.
64. Nies AT, et al. Organic cation transporters (OCTs, MATEs), in vitro and in vivo evidence for the importance in drug therapy. Handb Exp Pharmacol. 2011;201:105–67.
65. Tzvetkov MV, et al. The effects of genetic polymorphisms in the organic cation transporters OCT1, OCT2, and OCT3 on the renal clearance of metformin. Clin Pharmacol Ther. 2009;86(3):299–306.
66. McGuinness ME, Talbert RL. Phenformin-induced lactic acidosis: a forgotten adverse drug reaction. Ann Pharmacother. 1993;27(10):1183–7.
67. Owen MR, Doran E, Halestrap AP. Evidence that metformin exerts its anti-diabetic effects through inhibition of complex 1 of the mitochondrial respiratory chain. Biochem J. 2000;348(Pt 3):607–14.
68. Searle GL, Siperstein MD. Lactic acidosis associated with phenformin therapy. Evidence that inhibited lactate oxidation is the causative factor. Diabetes. 1975;24(8):741–5.
69. Williams RH, Steiner DF. Summarization of studies relative to the mechanism of phenethylbiguanide hypoglycemia. Metabolism. 1959;8(4 Pt 2):548–52.
70. Stumvoll M, et al. Metabolic effects of metformin in non-insulin-dependent diabetes mellitus. N Engl J Med. 1995;333(9):550–4.
71. Graham GG, et al. Clinical pharmacokinetics of metformin. Clin Pharmacokinet. 2011;50(2):81–98.
72. Huang X, et al. Important role of the LKB1-AMPK pathway in suppressing tumorigenesis in PTEN-deficient mice. Biochem J. 2008;412(2):211–21.
73. Appleyard MV, et al. Phenformin as prophylaxis and therapy in breast cancer xenografts. Br J Cancer. 2012;106(6):1117–22.
74. Lea MA, et al. Addition of 2-deoxyglucose enhances growth inhibition but reverses acidification in colon cancer cells treated with phenformin. Anticancer Res. 2011;31(2):421–6.
75. Caraci F, et al. Effects of phenformin on the proliferation of human tumor cell lines. Life Sci. 2003;74(5):643–50.

76. Orecchioni S, et al. The biguanides metformin and phenformin inhibit angiogenesis, local and metastatic growth of breast cancer by targeting both neoplastic and microenvironment cells. Int J Cancer. 2015;136(6):E534–44.
77. Jiang W, et al. Repurposing phenformin for the targeting of glioma stem cells and the treatment of glioblastoma. Oncotarget. 2016;7(35):56456–70.
78. Dilman VM, Anisimov VN. Effect of treatment with phenformin, diphenylhydantoin or L-dopa on life span and tumour incidence in C3H/Sn mice. Gerontology. 1980;26(5):241–6.
79. Shackelford DB, et al. LKB1 inactivation dictates therapeutic response of non-small cell lung cancer to the metabolism drug phenformin. Cancer Cell. 2013;23(2):143–58.
80. Aoki M, et al. Kidney-specific expression of human organic cation transporter 2 (OCT2/SLC22A2) is regulated by DNA methylation. Am J Physiol Renal Physiol. 2008;295(1):F165–70.
81. Segal ED, et al. Relevance of the OCT1 transporter to the antineoplastic effect of biguanides. Biochem Biophys Res Commun. 2011;414(4):694–9.
82. Iczkowski KA, et al. Trials of new germ cell immunohistochemical stains in 93 extragonadal and metastatic germ cell tumors. Hum Pathol. 2008;39(2):275–81.
83. Hilgendorf C, et al. Expression of thirty-six drug transporter genes in human intestine, liver, kidney, and organotypic cell lines. Drug Metab Dispos. 2007;35(8):1333–40.
84. Zhang L, et al. NT1014, a novel biguanide, inhibits ovarian cancer growth in vitro and in vivo. J Hematol Oncol. 2016;9(1):91.
85. Cantrell LA, et al. Metformin is a potent inhibitor of endometrial cancer cell proliferation— implications for a novel treatment strategy. Gynecol Oncol. 2010;116(1):92–8.
86. Iglesias DA, et al. Another surprise from metformin: novel mechanism of action via K-Ras influences endometrial cancer response to therapy. Mol Cancer Ther. 2013;12(12):2847–56.
87. Sarfstein R, et al. Metformin downregulates the insulin/IGF-I signaling pathway and inhibits different uterine serous carcinoma (USC) cells proliferation and migration in p53-dependent or -independent manners. PLoS One. 2013;8(4):e61537.
88. Erdemoglu E, et al. Effects of metformin on mammalian target of rapamycin in a mouse model of endometrial hyperplasia. Eur J Obstet Gynecol Reprod Biol. 2009;145(2):195–9.
89. Tan BK, et al. Metformin treatment exerts antiinvasive and antimetastatic effects in human endometrial carcinoma cells. J Clin Endocrinol Metab. 2011;96(3):808–16.
90. Zhang Q, et al. Chemopreventive effects of metformin on obesity-associated endometrial proliferation. Am J Obstet Gynecol. 2013;209(1):24 e1–24 e12.
91. Hanna RK, et al. Metformin potentiates the effects of paclitaxel in endometrial cancer cells through inhibition of cell proliferation and modulation of the mTOR pathway. Gynecol Oncol. 2012;125(2):458–69.
92. Dong L, et al. Metformin sensitizes endometrial cancer cells to chemotherapy by repressing glyoxalase I expression. J Obstet Gynaecol Res. 2012;38(8):1077–85.
93. Zhang Z, et al. Metformin reverses progestin resistance in endometrial cancer cells by down-regulating GloI expression. Int J Gynecol Cancer. 2011;21(2):213–21.
94. Mu N, Wang Y, Xue F. Metformin: a potential novel endometrial cancer therapy. Int J Gynecol Cancer. 2012;22(2):181.
95. Wang Y, et al. Mechanism of progestin resistance in endometrial precancer/cancer through Nrf2-AKR1C1 pathway. Oncotarget. 2016;7(9):10363–72.
96. Wu B, et al. Metformin inhibits the development and metastasis of ovarian cancer. Oncol Rep. 2012;28(3):903–8.
97. Yasmeen A, et al. Induction of apoptosis by metformin in epithelial ovarian cancer: involvement of the Bcl-2 family proteins. Gynecol Oncol. 2011;121(3):492–8.
98. Liao H, et al. Luteinizing hormone facilitates angiogenesis in ovarian epithelial tumor cells and metformin inhibits the effect through the mTOR signaling pathway. Oncol Rep. 2012;27(6):1873–8.
99. Rattan R, et al. Metformin attenuates ovarian cancer cell growth in an AMP-kinase dispensable manner. J Cell Mol Med. 2011;15(1):166–78.
100. Rattan R, et al. Metformin suppresses ovarian cancer growth and metastasis with enhancement of cisplatin cytotoxicity in vivo. Neoplasia. 2011;13(5):483–91.

101. Li C, et al. LY294002 and metformin cooperatively enhance the inhibition of growth and the induction of apoptosis of ovarian cancer cells. Int J Gynecol Cancer. 2012;22(1):15–22.
102. Gwak H, et al. Metformin induces degradation of cyclin D1 via AMPK/GSK3beta axis in ovarian cancer. Mol Carcinog. 2017;56(2):349–58.
103. Patel S, Singh N, Kumar L. Evaluation of effects of metformin in primary ovarian cancer cells. Asian Pac J Cancer Prev. 2015;16(16):6973–9.
104. Chan DK, Miskimins WK. Metformin and phenethyl isothiocyanate combined treatment in vitro is cytotoxic to ovarian cancer cultures. J Ovarian Res. 2012;5(1):19.
105. Erices R, et al. Metformin, at concentrations corresponding to the treatment of diabetes, potentiates the cytotoxic effects of carboplatin in cultures of ovarian cancer cells. Reprod Sci. 2013;20(12):1433–46.
106. Shank JJ, et al. Metformin targets ovarian cancer stem cells in vitro and in vivo. Gynecol Oncol. 2012;127(2):390–7.
107. Gotlieb WH, et al. In vitro metformin anti-neoplastic activity in epithelial ovarian cancer. Gynecol Oncol. 2008;110(2):246–50.
108. Hijaz M, et al. Preclinical evaluation of olaparib and metformin combination in BRCA1 wildtype ovarian cancer. Gynecol Oncol. 2016;142(2):323–31.
109. Algire C, et al. Metformin attenuates the stimulatory effect of a high-energy diet on in vivo LLC1 carcinoma growth. Endocr Relat Cancer. 2008;15(3):833–9.
110. Phoenix KN, et al. Dietary energy availability affects primary and metastatic breast cancer and metformin efficacy. Breast Cancer Res Treat. 2010;123(2):333–44.
111. Jackson A, Zhong Y, Zhou C, Kilgore J, Makowski L, Gehrig P, Bae-Jump V. Metformin had increased efficacy under obese conditions in a novel genetically engineered mouse model of serous ovarian cancer. Annual meeting of the society of gynecologic oncology annual meeting, 2014.
112. Makowski L, et al. Obesity increases tumor aggressiveness in a genetically engineered mouse model of serous ovarian cancer. Gynecol Oncol. 2014;133(1):90–7.
113. Wysham, W., Zhong, Y, Dickens, HK, Malloy, KM, Han, X, Guo, H, Zhou, C, Makowski, L, Bae-Jump, VL. Increased efficacy of metformin corresponds to differential metabolic effects in the ovarian tumors from obese versus lean mice. 47th annual meeting of the society of gynecologic oncology, Mar 2016, San Diego, CA.
114. Litchfield LM, et al. Hyperglycemia-induced metabolic compensation inhibits metformin sensitivity in ovarian cancer. Oncotarget. 2015;6(27):23548–60.
115. Zhang Q, et al. CGRRF1 as a novel biomarker of tissue response to metformin in the context of obesity. Gynecol Oncol. 2014;133(1):83–9.
116. Siegel R, Naishadham D, Jemal A. Cancer statistics, 2013. CA Cancer J Clin. 2013;63(1):11–30.
117. Siegel RL, Miller KD, Jemal A. Cancer statistics, 2016. CA Cancer J Clin. 2016;66(1):7–30.
118. Ko EM, et al. The complex triad of obesity, diabetes and race in type I and II endometrial cancers: prevalence and prognostic significance. Gynecol Oncol. 2014;133(1):28–32.
119. Setiawan VW, et al. Type I and II endometrial cancers: have they different risk factors? J Clin Oncol. 2013;31(20):2607–18.
120. Schmandt RE, et al. Understanding obesity and endometrial cancer risk: opportunities for prevention. Am J Obstet Gynecol. 2011;205(6):518–25.
121. Secord AA, et al. Body mass index and mortality in endometrial cancer: a systematic review and meta-analysis. Gynecol Oncol. 2016;140(1):184–90.
122. Renehan AG, et al. Body-mass index and incidence of cancer: a systematic review and meta-analysis of prospective observational studies. Lancet. 2008;371(9612):569–78.
123. Chia VM, et al. Obesity, diabetes, and other factors in relation to survival after endometrial cancer diagnosis. Int J Gynecol Cancer. 2007;17(2):441–6.
124. Calle EE, et al. Overweight, obesity, and mortality from cancer in a prospectively studied cohort of U.S. adults. N Engl J Med. 2003;348(17):1625–38.
125. Steiner E, et al. Diabetes mellitus is a multivariate independent prognostic factor in endometrial carcinoma: a clinicopathologic study on 313 patients. Eur J Gynaecol Oncol. 2007;28(2):95–7.

126. Arem H, et al. Prediagnosis body mass index, physical activity, and mortality in endometrial cancer patients. J Natl Cancer Inst. 2013;105(5):342–9.
127. Ward KK, et al. Cardiovascular disease is the leading cause of death among endometrial cancer patients. Gynecol Oncol. 2012;126(2):176–9.
128. Bokhman JV. Two pathogenetic types of endometrial carcinoma. Gynecol Oncol. 1983;15(1):10–7.
129. Currie CJ, et al. Mortality after incident cancer in people with and without type 2 diabetes: impact of metformin on survival. Diabetes Care. 2012;35(2):299–304.
130. Nevadunsky NS, et al. Metformin use and endometrial cancer survival. Gynecol Oncol. 2014;132(1):236–40.
131. Ko EM, et al. Metformin is associated with improved survival in endometrial cancer. Gynecol Oncol. 2014;132(2):438–42.
132. Becker C, et al. Metformin and the risk of endometrial cancer: a case-control analysis. Gynecol Oncol. 2013;129(3):565–9.
133. Ko E, Stürmer T, Hong JL, Castillo WC, Bae-Jump VL, Jonsson Funk M. Metformin and the risk of endometrial cancer: a population-based cohort study. Annual meeting of the society of gynecologic oncology annual meeting, 2014.
134. cancer.org, http://www.cancer.org/cancer/ovariancancer/detailedguide/ovarian-cancer-survival-rates. 2014.
135. Sankaranarayanan R, Ferlay J. Worldwide burden of gynaecological cancer: the size of the problem. Best Pract Res Clin Obstet Gynaecol. 2006;20(2):207–25.
136. Markmann S, Gerber B, Briese V. Prognostic value of Ca 125 levels during primary therapy. Anticancer Res. 2007;27(4a):1837–9.
137. Protani MM, Nagle CM, Webb PM. Obesity and ovarian cancer survival: a systematic review and meta-analysis. Cancer Prev Res (Phila). 2012;5(7):901–10.
138. Yang HS, et al. Effect of obesity on survival of women with epithelial ovarian cancer: a systematic review and meta-analysis of observational studies. Int J Gynecol Cancer. 2011;21(9):1525–32.
139. Olsen CM, et al. Obesity and the risk of epithelial ovarian cancer: a systematic review and meta-analysis. Eur J Cancer. 2007;43(4):690–709.
140. Lubin F, et al. Body mass index at age 18 years and during adult life and ovarian cancer risk. Am J Epidemiol. 2003;157(2):113–20.
141. Engeland A, et al. Height and body mass index in relation to total mortality. Epidemiology. 2003;14(3):293–9.
142. Bodmer M, et al. Use of metformin and the risk of ovarian cancer: a case-control analysis. Gynecol Oncol. 2011;123(2):200–4.
143. Romero IL, et al. Relationship of type II diabetes and metformin use to ovarian cancer progression, survival, and chemosensitivity. Obstet Gynecol. 2012;119(1):61–7.
144. Kumar S, et al. Metformin intake is associated with better survival in ovarian cancer: a case-control study. Cancer. 2013;119(3):555–62.
145. Brenner DE, Hawk E. Trials and tribulations of interrogating biomarkers to define efficacy of cancer risk reductive interventions. Cancer Prev Res (Phila). 2013;6(2):71–3.
146. Fabian CJ, et al. Breast cancer chemoprevention phase I evaluation of biomarker modulation by arzoxifene, a third generation selective estrogen receptor modulator. Clin Cancer Res. 2004;10(16):5403–17.
147. Patel KR, et al. Clinical pharmacology of resveratrol and its metabolites in colorectal cancer patients. Cancer Res. 2010;70(19):7392–9.
148. Heymach JV, et al. Effect of low-fat diets on plasma levels of NF-kappaB-regulated inflammatory cytokines and angiogenic factors in men with prostate cancer. Cancer Prev Res (Phila). 2011;4(10):1590–8.
149. Simoneau AR, et al. Alpha-difluoromethylornithine and polyamine levels in the human prostate: results of a phase IIa trial. J Natl Cancer Inst. 2001;93(1):57–9.
150. Hadad S, et al. Evidence for biological effects of metformin in operable breast cancer: a pre-operative, window-of-opportunity, randomized trial. Breast Cancer Res Treat. 2011;128(3):783–94.

151. Bullwinkel J, et al. Ki-67 protein is associated with ribosomal RNA transcription in quiescent and proliferating cells. J Cell Physiol. 2006;206(3):624–35.
152. Joshua AM, et al. A pilot 'window of opportunity' neoadjuvant study of metformin in local-ised prostate cancer. Prostate Cancer Prostatic Dis. 2014;17(3):252–8.
153. Laskov I, et al. Anti-diabetic doses of metformin decrease proliferation markers in tumors of patients with endometrial cancer. Gynecol Oncol. 2014;134(3):607–14.
154. Schuler KM, et al. Antiproliferative and metabolic effects of metformin in a preoperative window clinical trial for endometrial cancer. Cancer Med. 2015;4(2):161–73.
155. Sivalingam V, et al. A presurgical window-of-opportunity study of metformin in obesity-driven endometrial cancer. Lancet. 2015;385(Suppl 1):S90.
156. Sivalingam VN, et al. Measuring the biological effect of presurgical metformin treatment in endometrial cancer. Br J Cancer. 2016;114(3):281–9.
157. Soliman PT, Broaddus RB, Westin S, Iglesias D, Munsell MR, Schmandt R et al. Phase 0 study: prospective evaluation of the molecular effects of metformin on the endometrium in women with newly diagnosed endometrial cancer. Society of gynecologic oncologists annual meeting on women's cancer, society of gynecologic oncologists, 2013; p S15.
158. Mitsuhashi A, et al. Effects of metformin on endometrial cancer cell growth in vivo: a preop-erative prospective trial. Cancer. 2014;120(19):2986–95.
159. Staley, S., Roque, DR, Schuler, KM, Rambally, BS, Sampey, B, Everett, Thakker, D, Gehrig, PA, O'Connor, S, Makowski, S, VL Bae-Jump Molecular and metabolic differences of treat-ment responders versus non-responders in a phase 0 clinical trial of metformin in endometrial cancer. 47th annual meeting of the society of gynecologic oncology, Mar 2016, San Diego, CA.
160. Soliman PT, et al. Prospective evaluation of the molecular effects of metformin on the endo-metrium in women with newly diagnosed endometrial cancer: a window of opportunity study. Gynecol Oncol. 2016;143(3):466–71.
161. Khawaja MR, et al. Phase I dose escalation study of temsirolimus in combination with metformin in patients with advanced/refractory cancers. Cancer Chemother Pharmacol. 2016;77(5):973–7.
162. Miranda VC, et al. Phase 2 trial of metformin combined with 5-fluorouracil in patients with refractory metastatic colorectal cancer. Clin Colorectal Cancer. 2016;15(4):321–328.e1.
163. Braghiroli MI, et al. Phase II trial of metformin and paclitaxel for patients with gemcitabine-refractory advanced adenocarcinoma of the pancreas. ECancerMedicalScience. 2015;9:563.
164. Goodwin PJ, et al. Effect of metformin vs placebo on and metabolic factors in NCIC CTG MA.32. J Natl Cancer Inst. 2015;107(3):djv006.
165. Mitsuhashi A, et al. Phase II study of medroxyprogesterone acetate plus metformin as a fertility-sparing treatment for atypical endometrial hyperplasia and endometrial cancer. Ann Oncol. 2016;27(2):262–6.
166. Soliman PT, Westin SN, Iglesias DA, Munsell MF, Slomovitz BM, Lu KH, Coleman RL. Phase II study of everolimus, letrozole, and metformin in women with advanced/recur-rent endometrial cancer. J Clin Oncol. 2016;34:5506.

Appendix

Gynecologic malignancies, especially endometrial and ovarian cancers are among the most important and most severely affected by obesity. This volume of Energy Balance and Cancer, written by the world's leading experts in this field, is arranged to provide a transdisciplinary assessment of the pertinent issues, results of relevant research on mechanisms, and control, strategies for dealing with affected patients and improving outcomes and future research needs. The volume comprehensively covers the epidemiology linking obesity to endometrial and ovarian cancer as well as the public awareness of this critical problem. Subsequent chapters explain biologic aspects of linkages between energy balance and gynecologic malignancies. The volume further outlines strategies to disrupt the linkage between obesity and gynecologic malignancies and concludes with a series of chapters focused on management strategies for obese patients with gynecologic malignancies.

This volume provides a valuable resource for all physicians, scientists and other transdisciplinary investigators and practitioners interested and involved in energy balance and cancer. It should be a particularly useful guide to optimize outcomes for all practitioners dealing with patients with gynecologic malignancies challenged by energy balance issues. Moreover, it should serve as a useful guide to students and investigators interested in conducting further research on defining and disrupting the important linkage between energy balance and gynecologic malignancies.

© Springer International Publishing AG 2018
N.A. Berger et al. (eds.), *Focus on Gynecologic Malignancies*, Energy Balance and Cancer 13, DOI 10.1007/978-3-319-63483-8

Index

© Springer International Publishing AG 2018
N.A. Berger et al. (eds.), *Focus on Gynecologic Malignancies*, Energy Balance
and Cancer 13, DOI 10.1007/978-3-319-63483-8

Printed in the United States
By Bookmasters